The Modern
Parents'
Guide
to Baby
and
Child Care

The Modern Parents' Guide to Baby and Child Care

Violet Broadribb, R.N., M.S. & Henry F. Lee, M.D.

J. B. LIPPINCOTT COMPANY
Philadelphia and New York

U.S. Library of Congress Cataloging in Publication Data

Broadribb, Violet.
  The modern parents' guide to baby and child care.

  Bibliography: p.
  1. Infants—Care and hygiene. 2. Children—Care and hygiene. I. Lee,
Henry F., birth date   joint author. II. Title. [DNLM: 1. Child care—
Popular works. 2. Infant care—Popular works. 3. Pediatrics—Popular
works. WS 113 B863m 1973]
RJ61.B83   649'.1   73–4302
ISBN–0–397–00757–4

Contents

Introduction

We are living in a rapidly changing world—and change implies learning to adjust. Older people point out, "Things are so different now." *Things* are different. Babies are not. In all of recorded history babies have not changed. There is no evidence that the basic responses of the newborn are any different now from what they were thousands of years ago.

Then why a new book on baby and child care? Hasn't everything important been said?

We wrote this book partly because *so much* has been said—in books, magazines, newspapers, and on radio and television. Conscientious parents are baffled by conflicting advice, upset by reports of new scientific developments, frightened by the many pronouncements on child behavior and discipline. Uncertain whether they are doing things just right for their children, parents become anxious. Next to physical illness the most frequent thing that brings parents to their child's doctor can be summarized in one word: uncertainty. Doubt and uncertainty lead to weak responses; this is the source of more problems with children than any other factor in family relationships.

And yet most parents are inherently right in their natural

responses to their child, as long as they aren't confused by too many directives. For the implication that there is only one right way to treat children is nonsense. There are many ways. There are many happy, successful people who were reared by only one parent, who had no pets, little space for play, and very little in the way of material things, but who received plenty of love. We want to set out the ground rules for dealing with a child with common sense, love, a sense of humor, and a minimum of anxiety.

We wrote this book primarily because the world *is* changing so much—because though children are born with the same capacity for healthy development, it is far from easy to adapt today's society to their needs and potentials. The family unit itself has changed. Most often it is no longer made up of three generations; grandmother is not available either as baby-sitter or comfort-giver. And yet often the mother works. Who, then, can help with the child? How does a young couple combine college or graduate school with having a baby? If there is only one parent, can that parent work outside the home and leave the greater part of the child's care to others? What of the child who grows up in a home without a father?

Some mothers work to supplement the family income, some to provide the whole income. Others work because they have skills and knowledge needed and valued by society, and because they find personal fulfillment in the business and professional world. There is no evidence that a mother's desire for outside employment indicates a lack of parental love or responsibility. The question to be considered is not whether she should work outside the home—she already does and will continue to do so—but how she can best carry the responsibility for two jobs. Our responsibility in this book is to give her all the help we can: to suggest special ways to make things run more smoothly, to give hints for the use of work-saving aids, and to emphasize that the day for considering a mother more motherly when she makes a martyr of herself is long past. Children will love and trust her more, will build their own personalities on hers, when they sense that she respects herself as much as she does others.

For let's make one thing clear from the start. You as parents have rights and needs of your own. Certainly you must be concerned with your child, but you must also maintain your own healthy personalities.

The second part of the book is devoted to the health problems of babies and children—to the prevention, recognition, and treatment of common ailments. Just as you wish to know more about your own medical problems than what they are called, you will not be satisfied to be told merely that your child has an allergy or bronchitis or diabetes or warts but will want to know more about what each condition means. The more you understand about the common illnesses of childhood, the less threatening most of them will seem.

We have tried to answer those questions that come up most frequently at home and in the doctor's office, to provide up-to-date medical information, and to present those ideas of child care which seem to us most valid in today's world. But this is not a do-it-yourself diagnostic and treatment manual from which you might expect to make the correct diagnosis among dozens of possible ailments and determine the proper dosages of medications. We are not trying to take the place of your child's doctor but rather to enable you to work better with him for your child's benefit. You will need the doctor from time to time, and this book will help you to decide when to call him and to understand what he does and what he does not do.

First aid treatment for emergencies is presented in a section printed on yellow paper at the end of the book for quick reference.

We have written from the vantage point of long experience with children. Each year in your child's life brings new developments. If we can help you to understand why he is as he is at that particular moment, it will be easier for you to find joy and satisfaction in helping him grow into a strong, confident adult.

In order to avoid constantly referring to your child as "he or she," we shall use the male pronoun unless we are dealing with a problem peculiar to girls. If we seem, most often, to address the child's mother, it is not because child care is solely the province of mothers but because mothers are more often the book readers in this field—and if you, the mother, are doing the reading, the least we can do is address you directly.

15

PART ONE
Infant and Child Care

1

The Very Beginning of Life

LIFE BEFORE BIRTH

Let's start your knowledge of your child with his beginning; it could help you become a better parent.

A baby is actually 9 months old before he is born. Even though he starts life as a single cell just barely visible without a microscope, he already possesses all the inherited characteristics he will ever have.

This is not to say that this future human being will never change or develop. Many things happen to a new life, either before or after birth, that modify or affect inheritance. Environmental conditions can have a profoundly favorable or unfavorable effect. But the fact remains that a single cell contains the complete blueprint for its development right from the start. The color of the eyes and hair, the shape of the nose, even the basic character are determined; fortunately, the personality can grow and change.

Interestingly, the father alone determines the sex of the child, for in his sperm are both male and female potentials while the mother's egg has only female. Once conception has occurred, nothing can change the sex of the unborn child. It is ironic that many women have been blamed, and even divorced, because they have not produced sons.

THE EMBRYO: FIRST THREE MONTHS

After the egg is fertilized it starts to grow, although at first it is just a mass of undifferentiated tissue. But what a potential that tiny blob of tissue has! Soon the embryo, as it is called in this early stage, attaches itself to the lining of your uterus, or womb, and begins building a lifeline, called the placenta, between your blood system and its own. For even as an embryo, the child-to-be has its own blood system. It absorbs nourishment and oxygen from your circulation through the walls of its own blood vessels, and it gets rid of its wastes into your system, but its blood is its own, and its blood type may even be different from yours.

What is going on in your body is far more intricate than the wildest concoction of engineers and chemists. Nothing else you create in a lifetime will approach this marvel of complexity and rapid growth.

During the first weeks in the uterus, all the body parts of the embryo form and start to develop. The heart begins to beat at about the third week, although at this very early stage it is still a tiny hollow tube without chambers.

At the end of the first 4 weeks, the embryo is about ¼ inch long, its head constituting about a third of its size. The digestive system is beginning to form, as well as a backbone which ends in a taillike appendage. No eyes, nose, or ears are visible, but budlike projections have started to appear as the beginnings of arms and legs.

At the end of the eighth week, the embryo weighs about $\frac{1}{30}$ ounce and is 1⅛ inches long. The umbilical cord has developed, and the features of the face are forming, although the eyelids are fused together. The taillike process has disappeared, and arms, legs, feet, hands, toes, and fingers are developing, as well as internal organs.

At the end of the twelfth week, the fetus, as the baby-to-be is now called, weighs about 1 ounce and is approximately 3 inches long. The limbs are fully formed, with membranelike fingernails and toenails. Tooth buds are starting to form in the jaw, and the eyes, although still closed, are almost fully developed.

At this point the fetus has completed the most critical period of life, for it is while body parts and organs are being formed that deformities and malformations can occur. However, malformations are almost never caused by physical injury to you, because the unborn child is floating in a bag of fluid which acts as protection.

The developing fetus is also protected from infections by whatever immunities you have built up. But if you lack immunity against certain viruses, they may, under certain conditions, be capable of passing from you to the baby-to-be. In this way serious injury may occur in the developing child while you yourself have only a minor illness—as is well known in the case of German measles (rubella).

Many drugs which may be beneficial for you are capable of harming your developing baby. That is why you should always ask your doctor before you take *any* kind of medicine, even aspirin, especially during the first months of pregnancy. After the critical first 3 months when the body parts have become formed, damage by virus or medicines is much less likely to occur, but you should never take anything during pregnancy without your doctor's permission.

THE FETUS: FOUR TO NINE MONTHS

From now on, the fetus grows and develops at a rapid rate. At the end of the fourth month, it weighs about 4 ounces and is about 6½ inches long. The skin is covered with fine downy hair; the heartbeat is strong, the muscles active, the bones are formed, and the sex is now evident.

At the end of the fifth month, the baby-to-be weighs about 8 ounces and is about 10 inches long. At the end of the sixth month, he weighs about 24 ounces and is about 12 inches long. He can now open his eyes, and eyelashes are forming.

At the end of the seventh month, he has doubled his sixth-month weight and is about 15 inches long. A month later, at the termination of the eighth month, he weighs 4 to 5 pounds and is 16½ to 18 inches long.

20

Somewhere between the sixteenth and twentieth week, your baby-to-be will actively announce his presence to you. At first you may feel only a fluttering movement, the so-called quickening. Soon the movements become strong and forceful, keeping you well aware of his existence. Some unborn move less strongly than others, but a healthy occupant of the uterus is never a passive, unresponsive passenger.

True, he sleeps 20 or more hours out of the 24, just as he probably will do as a newborn, but when he is awake, he is very busy. He turns about, sometimes upside down, and stretches and kicks, strengthening his arm and leg muscles in the process; these are not purposeful but rather reflex movements. Late in pregnancy he may sometimes change his position for one more comfortable, and you may feel he is turning cartwheels!

Deep inside you he yawns, hiccups, and may suck his thumb. Although his lungs have not expanded and he does not yet breathe, his actions constitute practice in breathing and swallowing.

His hearing is developed before birth, and he may make startled movements at loud or unusual noises from the world outside. Your heartbeat is a constant rhythmic sound to him, and probably the gentle rocking he receives as you move about adds to his comfort.

Although he does respond to discomfort, it is a mistake to credit him with reasoning ability or emotional responses. All purposeful activities, including emotional responses, are built up and developed through previous experiences. Since the child before birth has had no experience with independent living, he cannot respond to situations that have no meaning for him. As a matter of fact, even after he is born, his responses will be purely physical; he will cry because of the physical pain of hunger and be soothed by the familiar physical feeling of being held close and gently rocked.

Because the fetus has not lived in a world of color, music, and art, your enjoyment of these cannot influence him; nor can your enjoyment of strawberries during pregnancy produce "strawberry marks" on his skin. Your discontent, anger, or fear cannot mark him in any way.

Your reactions cannot influence or mark him for two reasons. First, your nervous system is not his. He is a separate being, his only connection with you the umbilical cord. Second, his own nervous system is immature. He would not be able to understand such reactions even if they did reach his consciousness.

The only way you can mark him is in the sense that he may have inherited certain personality traits from you. Hereditary traits are not the only shapers of a child's personality; they may not even be the most important factors. His environment after he is born—the way he is treated by his parents, especially his mother—will greatly influence him. Nevertheless, every experienced pediatrician knows that babies come into this world with definite personalities, some placid and easygoing, others forceful and hyperactive.

READY FOR BIRTH

An infant born after 5 months of pregnancy may breathe for a few minutes, but he is too immature to survive. Born at 6 months, he has about a 10 percent chance of survival, if given the most careful and skilled care. At 7 or 8 months his chance is greatly improved, although he will still need special care.

The full-term infant obviously has the best chance of all, but there are certain unfavorable conditions which at times may make continued fetal living a hazard for mother or child or both. In these cases induced labor or Cesarian section a few days or weeks early can be lifesaving.

During the final weeks before birth the baby lays down the layer of fat under the skin that gives him his chubby appearance. This is also the period when he stores up iron for use during his first weeks. He does not grow as rapidly in size after the eighth month, but he continues to develop the ability to maintain life.

As the time for birth draws near, the baby fills most of the available space and can no longer move about freely. What actually triggers the onset of labor is not completely understood. Shortly before birth, painless contractions of the uterine muscle help the fetus to assume the position that will make the exit from the uterus easiest; for most infants this is a head-down, chin-on-chest position.

He has now reached the stage where he is ready to begin his own separate life as your baby, the ultimate expression of your creativity as a woman. Life holds many other pleasures, but it is doubtful if anything else can compare to this.

YOUR PART IN PREGNANCY

The knowledge that a new life has been conceived can be a cause of great joy. But it takes 40 weeks of routine living for this process of creation to be completed and the finished product to appear. And so, even though you longed for pregnancy and are delighted to be part of the act of creation, it is inevitable that sometime during those 280 days you will have moments of boredom or twinges of regret.

There probably will be times when you deplore your ungainly figure and sense a change in the attitude of those you meet as you walk up the street or go to your place of business. You may miss the approving glances you used to receive.

Don't feel guilty; your reactions do not mean that you are rejecting your baby. Certainly some women do, and they are in need of expert help; but the average woman during the first months of pregnancy turns her thoughts naturally to herself, adjusting to the situation and adapting to her new role. Just remember that negative feelings do not apply to your baby as a *person*. After all, he is hardly a reality to you as yet. Most women do not become conscious of the fetus as an individual until it starts to move, and many do not have strong feelings of motherhood until they actually hold their baby in their arms. Sometimes the maternal feeling comes even later.

Even those occasional women who initially resent their condition usually come to accept it, and eventually they too feel the joy and profound satisfaction of motherhood.

All expectant mothers have one thing in common: they need

23

to learn how to live in the best possible physical, emotional, and mental health for their own sake and their child's.

PRENATAL MEDICAL CARE

In large communities prenatal care and delivery are usually the province of an obstetrician, a doctor who specializes in maternity work. You can also get good care in hospital prenatal clinics and public health centers. Your choice will be made largely according to your financial ability and the facilities available in your community.

If you have as a family doctor a general practitioner who takes maternity patients, you know he has had training in maternity care and has the added advantage of knowing you and your family. Present medical knowledge is so great, however, that specialization has become almost a necessity whenever any unusual problem is present, and general practitioners often prefer to leave all obstetrical practice to specialists.

Unless the doctor has cared for you before, he will need to get a complete medical history from you. At your first visit he will give you a physical checkup and also make both an external and internal pelvic examination.

It is natural to feel rather shy about your first prenatal visit to a doctor. Some young women who have never had a pelvic examination dread the idea and may even postpone the first visit because of their fear, but there is nothing to be afraid of. The examination is painless, and the doctor's approach is matter-of-fact enough to put you completely at ease.

If your first visit comes 10 days or more after your first missed period, a laboratory test can confirm your pregnancy; the test is accurate in over 95 percent of cases. Without the test the doctor cannot be certain that you are pregnant until the sixth or eighth week, but you should not wait that long to be checked. The first 3 months of pregnancy are too important.

If you have questions about anything related to pregnancy or childbirth, ask them. Your doctor would much prefer that you ask him rather than rely on stories you hear from others.

During this visit, or perhaps the following one, he will discuss your general care during pregnancy, adapting it to your own particular needs. He will also help you estimate your probable date of delivery.

HOW DELIVERY DATE IS ESTIMATED. As we have said, the total period of pregnancy is generally 40 weeks, or 280 days. Calculation is made by adding 7 days to the first day of the last menstrual period and counting back 3 months. For example, if the last period started March 1, adding 7 days and counting back 3 months will give you a probable due date of December 8. But only a small percentage of babies arrive precisely on their due date.

PRENATAL CLINICS AND CENTERS. If you choose to have care at a clinic or center, you will find the same kind of scheduling. All examinations will be carried out under the supervision of a competent obstetrician. The services of a nutritionist are available, as well as those of social workers if these are needed.

For the mother who must bring her older children with her, some clinics provide supervised play areas. Many clinics sponsor discussion groups in which mothers can express common problems and share ideas under responsible leadership. Unfortunately, not all centers have been able to provide these services.

The working mother may find it difficult to attend prenatal clinics, for they are usually held during working hours. But some cities now have prenatal clinics during evening hours for the convenience of mothers who work. Ask your health department whether there is an evening clinic in your city.

PARENTHOOD CLASSES. In most communities there are classes for expectant mothers, and many have evening classes that fathers are expected to attend as well. Information about such classes can be obtained from your doctor or clinic or from the public health department.

At these classes you will discuss not only your nutrition and maternity clothing but also the preparation for labor and delivery and the care of the newborn. You may learn exercises to practice during pregnancy and delivery, including deep breathing and relaxation for use during labor.

If the classes are held in the hospital, a tour of the maternity department will probably be included. In fact, tours for prospective maternity patients are arranged in many hospitals, whether or not classes are held there.

OTHER AVAILABLE SERVICES. An increasing number of registered nurses are taking additional training in obstetrics to acquire midwifery certificates. These midwives perform normal deliveries in the hospital, with an obstetrician on call for any complication. Women who have been so fortunate as to live where this service is available have been well pleased with it.

County health nurses are usually available in any community. A health nurse is most useful in helping to prepare for the coming child and in finding solutions to special problems. A phone call or letter to the county or state health department will bring information concerning available health nurse service.

The pregnant schoolgirl, whether married or unmarried, should not hesitate to consult the school nurse for information and help. Frequently the school nurse is the person who can best understand her problems and who will know how to obtain the services she needs.

WHAT TO DO ABOUT DAILY LIVING

Although a number of changes occur in your body during pregnancy—the most obvious, of course, the enlargement of your abdomen and breasts—it is a mistake to consider normal pregnancy a time of poor health or physical weakness. After their first period of adjustment, most women feel healthier than they ever have before. But there are changes to make in your daily living.

The suggestions that follow are for the comfort and wellbeing of the average woman. If your doctor tells you to do anything different from the instructions given here, remember he knows you personally and has your individual welfare in mind.

Now for the questions most commonly asked:

I am fond of outdoor activities; must I give them up now? How must I change my previous habits?

Exercise and fresh air are very important during pregnancy. The muscle tone you maintain will be of help during delivery. Generally speaking, you should continue the activities you have been accustomed to, except for the really strenuous sports. If you are in doubt as to what is too vigorous, ask your doctor. The important thing is to avoid overfatigue.

If you have never been an active person, this is not the time to begin active sports. A daily walk may be enough, in addition to any exercise your doctor recommends.

If you have a job that keeps you active, or are a homemaker with plenty of household activity, you may prefer to use your time outdoors for rest and relaxation.

I want to continue working for as long as I can.
Any suggestions?

If you ask five people what they think about holding down a job during pregnancy, you can be sure you will get five different answers. Much depends on the kind of work you do and your own general condition. Many women do work right up to the time the baby is expected, though it is usually a better plan to have the last 3 or 4 weeks to get things organized for after the baby arrives.

Most women wonder what it's going to be like to work during the later stages. The truth is that the first 3 months are likely to be the hardest. In the early weeks your body is making many drastic and truly marvelous adaptations to prepare itself. It will generally do a splendid job, but nevertheless there will be ups and downs.

During the early weeks you don't *look* pregnant, and so your boss may not be very sympathetic. Perhaps you lost your breakfast and your stomach feels like a pair of old jeans that someone is wringing out—but you're supposed to be bright and happy at 9 A.M. at the office. Be as tough on yourself as you can. Tell yourself that, like seasickness, your nausea is only temporary. It's the truth.

Don't try to solve all future problems and make all arrangements in a day. Take your time, for you do have time. A little later, when you begin to bulge, you're going to find people more helpful. The more you bulge, the more helpful they get. Enjoy it.

Strangely enough, you won't need as much help as you thought. As the bulge gets bigger your power increases. You'll feel better at the seventh or eighth month than you did at the second. You will wonder where all the energy comes from. But don't squander it; try to make the most of it and do some active planning.

If your doctor advises a little extra rest, take it here and there even if you don't feel the need. If your kind of work keeps you on your feet a great deal, there are ways to avoid getting too tired. Take a thermos of milk or coffee and a snack along for coffee break instead of going to the cafeteria. This will give you a chance to lie down in the rest room and relax. If you can't lie down, choose a comfortable chair and put your feet up on another.

Or think about taking your lunch to work so that you can have most of your lunch hour for resting. That will also help you avoid the noon-hour crowds.

Especially during the early months, you will find that you tire more easily than usual, and when people are tired they get tense and jumpy, worry over small matters, and lose their sense of humor. So call a halt. You really can afford to take a few minutes off to straighten yourself out. Take a minute or two between customers, letters, or appointments to relax. Take a really deep breath, let it go, and relax your whole body. Do this two or three times. If you can manage to sit for a moment and let yourself go limp, that will help. Let your mind relax, too; think of something pleasant for a few minutes. And always try to rest a little while when you first get home from work, before you start coping with supper.

Can you sleep late on your days off? Or slip away to bed early? Even if you don't fall asleep, you can relax your body while lying down.

I can't even relax at night when I go to bed. Any suggestions?
If you go to prenatal classes you will probably learn and practice relaxing. Here are some hints.

Lie down in the position you find most comfortable, or sit in a comfortable chair where you can spread out. Concentrate on each portion of your body. Close your eyes and try to let your face go limp. Let your jaw sag; relax your face muscles and neck. Sag your shoulders. Let your arms and legs go limp. Then relax your mind. Think about something monotonous, or fix your mind on some pleasant scene, perhaps something from childhood. You will find your tensions ebbing away.

If you find it hard to go to sleep at night, try relaxing this way. Instead of going over all your problems and worries, push them away and try to picture something you really enjoy seeing.

What can I do about housework while I am coping with pregnancy and a job?

The important thing is to space your work and conserve your energy. You may think you have been doing this all along, if you have worked and managed your home for some time. But things are different now. You have a growing baby sharing your energy reserves.

Here are some ideas other women have used to space out their housework and to have time for relaxing with their husbands.

SHOPPING. Try doing your shopping for the week on a day or evening when the stores are not crowded; avoid Friday night and Saturday. You want to keep out of crowds anyway to avoid picking up infections. Take your husband shopping with you, if you can, and make it a leisurely time. Buy staples like flour and sugar in large quantities to cut down on your weekly list. And see whether you can do all your shopping in one place: a supermarket will cut down on your running around. Keep an up-to-date shopping list in your kitchen so that you won't have to go back to the store for something you forgot.

MEAL PLANNING. Take an hour to sit with your husband and plan all your meals for the coming week. Then write everything you will need to buy on your shopping list.

Over the weekend or on one of your days off, prepare several main dishes and put them in the freezer. There are any number of casseroles that can be made ahead. Or fix a basic stew to which all you will have to add are vegetables when you are heat-

29

ing it. Breads, muffins, coffee cake, cakes, and pies can all be frozen and brought out when needed.

Salads, many main dishes, and many fruit desserts can be prepared the night before and kept in the refrigerator. Many women find it helpful to make tomorrow night's dinner as soon as they have cleaned up tonight's.

If you cook ahead, you will have time to relax and enjoy your family when you get home from work, for you will only have to add the last-minute touches to your meal. If your husband or older child gets home before you, he can take the dish out of the freezer.

There are excellent cookbooks available that explain how to cook now and serve later and that tell which food dishes can be kept refrigerated for 24 hours before serving and which can be frozen. They tell how to prepare and wrap dishes for freezing and offer menus for prepare-ahead dishes. A few of these are named in the reference list at the back of the book, but there are many others.

CLEANING. Try spreading your weekly cleaning over the week to make housekeeping easier. Use a squeeze mop on your kitchen floor in the evening after the dishes are done. While you are cleaning your kitchen, throw your clothes in the washing machine. But if washing means going to the basement, ask your husband to take this job on as part of his housework. If you take your clothes to a laundromat, make it an evening project.

Pick a different time and a lightweight vacuum sweeper to clean your floors and upholstered furniture. If your vacuum is heavy, ask your husband to take over.

Buy drip-dry maternity clothes to cut down on your laundry chores, and if you need new sheets get the no-iron variety. Sit on a high stool with a back while you are ironing. It will get you off your feet and make the job much easier.

Don't try to move heavy furniture or lift heavy objects. Let your husband be a real partner in the pregnancy, and save the heavy work for him if it must be done.

What about eating, smoking, an occasional drink?

Proper diet is vital for you and your baby. It is such an important subject that the next section is devoted to nutrition in pregnancy. But one point right now: When you first get home from work is a good time for a snack. It adds a little fuel when you need it and helps to keep your dinner appetite within bounds.

You certainly know by now that smoking is a health risk at any time. Smoking will not affect *you* any differently now than it would if you were not pregnant, but it can affect your child: More heavy smokers have premature babies than do nonsmokers, and prematurity presents a distinct hazard to the newborn. Furthermore, even full-term babies of heavy smokers are apt to be smaller than average. Your baby's chances for a good start in life are better, then, if you don't smoke. If you do, cut down, or, better still, stop entirely.

A healthy pregnant woman who is used to an occasional cocktail or glass of beer or wine will probably find only one reason to change her habits: Alcoholic drinks are quite rich in calories, so if you are gaining too fast you will find it is better to cut down here than on some more necessary food.

If you are used to a drink before dinner, and your doctor has approved, be sure that the snack you have when you get home from work includes some fluid—fruit juice or a glass of water. This will slow the rate at which your thirsty body will absorb the alcohol.

What if I have a cold or headache? Can I take a cold pill or an aspirin?

Take nothing without first getting your doctor's permission— even drugs you can buy without a prescription. The simplest medicine, including aspirin, may be harmful to your developing baby. Perhaps no harm will come of it, but the stakes are far too high to take a chance. Be safe and don't take *any* medicine without your doctor's approval.

My neighbor tells me there are certain months when I should not take a tub bath. Is this true?

Daily baths are especially refreshing and relaxing during pregnancy, for there is a tendency to perspire more than usual. Generally, you are allowed both tub and shower baths, whichever you prefer. But during your last few weeks of pregnancy, you may find climbing into a tub or shower rather difficult. At that point why not wait until you have someone with you to help you?

I have heard that special care should be given to the breasts. What is this special care?

Nothing at all special. Wash your breasts when you bathe, but use a soft turkish washcloth on your nipples so that they stand erect and tingle. During the last month of pregnancy your doctor may prescribe a special cream for massage. In the last months a colorless fluid called colostrum may ooze from the nipples. This can be washed off with soap and water or with cold cream or lanolin. If the fluid oozes onto your clothing, cover the nipples with squares of gauze or soft cloth. Some women have inverted (turned-in) nipples and worry about being able to breast-feed their babies. If this is your case, your doctor may suggest gentle massage. Other doctors prefer that inverted nipples be left alone, since the baby tends to draw them out as he nurses.

Is there any truth in the saying "for each baby, a tooth?"

No, pregnancy does not cause tooth decay, but it is good practice to have the dentist look your teeth over early in your pregnancy and do any required dental work at that point, to eliminate unnecessary pain later.

Should sexual intercourse be avoided during any or all of the nine months?

Sexual intercourse during pregnancy can do no harm to the baby. There is no reason to abstain unless your doctor tells you to—and he won't unless you have been staining during your pregnancy and he wants to take special precautions against miscarriage. But for any normal pregnancy, you and your husband can still enjoy each other.

What about maternity clothes?

During the first 3 or 4 months, there is seldom any need to wear

32

maternity clothes, although many women are so proud that they put on maternity dresses early. Maternity clothes were never so attractive as they are now.

MATERNITY GIRDLES. If you never wear girdles, there is no reason to start wearing one now; panty hose are fine for maternity wear. If some support during the later months of pregnancy will make you more comfortable, wear a girdle then.

But if you are in the habit of wearing a girdle, continue to do so: an ordinary two-way stretch for the first 2 or 3 months, and a two-way-stretch maternity girdle for the remaining months. Maternity girdles have extra back support and a low abdominal band for support of the enlarging abdomen.

BRASSIERES. Even if you have not been wearing brassieres, try one; as pregnancy progresses the breasts become larger and heavier, and you will find that a well-fitting bra will make you more comfortable and help prevent backache. Wearing a bra may also help prevent the tissue sagging often noticed after pregnancy. Much depends on the size of your breasts and the need for support.

If you wear a bra regularly, you will not need to change it until your breasts start to enlarge during the later months of your pregnancy. When you buy a new bra, get one with cups large enough to cover all the breast tissue and of a size to allow for breast growth. If you plan to breast-feed your baby, a nursing brassiere is good economy; these are well-fitting brassieres opening in the front.

When you go to the hospital to have your baby, take your bra. You will need to wear it for breast support after your baby is born whether you plan to breast-feed or not.

SHOES. You should wear low-heeled shoes, since change in body posture will cause high heels to throw your body off balance, possibly causing backache and leg cramps.

MINOR DISCOMFORTS OF PREGNANCY

Certain discomforts are called minor because their effects on a mother or her child are slight, but they can be most annoying and seem not at all minor to the person affected. So it is well for you to know which symptoms may be signs of trouble that should be reported at once and which you should regard as nothing more than a nuisance. First, the minor ones.

A *frequent desire to urinate* is usual during the first 3 or 4 months; it is caused by pressure of the enlarging uterus on the bladder. As the pregnancy continues, the need to urinate frequently subsides until the last month, when pressure comes again as the fetus drops lower in the abdomen.

Though the frequency is normal, it is annoying, especially when it interrupts your sleep. Don't cut down on your fluid intake to counteract it, however, because your body needs additional liquids during pregnancy. Try instead to drink most of your liquids early in the day, not at bedtime.

If the frequency is accompanied by a burning sensation or pain, or if your urinary output becomes scanty, tell your doctor right away, for this may indicate a medical problem, such as a urinary infection, that needs treatment.

Nausea and vomiting, either early in the day or at intervals during the day, trouble some pregnant women. These disturbances should stop as your body adjusts to its new functions.

To control early morning nausea, keep a few dry crackers at your bedside and eat them before you raise your head from the pillow; then rest for 15 more minutes or so. Try crackers and rest during the day for periods of nausea. Drink carbonated or fruit-flavored beverages instead of plain water. Do *not* use medicines bought over the counter at the drugstore for nausea. If your nausea is persistent and troublesome, tell your doctor.

Leg cramps frequently occur during the later months of pregnancy, especially when you are lying flat. They are caused by pressure of the enlarged uterus on the leg veins. Walking around in bare feet and stretching the leg, heel first, helps get rid of them, and daily baths and elevating the legs helps prevent them. Avoid constrictive clothing around the thighs or legs, above or below the knee, such as round garters or panty girdles with tight legs, and report persistent leg cramps to your doctor.

Backache may be troublesome but can be helped by low-heeled shoes, a properly fitting girdle, and good posture. If you work in an office, make sure you have a properly adjusted posture chair.

SIGNS AND SYMPTOMS THAT SHOULD BE REPORTED AT ONCE

Certain symptoms can be signs of impending trouble. They do not have to be danger signals, but they may be; so don't take chances. Besides, early discovery allows treatment before trouble really starts.

Report the following to your doctor as soon as they occur; don't just wait until your next appointment:

1. Vaginal bleeding or spotting
2. Swelling of face, ankles, arms, or legs
3. Severe, persistent headache
4. Severe abdominal cramps
5. Persistent vomiting
6. Vision trouble, dimness, or blurring
7. Absence of fetal movements for a period of 24 hours, after the time when they have been vigorous
8. Ruptured membranes, indicated by a sudden gush of fluid from the vagina
9. Burning sensation or pain when urinating (especially if there is a desire to urinate frequently in small amounts) or scanty urinary output
10. Persistent irritating vaginal discharge

SPECIAL PRECAUTIONS

By now you know that you should not take any form of medication during pregnancy without your doctor's permission. But you must be aware of two other possibilities of harm to your developing child: German measles (rubella) and Rh-negative blood.

Effects of German measles

Following a widespread epidemic of German measles in Australia in 1941, it was noted that a large number of babies were born with various defects, such as cataracts of the eyes, deafness, heart conditions, and mental retardation. Eventually it was dem-

35

onstrated that, when a woman has German measles during pregnancy, the virus passes across the placental barrier into the bloodstream of the developing fetus and may cause harm to the baby.

The greatest danger comes during the first 3 months of your pregnancy, when the baby-to-be's body is forming. Even during this period only about 15 to 25 percent of embryos exposed to German measles virus show harmful effects. But this is small comfort to the mother of a child who is affected—particularly when she knows she could have prevented the disease.

It is important that every woman develop an immunity to German measles *before* she becomes pregnant. Until quite recently the only way to accomplish this was by actually having the disease. German measles parties were even arranged so that many young girls could be exposed to a known case. (Because the disease itself is usually so mild, there was little hazard in this.) Unfortunately, "takes" were often disappointingly few.

Now, at last, a rubella virus vaccine makes it possible to protect every girl. It is safe and effective, but it must be given *before* there is any chance of pregnancy. Recommended ages are after age 1 and before puberty. It will not protect your expected baby if given after pregnancy has occurred. As a higher and higher percentage of children are immunized, the threat of German measles to unborn babies is becoming a thing of the past.

As you read this chapter, you are probably pregnant already, so it is too late to be vaccinated. But you can take precautions to avoid getting German measles. Keep out of crowds. Keep away from any child or adult who has a fever, rash, or swollen neck glands, even if you have had German measles before. Too many rashes look alike, and you cannot be certain that you really have had the disease.

If you have been exposed, however, tell your doctor, even if you are past the first 3 months of pregnancy. Do not take it for granted that you are immune.

The Rh factor

There is a blood type, called Rh-positive, which differs from all others by the presence of a substance known as the Rh factor. People who have this factor in their red blood cells are said to be *Rh-positive.* About 15 percent of people completely lack this substance; they are said to be *Rh-negative.*

If you are one of the 15 percent who are Rh-negative, and your husband is one of the 85 percent who are Rh-positive, there may be a problem, for you may have an Rh-positive baby. (There is no difficulty if you and your husband are both Rh-positive or both Rh-negative.) It is essential that your doctor know whether you are Rh-negative, and he will check this early in your pregnancy, for an Rh-negative mother and an Rh-positive baby-to-be may interact badly. It works like this:

The Rh factor is a protein substance that is foreign to the bloodstream of an Rh-negative person. If it is introduced there, it can bring about the production of substances called antibodies * that will chemically attack the Rh factor.

So if some of an Rh-positive baby's red blood cells leak into his Rh-negative mother's bloodstream through the placenta, her system will respond biologically by producing protective antibodies against the foreign substance. Then, when some of these antibodies in her blood leak *back* into the baby's bloodstream, they will attack his Rh substance. Because the baby's Rh material is part of his red blood cells, these blood cells will be destroyed.

As this process goes on, the infant is unable to manufacture red blood cells fast enough to make up for those that are eliminated. Finally he is born with a lack of red cells (anemia) that varies from mild to very severe, depending on the amount of his mother's antibodies.

FIRST-BORN AND THEREAFTER. It takes time for a mother's Rh-negative blood to build up antibodies to the blood of an Rh-positive baby. The antibodies begin to build up rather late in a first pregnancy, seldom in time to do the first-born any harm.

* See Chapter 12, Allergy, for a more detailed discussion of the production of antibodies.

But after the first pregnancy the antibodies persist in the mother's blood and may rise to much higher levels in a subsequent pregnancy. Then damage may occur. Even so, not *all* later babies are affected.

Testing the mother and the baby during pregnancy gives all the information needed to treat the occasional baby that is born with severe trouble.

In the past these babies were identified only after birth, and the only treatment was exchange transfusion by which small amounts of blood were drawn from the baby's umbilical vein at a time and replaced with Rh-negative blood until about 80 to 90 percent of the blood had been exchanged. Now doctors can tell whether the baby is affected before he is born, and an exchange transfusion can be given right after birth.

There is also a preventive material given to the Rh-negative mother immediately after the first delivery that is helping to make the problem obsolete.

The mother who visits her obstetrician as soon as she suspects she is pregnant and who faithfully keeps her prenatal appointments can confidently look forward to a successful pregnancy and delivery. Accidents can happen, of course, but keep in mind that the majority of newborn babies are healthy and active.

NUTRITION DURING PREGNANCY

For those of us who tend to eat too much, any excuse for eating to our heart's content is welcome. But "the expectant mother must eat for two" does not provide such an excuse. It is not that she must eat *enough* for two grown people but rather that she has to provide the *right kind* of nourishment for herself and her baby. The amount of food needed to supply the unborn baby's requirements for prenatal growth is not great.

On the other hand, the woman who has never had much interest in food may lose whatever interest she had if she bcomes nauseated at the beginning of the pregnancy.

DESIRABLE WEIGHT GAIN DURING PREGNANCY

No one can set a precise figure for the amount of weight any individual person should gain during pregnancy. A general recommendation for average weight gain is from 20 to 30 pounds. This takes into account the gain in weight due to pregnancy itself. By the time the baby is born, you will be carrying a baby weighing from 6 to 8 pounds, a placenta, and the amniotic fluid surrounding the baby. Your uterus will be several times heavier than normal. Your blood volume will have increased. All of these additional weights due to pregnancy add up to 14 pounds or more.

If you were underweight before pregnancy, you will need to increase your food intake to provide sufficient nutritional elements for yourself as well as for your child. Premature births and babies of low birth weight are more frequently born to mothers who fail to gain an average amount of weight during pregnancy, and the premature or very small baby is less well equipped to cope with life in the world he has entered.

Some women purposely limit their food intake drastically during pregnancy in order to have a small baby at birth. This is a *very* unwise thing to do unless you are on a special diet under a doctor's orders.

If you were overweight before pregnancy, you will still need to provide essential nutrients for your developing baby, but you can very well cut down on nonessential foods.

The *adolescent* expectant mother needs special consideration, for she herself is still developing. Unless she is already grossly overweight, she should be expected to gain more weight than the older woman, because she needs to provide elements for her own continuing growth as well as that of her child.

EFFECT OF MATERNAL NUTRITION ON THE FETUS

There has been a great deal of study of the effect of maternal nutrition on the developing infant. Although there have been many promising leads, it has been difficult to come up with positive proof that the mother's nutritional state has any specific bad effects except for an increase in the number of miscarriages and premature births.

Babies born deformed have been found to lack certain nutritional elements in their systems. We cannot be sure, however, that this results from a deficiency in the mother. It is possible that something in the developing fetal system went wrong, preventing the proper use of the maternal supply.

But one thing can be positively stated: Your developing child cannot make use of needed food elements if they are not made available to him. And we know from laboratory studies that animal mothers whose diet during pregnancy is lacking in important elements have a larger number of deformed offspring than do mothers whose diet is adequate.

Most people cannot be confident that they instinctively eat correctly. Many adolescents find acceptance of group habits much more important than concern about the future. Yet when we consider the large number of teen-age mothers, we realize the importance of the establishment of good eating habits early in life. Young women will be doing their future babies a great favor if they build up their own bodies now.

Your body makes an effort to supply the nutritional elements needed by the new life growing within it. But common sense tells us that no stores can be taken from an empty warehouse. If your diet was poor before pregnancy, the nutritional elements will not be there to be used and the baby will have to compete with you for what is available. Without question, a baby's best interest will be served if he is fortunate enough to have a mother who developed good nutritional habits long before he came along.

Everyone who has gone to school has had some teaching concerning the kinds of foods needed for good health. Unfortunately rules may be too arbitrary—"so much meat, so many citrus fruits"—without giving alternatives for the family whose budget just will not stretch that far. Some people cannot afford the food needed for health. Many others simply do not bother to take the time to prepare it.

Nutritionists employed by state, county, or city health bureaus can be helpful in food planning. A brief list of books and pamphlets on meal planning is given at the end of the book.

WHAT IS A WELL-BALANCED DIET FOR PREGNANCY?

If you are of normal weight, you will need little extra food during pregnancy. But you may need to increase the proportion of some kinds of foods in your diet.

PROTEIN. This is the most important food; it is essential for the developing infant before birth and throughout life. In addition, you will also need a good supply for the growth and repair of your own body. The best sources of protein are meat, fish, milk, eggs, and cheese. Other good sources are dry beans, lentils, soybeans, chick-peas (garbanzos), and peanut butter.

VITAMINS. An ample supply of vitamins can be obtained in a well-balanced diet, with the exception of Vitamin D. This can be supplied through irradiated milk or margarine, but you would need a quart of fortified milk daily or five tablespoons of vitamin-D-fortified magarine for a sufficient amount. Vitamin C may also be low unless special attention is given to citrus fruits and tomatoes. Because an adequate supply of all vitamins is so important, most obstetricians prescribe a basic formula polyvitamin preparation for the expectant mother.

MINERALS. The most important minerals are iron, iodine, and calcium.

Studies have shown that the majority of women of child-bearing age in the United States do not have enough iron in their systems and are often somewhat anemic. It is important that you have enough to supply your baby as well as yourself. Your doctor will check the iron level of your blood early in pregnancy and see to it that you get enough, either from your food or from a mineral supplement.

Iodine is important for the body tissues, but any lack in your diet can easily be remedied by using iodized salt for seasoning.

Calcium is essential for bone building, for both mother and baby. Milk (and milk products) is the usual source of calcium.

41

Foods that should be eaten every day

To meet the requirements of a well-balanced diet in pregnancy, the kinds of food listed below are necessary.

Milk. You should have three to five 8-ounce glasses a day. Before you say, "But I could never drink that much milk," remember that you don't have to *drink* it all. Count the milk used in cooking, in sauces, poured over cereal, put in puddings, and contained in cottage cheese, yogurt, and ice cream. If you have not tried yogurt, you will find the sweet, tangy taste of the fruit-flavored preparations a pleasant surprise. If you can't get fruit-flavored yogurt, mix slightly tart jam or jelly with the plain variety.

Meat, fish, eggs, cheese, cottage cheese, dried beans, peas, and nuts. Eat a total of 6 to 10 ounces daily. That's three or four ordinary portions. Three ounces of meat is about the size of an ordinary cooked hamburger. One ounce of meat (cooked) is approximately the equivalent of 1 egg, 1 ounce of cheese, or 2 ounces of cottage cheese (about 2 rounded tablespoons). You can substitute ⅓ cup of dried beans, peas, or lentils—or 2 tablespoons of peanut butter—for 1 ounce of meat.

Peanut-butter sandwiches and toasted cheese sandwiches make pleasant ways to add protein. If you enjoy eating liver, oysters, or kidneys, they are good sources of both protein and iron.

Fruits and vegetables. Twice a day you should eat fruit and vegetables high in vitamin C: oranges, lemons, limes, grapefruit, tomatoes, and strawberries. One orange, ½ grapefruit, 1 medium-size tomato—or 4 ounces of their juices—equals a serving, as does 1 cup of strawberries.

Two other servings of fruit should also be part of your daily diet. Cooked or dried fruits are as useful as raw ones. If you are gaining weight too fast, check the amount of sugar in your fruit. Eat the sweet fruits plain; their flavor will come through better.

You need at least two servings of vegetables daily, including one of the deep yellow or deep green vegetables for vitamin A: carrots, sweet potatoes or yams, broccoli, yellow (winter) squash, spinach, kale, endive, parsley, and other such greens. If you find spinach too bland, try the tangy flavor of mustard or turnip greens or collards. If you don't want the job of cleaning them, use the canned or frozen varieties; they are surprisingly good.

Bread and cereals. Four or five servings are recommended. One serving can consist of 1 slice of bread or ½ cup of cooked cereal. If you are counting calories, don't forget to count whatever you add to your cereal—butter, margarine, sugar, or fruit. Count ½ cup of rice, macaroni, or spaghetti as a serving.

Fats. Two or three tablespoons of margarine or butter or salad oil are suggested.

FOOD RESTRICTIONS

Unless you are in the habit of using excessive salt (sodium chloride) you will not need to reduce your intake. The doctor may ask you to cut back if your ankles tend to swell, indicating excess fluid in your tissues. If you do need to limit your intake of salt, you won't find it as hard as you might think; reaching for the salt shaker may be largely habit. You will discover the true flavor of foods when you try them with less salt. If salt is to be restricted, you should also omit such salty foods as canned nuts, pretzels, and ham.

Counting calories is certainly one of the games of American women, yet many of them might be hard put to tell exactly what they are counting. A calorie is a unit of measurement of the energy value of food. It takes a certain number of these units to maintain the energy needed for all body functions and activity. Food eaten in excess of this need is stored in the body as fat. When too few calories are taken in, the body uses its stores and weight is lost.

A pregnant woman needs more calories than are normally used in order to support both herself and her child, but how many more depends on many factors, including her nonpregnant weight, her height, her age, and her activity level.

Calorie counters are available in bookstores, supermarkets, libraries, and popular magazines and often contain tables of dietary allowances for people of different ages, heights, and activity levels. In the United States these tables are based on the recommended dietary allowances prepared by the National Research Council of the National Academy of Science. The Council revised the tables in 1968 to meet current living conditions in the United States, lowering the calorie allowance because Americans generally appear to be less active today.

The report stresses the fact that all recommended allowances, with the exception of that for iron, can be met by the average American diet. Of course, those persons whose diets are lopsided because of fads, sickness, or economic hardship do not fit the average picture.

WHAT TO BUY FOR THE BABY *

Part of the fun of having a baby is getting things ready, but it can be bewildering as well. Look in any baby department and you will see the enormous variety of nursery furniture, baby clothes, and supplies.

How much you spend depends on you. If this is your first baby, you'll spend more than you will for the second or third. If your family or friends have equipment to offer, accept it. Your baby will outgrow clothes and furniture so fast that it is silly to put money into things you need so briefly.

Just remember, the looks of the clothes and furniture is important only to you. Your baby won't care about ruffles or a silk-lined bassinet; he will do just as well with a diaper and a bureau drawer.

FURNITURE

Though many families do not set up a special room as a nursery, it is good if your baby can sleep in a separate room from his parents—to allow all three of you a better chance for a good night's sleep. Wherever he sleeps, he needs his own bed. As a matter of fact, all a small baby needs in the way of furniture is something in which to sleep. This can be almost anything

* A list of basic layette needs appears at the end of this section.

that will give him room to stretch and breathe. In 3 or 4 months, however, he will need room to turn over and roll about. Later he will need even more room to sit up, creep around, and stand.

BABY CRIB AND BASSINET. A regular-size crib with deep sides is a good investment from the start, but if you cannot afford one, start off with a smaller crib (borrowed if possible); it has the advantage of being moved around more easily.

A bassinet is fine, and useful as well. If you buy or borrow one, try to get one with as few dust-catching bows and ruffles as possible. A lined clothes basket makes a very good bassinet at little cost. You can make a mattress by folding an old blanket to size and stitching it into a pad. If possible get a zippered plastic cover to protect the mattress. Don't use a pillow. The baby needs a firm surface to lie on. The entire basket needs some kind of a padded lining. Quilted pads or a folded blanket work well. But the lining must be tied firmly to the basket at top, bottom, and sides. There should be no sagging material for your baby to get his face into.

If you buy or borrow a crib, make sure it is good and strong, with closely spaced spindles and a drop side (or sides) that works well but will not fall down unexpectedly.

The portable cribs on the market have several advantages. They can be rolled through doorways easily. The crib bottom can be raised to make a convenient dressing table or lowered to become an excellent playpen. They are made of sturdy hardwood, with spindles 3 inches apart, and they can be folded for compact storage. The drop sides have a safety catch to discourage older children from lowering them.

Larger cribs have adjustable bottoms, high at first so that you can easily reach the tiny baby, lower as he grows so the sides protect him when he pulls himself up.

There should be 12 spindles on each side of a standard crib. This gives a 3¼-inch gap, small enough so that no head can get caught. Most modern cribs have this safety feature. Check the safety catches on the drop sides to see if they are really "child-proof." A useful feature of most cribs is the plastic covering the top rail, making a safe teething rail for the baby to gnaw on.

If you are repainting an old crib, be sure to use a nontoxic, lead-free paint. Don't *ever* use leftover outdoor paint. And again, if you are working with an old crib, put a safety catch on the drop side and check the space between spindles; you can use plastic side liners if the spaces are too wide.

BEDDING. *Mattresses* of foam rubber or cotton felt are ideal. Most new crib mattresses come with a waterproof covering. If yours doesn't, you can buy a zippered plastic mattress cover or you can sew your own. But beware of loose sheet plastic in your baby's crib, bassinet, or carriage. No loose plastic sheeting should ever be within a baby's (or toddler's) reach. *Never* use the bag your dry cleaning comes in: your child can smother.

Sheets, fitted cotton-knit ones, are very nice for the bassinet, carriage, or small improvised crib. They stay in place in spite of the baby's turning and squirming, they are warm and soft, and they are convenient; they wash and dry easily and do not need to be ironed. A cotton receiving blanket or large diaper may also serve as a sheet, provided it is large enough to tuck under at sides and top. A quilted or flannel-back pad to slip under the baby will help in keeping the bottom sheet dry.

Perhaps someone has given you one of the cotton-knit fitted top sheets. These are also useful; otherwise, the receiving blanket serves well. As your baby gets more active, it may be difficult to keep him under any covering. That is when coveralls or sleepers are helpful.

Blankets such as thermal crib blankets are easily washed, very light in weight, yet warm and comfortable. They are 100 percent cotton and do not shrink. Other blankets of synthetic fibrics also wash well without shrinkage. You will also want some small cotton "receiving blankets." These can be cut from an old soft blanket or made from cotton flannelette.

In cold climates, sleeping bags are handy for night use, keeping your baby warm even when he has kicked the covers off.

PLAYPENS. A playpen is useful for the older baby between 6 months and 1 year who is beginning to cruise about by one means or another. If you buy a wooden playpen, make sure it has no hinges or cracks that can catch and pinch little fingers.

Playpens with mesh sides are very popular. They are light-weight and easy to move. Those with a fairly fine mesh are firmer and have less tendency to sag if older children pull or climb on the sides.

Proper use of a playpen is very important and has many psychological implications (see The Playpen Versus Freedom in Chapter 3).

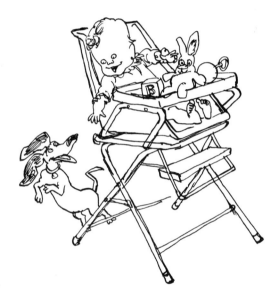

HIGH AND LOW CHAIRS. You can bring your baby to the family table as soon as he enjoys sitting in a high chair. Usually this will be about 7 to 9 months. But you should never leave him alone in a high chair for long; even harness straps do not always keep a small baby from slipping through or stop the young explorer from falling out. (A folded diaper tied around the baby's middle and through the back of the chair often works better than the best of harnesses.) So if you are going to use a high chair, limit its use to when the baby is eating with the rest of the family and you can keep an eye on him.

If you want a high chair, look for one with a wide base, a latch for the tray, and a heavily constructed frame. Try tipping the chair yourself to see how safe it would be.

There is a convertible high chair on the market with adjustable legs to allow conversion to a low-chair set with a baby table. This is a sturdy, wide-based high chair with vinyl cushions and sides and an adjustable footrest. The convertible high chair allows your older baby or toddler to sit on a level with the rest of the family at meals but can be lowered easily to the low table-chair arrangement.

There are also low tables with inset seats that are very satisfactory if the child eats most of his meals alone. In each case, the table top holds him in and gives him a surface for eating and playing. You can buy simply the low table-chair or the combination.

Use of a high chair can be important in integrating the baby into the structure of family life.

Toilet-Training Chair and Toilet Seat. The old standby wooden potty chair still has a place in the nursery. One model comes with a plastic seat and removable potty for easy cleaning.

Training chairs also come in lightweight plastic with comfortable backs. These are easy to keep clean and odor-free. Another advantage is that they resemble a real toilet, perhaps making the transition easier later. Some of these have detachable seats that can be placed over a regular toilet seat. Small toilet seats for this purpose can also be bought without the chair. However, many toddlers are afraid of flush toilets and adjust better to the low potty chair.

Bathtub and Dressing Table. Of course you can bathe your baby in any sort of container large enough for him to splash around. But the regular family tub makes bathing a small baby quite difficult.

A molded plastic portable tub is ideal for bathing a baby. It comes simply as an oblong tub or with useful added features. It is deep enough to immerse the baby but shallow enough to allow you to hold him comfortably with one hand while washing him with the other.

A tub that has a wide edge on which to rest your arm while supporting the baby is helpful. Some models also have a removable "security sling" which holds a tiny baby securely while he is in the water.

Any table you already own can double nicely as a dressing table; just pick one at which you can sit or stand comfortably. Or you can buy one of the baby dressing tables with padded tops, drawers, and hanging or closet space below for your baby's clothes. These tables can be folded to chest size when not being used for dressing.

DIAPER PAIL OR CONTAINER. A diaper service will furnish its own containers, but if you are not using a service you will need a pail with a cover for wet and soiled diapers.

INFANT SEAT. The lightweight baby seats you see mothers using are certainly convenient. Your baby will even like one in his crib because his head can be raised to various levels so that he can look around.

Infant seats come in many styles and prices. One precaution: Don't leave your baby unattended in one on a table, counter, or any other elevated surface. He may wriggle out or tip over, even though there is a safety strap. If you have to leave him alone, put him and the infant seat inside his crib or on the floor.

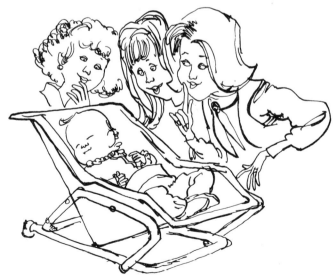

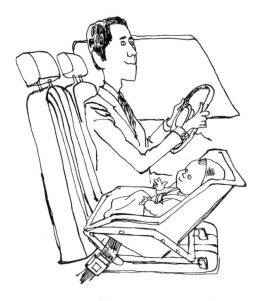

STROLLERS OR CARRIAGE AND CAR BED.   Strollers come in varying shapes, sizes, and prices. They can be adjusted to a flat position for the very young baby, and some convert into carriages, car beds, or walkers. Many have a wire shopping basket attached. They can be folded up and put in the car, ready for use when you arrive at your destination.

Carriages are not used as much as formerly in this country, since the stroller is much easier to handle. However, if you have been given or loaned a carriage, you can use it until the baby can sit alone and starts climbing about.

Back-pack toters offer another useful way of getting around with a baby. Your hands are left free, and the baby's weight is evenly distributed. Babies seem to love them. After all, the custom of carrying a baby around on the mother's back is nearly as old as man himself.

A car bed has a unique advantage; it can double as a crib or bassinet. Lightweight and easily carried, it is quite versatile.

As your baby grows older, he will need a travel seat if he rides much in a car. Make sure you get one with a safety cushion headrest to protect against whiplash. It should have a harness strap as well as a safety rail around the seat, and there should be some way of making the seat secure, whether it is placed on a car seat or rests between the seats. Chapter 17 suggests some effective models.

OTHER BABY FURNITURE. Jump seats have become popular, and walkers seem to have come back in favor. Of course you don't want to leave your baby in his jump seat or walker all the time. A healthy baby will get up and walk independently when he is ready.

CLOTHING

Your baby will grow very fast during his first year, and he will quickly outgrow his clothes. Generally speaking, a 6-month or even 1-year size is the best to buy for a newborn baby.

SHIRTS. Long-sleeved, short-sleeved, or sleeveless shirts? Snapped on or tied or pulled over the head? The temperature has much to do with regulating your baby's clothing. On really hot days he does best by going shirtless.

Snap-on or pullover? Many babies seem frightened by clothing pulled over their heads, and their mothers find the double-breasted snap-on or tied shirts easier to put on. If you do use a pullover, look for one that has a stretch neckline.

Also look for a seamless nonbinding underarm. Shirts with diaper tabs are handy if you use cloth diapers.

GOWNS AND PAJAMAS. Footed pajamas made of a stretch-knit material are very popular with mothers—and babies as well. They have snap fastener openings down the front and legs for easy changing. They come in several colors and are just fine for sleeping, sitting, crawling, or just kicking. The stretch fabric makes them an easy fit for a long time.

Many mothers like the long cotton-knit gowns for their young babies. These have mitten sleeves and drawstring hems at the bottom. Keep in mind that your baby will rather quickly outgrow a gown.

Sophisticated sacque sets—dainty knit cotton sacques with plasticized panties to match—are nice for dress-up.

Out-of-Doors Wear.   In cold weather, a light but warm acrylic or wool blanket does nicely as an outside wrap over the baby's regular clothing.

Bonnets and booties are nice but difficult to keep on.

Diapers.   Diapers nowadays come in a bewildering assortment of materials, shapes, and sizes. Fortunately, babies use them in the same old way.

Disposable diapers come in two main styles. One has a waterproof backing and needs just an old-fashioned safety pin to keep them in place. The other fits nicely into a reusable panty that snaps on, eliminating the safety pin. Mothers show enthusiasm for both styles. It is, of course, more expensive to use disposable diapers than to reuse cloth ones—about the same as the cost of a diaper service. A large plastic bag can hold used diapers for disposal with the rest of the household rubbish.

Some mothers like to use disposable diapers just for traveling; others are happy to use them all the time. But some babies develop skin reactions to the waterproof backing. This covering protects outer clothes and bedding but prevents air circulation from drying the diaper itself, so the baby is actually much wetter inside the diaper than he otherwise would be. Some babies' skins just can't stand being so wet. Overnight sleeping in plastic-backed diapers or waterproof pants is the commonest single cause of diaper rash.

Prefold cloth diapers made of soft cotton gauze come ready-shaped to fit your baby. Some have a gentle stretching action that allows them to fit better to your baby's movements.

Regular rectangular diapers that are folded to fit are preferred by many mothers because the baby does not outgrow these as he does the ready-shaped ones.

Waterproof Pants.   Waterproof pants do a good job of keeping the baby's clothes dry. Most are made of soft vinyl or waterproof nylon and come in pull-on or snap-on styles. If you wish, you can find waterproof pants with striped or colored coverings, or even with lace and ribbon. All are washable and retain their softness.

But again we warn that some babies develop severe diaper rash from waterproof pants. So, particularly in hot weather, leave them on for short periods only.

FORMULA EQUIPMENT

If you do not plan to breast-feed your baby, you can buy his nursing equipment at the same time you get his layette ready.

The plastic bottle, easily sterilized and square-sided for better handling, has become a favorite.

Some mothers find that a disposable nurser simplifies bottle feeding. This is a plastic bottle containing a presterilized, disposable plastic formula sac. The idea is that after the baby has nursed the formula sac is discarded, and the bottle doesn't need washing. But if you make your own formula, you will have to boil it before pouring it into the sac.

There are moderately priced electric sterilizers, as there are regular sterilizers. Or you can make your own (see Chapter 3).

Basic needs

Following is a list of the minimal basic needs for the first 3 months. Once you have these, you can suit your fancy to your purse.

CLOTHES AND BEDDING

4–6 shirts, sleeved, short-sleeved, or sleeveless (according to temperature, climate, time of year)

3–4 gowns or coveralls (footed pajamas)

4–6 small cotton blankets ("receiving blankets")

3–4 pair waterproof pants

4–6 dozen cloth diapers, or packs of disposable diapers as needed *or* (if a diaper service is to be used) 1 dozen cloth or disposable diapers for emergencies

Diaper pins

4–6 waterproof pads for under baby

Crib blankets as needed

3–6 cotton-knit sheets

Sweater (1-year size) or shawls (optional)

Booties (optional)

BATH SUPPLIES

1 bathtub
Table or shelf for bathtub and bath supplies
3–4 soft washcloths
3–4 large soft bath towels
Mild soap
Mild unmedicated baby oil or petroleum jelly
Cotton
Fingernail scissors

FORMULA SUPPLIES

8–12 8-oz. nursing bottles (plastic or glass) *or* 1 set of disposable nursers
6 or more nipples and bottle tops
Sterilizer kit or electric sterilizer (if not using disposable bottles)
Bottle brush

FURNITURE

Crib, bassinet, or basket
Car bed or baby toter
Utility bag for traveling
Diaper pail

PLANNING FOR THE BIG EVENT

What method of childbirth for you? Let your own feelings decide. If you want to be mentally alert and conscious through labor and delivery, because you feel you want to savor in its entirety this the greatest moment of your life, there are methods that allow you that privilege. But not every pregnant woman feels this way, and no woman should feel shame or guilt if she cannot or does not wish to be fully alert during the birth—just as no woman should feel smug or superior because she chose and was able to carry out such a program.

Dr. Helen Wallace has stated the matter well:

It is important for some women to be conscious in labor, to
see the delivery if possible, to view the infant immediately
after being delivered and to "room-in" with the infant and to
breast feed as part of the adaptive sequence. It is equally important for those who cannot tolerate the investment, the in-
timacy and the unknown demanded of them, to be exposed
only to the limit of tolerance.*

NEW METHODS OF CHILDBIRTH

Two approaches to childbirth that many women have found
satisfying are the natural childbirth method and the psychoprophylactic method. A brief description of each will help you
to decide whether you would like to learn about either or both.
A brief list of references concerning both methods is included at
the end of the book.

Natural childbirth

Early in the 1930s, an English obstetrician, Dr. Grantly Dick-
Read, took issue with the age-old belief that women must bear
children in pain. He reasoned that much pain is caused by tension due to fear, especially fear of the unknown. Women, he
found, were nearly totally ignorant of the process of birth—and
steeped in traditions and folk tales about the terrors of childbirth.
It was only human for older women to tell the younger how
very brave *they* had been, and to embellish the truth somewhat
in the process. Also, some of them had known the terror of
being handled by midwives and neighbors who did not know how
to deal with the complications of childbirth, or by doctors who
knew little more.

Dr. Read believed that when women were taught the orderly
process of pregnancy, labor, and delivery, their fear of the unknown would disappear. His method of natural childbirth con-
sists of education about childbirth, as well as practice throughout

* Helen Wallace, *Health Services for Mothers and Children* (Philadelphia:
W. B. Saunders Co., 1962), p. 125.

pregnancy in learning how to relax the entire body.

When labor starts, the muscles of the uterus tense and relax in a rhythmic fashion. These contractions, as they are called, are entirely involuntary; they can neither be started nor stopped by the patient. But fear of pain will cause the patient to tense other muscles which work against the muscles of the uterus. When the woman has learned through repeated practice to relax her body, she will almost automatically relax during labor contractions, thus letting the uterus do its work without interference and with little pain. Therefore the patient is able to go through the experience awake, fully realizing all that is going on. And she can always request a pain reliever if she needs one.

The Read method also stresses the father's role in preparing for childbirth. Both prospective parents attend a series of classes in which the anatomy of childbearing organs and their function is taught. They learn about the stages of labor and the way the mother can cooperate and work with the normal labor process. They practice exercises that will tone up the muscles used in labor, the husband assisting the wife and learning how he can be of greatest help when labor begins. In other words, the aim of the program is to help the mother help herself and give her confidence.

The Read method, described in *Childbirth Without Fear*, emphasizes the exaltation and gratification experienced by a mother who has been alert and cooperative through the birth and who is awake to see and feel her baby being born.

Psychoprophylactic childbirth

A method differing slightly from the Read concept, but having the same goal of active participation in the birth of the baby, was developed by Dr. Fernand Lamaze in France. The Lamaze method is a psychoprophylactic one, based on the Pavlov method of "conditioning" to eliminate any consciousness of pain. Considerable emphasis is put on learning breathing techniques to be used during contractions, with complete relaxation between contractions.

Evaluation

Both the Read "childbirth without fear" and the Lamaze "childbirth without pain" teach that, because fear increases the perception of pain, a knowledge of what is happening helps diminish the fear. They also believe that tension that works against the normal progress of labor can be greatly reduced in a cheerful and calm atmosphere, particularly with a helpful husband to assist the mother. The aim of both methods is to allow the mother to experience childbirth as a wonderful, exhilarating, memorable event, a time of enjoyment rather than fear—and women all over the world can testify to their success. As a matter of fact, people who have used one of these methods tend to become so enthusiastic that they assume it is the ideal method for everyone.

This is not so. In the first place, many things can keep the delivery from being a simple straightforward affair. A baby may be in the wrong position and need to be turned; he may need help by use of forceps. Or the surgeon may tend to make a small cut in the mother's vaginal outlet before the baby's head is delivered to prevent tearing of the perineal tissues. Such procedures require some form of anesthesia.

People also differ in their consciousness of pain. Some experience very little; others have pain near the limits of endurance and need relief. If such help is needed, the mother should realize that her physician understands her particular case and should leave the management in his hands, regardless of the method used.

The current trend in relieving the discomfort and pain of labor and delivery is one of moderation, with the obstetrician watching out for his patient's needs. There are sedatives, pain-relieving medicines, and anesthetics that can safely be used without harm to either mother or child.

A woman who has been emotionally well prepared for labor by her physician is usually relaxed and may require very little medication.

THE HUSBAND'S PART IN THE ACTUAL BIRTH

In the past the husband was ushered into the waiting room when his wife entered the labor room. Now most hospitals will allow your husband to stay with you until you are taken to the delivery room if you wish it (though he may still find himself spending much of his time in the corridor while the doctor or nurse examines you). Whether your husband stays with you during your labor depends on how you both feel about it. You may find he provides much support and encouragement.

A number of married couples, but by no means all, would like to be together even in the delivery room. If your husband wishes to stay with you during delivery and your doctor agrees, he will be helped to scrub and gown under the nurse's direction and then be shown where he may sit at the side of the delivery table. Hospitals that are permissive about this allow your husband to stay only if you are awake. The only reason for his presence, they feel, is to give you support.

ROOMING-IN

Rooming-in is the term used when provision is made for your baby to stay at your bedside in his own crib during the daytime hours. If you have decided to breast-feed your baby on a demand schedule—whenever he is hungry—you will probably have to use rooming-in. It does provide a way for you and your husband to learn to care for your baby from the start. But if your hospital doesn't have such facilities, or if you prefer to use your few days in the hospital for resting, be assured that your baby will do very well in the nursery and that you will see and hold him often.

WHAT TO TAKE TO THE HOSPITAL

You will want to have a small suitcase or overnight bag packed and ready in advance of your due date just in case labor starts early. And have a list of taxi numbers by the phone in case you are alone when the time comes.

Your hospital may send you a list of articles to bring—for

yourself and for the baby. But just in case it doesn't, here are the most important things.

NIGHTGOWNS OR PAJAMAS. You will wear hospital gowns in the labor room and in the recovery room, and you can wear them throughout your hospital stay. But a gown or pajamas of your own will give a cheerful lift to hospital life. Pack a couple.

BATHROBE AND SLIPPERS. You will spend much of your time out of bed.

CLOTHING TO WEAR HOME. Don't forget to take clothes to wear home. You will want clean underclothes and a dress that fits your now normal figure.

TOILET ARTICLES. Pack your comb, brush, toothbrush and toothpaste, underarm deodorant, and whatever cosmetics you think you must have. The hospital will supply boxes of cleansing tissue.

NURSING BRASSIERE. You will need to wear one when your milk starts to come in. Whether you intend to breast-feed your baby or not, a brassiere will keep you more comfortable. Better take a couple.

SANITARY BELT. Some hospitals furnish a belt for wear there; others do not. (They all furnish sanitary napkins.) In any case, take one along to wear going home.

WRISTWATCH. This is an important asset. Don't take a small clock; it may get knocked off your bedside table.

MONEY AND WRITING SUPPLIES. Take a little change if you want to buy a newspaper. Paper and pencil are handy for taking notes on the baby's care, but don't expect to have much time for letter writing.

CLOTHING FOR THE BABY TO WEAR HOME. You will need 2 or 3 diapers, 4 large safety pins, a pair of waterproof pants, a shirt or gown, a wrapping blanket, and other clothing according to the season—sweater, bunting, warm blanket. Booties are pretty, but don't expect them to stay on.

FORMULA CONTAINER. If your baby is on a formula, the hospital will probably send enough formula home with you to last for the next few feedings. Usually this will be given to you in a sterile jar. Ask whether you need to bring a sterile container or nursing bottles.

ARRANGEMENTS FOR AFTER YOU COME HOME

Diaper service

If you are planning to use a diaper service, the arrangements should be made in advance. Find out what the company provides, what the cost will be, and arrange for service to be started when you are ready to bring the baby home, giving the approximate date. Then all you need do is call later to give the exact day for service to start.

Help in the house

In the hospital, you will be encouraged to get up and about early, and you will be ready to go home a few days after a normal delivery. During your short stay in the hospital, your husband can look out for himself well enough, so you will have a problem only if you have children at home. If you happen to live in or near a college town you might try calling the student employment office. Colleges and universities often have students eager for part-time work, and you may even find a student willing to live in, if you feel you need one. Perhaps a relative can come in, or you can hire a housekeeper.

Some communities have homemakers who care for the children if there is no other care for them and no money to buy help. Unfortunately these are not available everywhere. Day care centers also care for children on a temporary basis; all that is needed is someone to take the children back and forth. Sometimes a friend will take the children into her own home for the short time necessary.

If your children are going to be cared for by someone outside of their own home, make sure they get to know the place and the person who will take care of them before you go to the hospital. It is important that they understand what is happening

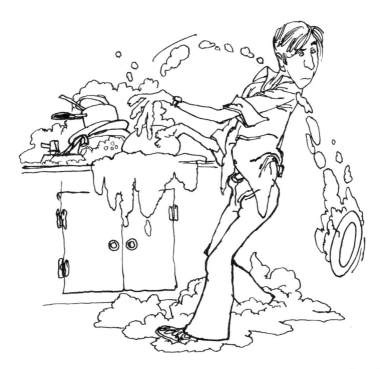

as much as they are able, so that they will not feel abandoned by you in favor of the new baby.

After you come home you will need some help for a week or more, whether you have other children or not. You may decide to care for your baby yourself and leave the housework for someone else. But if you can't get help with the housework, ignore it—it will keep for another day. Or let your husband help as much as he wants. After all, he has a part in all this, and rare is the husband who will not put forth the extra effort needed in his pride over *his* new child.

Arrangements for the working mother

If you are going back to your job, who will care for your baby during working hours? There are several alternatives to consider and look into: use of a day care center, care in a private home, someone to come into your home by the day, or someone to live in.

You will have to consider which type of care will best fit your situation. Another important factor is the availability of the particular kind of care you would like to use. Child care facilities are discussed in some detail in Chapter 4. Consider the advantages and disadvantages of each from the standpoint of your own situation and then investigate thoroughly before making your final choice.

Preparing older children for the baby

The coming of a new child into the family will mean many adjustments for the older children as well. If an older child is told right from the start about all that is happening, he feels as if he too is a partner in this adventure. Of course the toddler is too young to know the meaning of time; since he will expect the baby to appear immediately, don't tell him about it until a week or two before your delivery date. The special problems concerning the toddler's adjustment to a new baby in the family are discussed in detail in Chapter 4.

The child of 6 years or older will enjoy following your pregnancy. He will appreciate being told how the baby came to be in your abdomen and how he is growing. As the baby grows, let him feel it kicking.*

The older child may feel some jealousy when the baby comes home and requires a great deal of attention from you. He may feel unloved and left out. It will help if he is included from the beginning in the baby's care and allowed to hold the baby (under supervision, of course), help hold the bottle, and gather articles for his bath. And when visitors bring gifts to the baby make sure there is something for your older child as well, even if you have to keep a few small toys in store for that purpose.

Parents can work together to find time to give to the older child. Perhaps his father can take over the baby's bath or formula feeding, or just rock him, while you devote some special time to your older child.

* For help in telling him about the baby, see Andrew C. Andry and Steven Schepp, How Babies Are Made.

2
The Birth Experience

THE MATERNAL EXPERIENCE OF CHILDBIRTH

Everyone has been growing tired of waiting for the baby to appear. But now it is time—time for him to start a life of his own.

Signs of readiness for birth are usually present during the last month of pregnancy, particularly with the first-born. Sometime during the ninth month the event called *lightening* occurs. Before this, your baby was high in your abdomen. As he grew larger he pressed against your diaphragm, perhaps causing you to be short of breath. Shortly before he is ready to be born, he will drop lower in the pelvis, relieving the pressure on your rib cage. Although this shows that the period of pregnancy is coming to an end, it is not possible to predict accurately the length of time between lightening and the start of the birth process.

UTERINE CONTRACTIONS

Throughout pregnancy the muscles of the uterus have tightened and relaxed. This has not disturbed your baby in his roomy "bag of waters," and you have not felt these contractions. But as the birth date nears, these contractions become stronger, although still without discomfort to you. Your baby is now nearly filling the space inside his fluid sac, and the contractions help him get into a position for birth.

Sometimes a mother does feel these mild contractions and takes them for true labor contractions. Actually, it is not always possible to be sure whether this is *false labor* or the beginning of an early labor. If this happens to you, try a change of position, such as walking around. If the contractions diminish, it is false labor; if the contractions continue fairly regularly and increase in severity, notify your doctor. Don't feel embarrassed if you are wrong. Plenty of people think they are in labor when they are not.

Labor commences

At this time the contractions are strong and regular. They are usually felt first as a tightness in the lower back, then in the front of the lower abdomen, somewhat like menstrual cramps. Their purpose is to open or dilate the cervix of the uterus enough to permit your baby to pass into the birth canal.

The first indication that labor will soon commence may be a break in the amniotic sac, the bag of waters surrounding the baby. You will have a sudden gush of fluid from the vagina. This rupture of the membranes may occur just before your labor starts or any time before the actual birth. Or it may not happen spontaneously at all; in that case, the doctor will rupture the membranes to assist in the progress. In either case you will feel nothing except the rush of fluid. The so-called "dry birth" or "dry labor," meaning the membranes have ruptured early, has no effect on the process of labor and delivery.

Another indication that labor will soon begin is the mucus show. As the cervix begins to open, a plug of mucus mixed with a little blood passes out of the vagina. This may be the first sign. However, many women get neither signal before contractions commence. They just go into labor.

Once started, contractions become regular and more frequent. It is well with the first pregnancy to wait until several contractions have occurred and to time their frequency and length before calling the doctor or the hospital. That is, of course, unless the membranes have ruptured. If you have experienced the sudden release of fluid, notify your doctor promptly.

How to time contractions

Your doctor will ask you how often the contractions are coming. Time them by counting the minutes from the beginning of one to the start of the next. They may be anywhere from 4 to 15 minutes apart at first. Check twice or three times to see if they are coming at regular intervals.

Your doctor will also want to know how long a single contraction lasts. If you have a watch with a second hand, count the seconds from the time you first feel the tightening in your back or abdominal muscles until the muscles relax. If you do not have a watch with a sweep second hand, count from 1 to 60 at a slow rate (saying *thousand* after each number to space your counting).

If this is your first baby, the doctor may suggest that you wait until contractions become frequent, perhaps 5 minutes apart, before coming to the hospital. You probably will find daytime waiting more pleasant if you stay up and about; at night try to get some sleep between contractions. Unless it is very early in labor, you will do better not to eat solid food, because labor sometimes is accompanied by nausea and vomiting, and this can be aggravated by food in the stomach. But you may drink water and clear liquids as you wish. If your labor is long and dilatation of the cervix slow, the doctor may allow you to have some light food also.

ENTERING THE HOSPITAL

Again we say notify your doctor at once if the "bag of waters" breaks, whether or not contractions follow. It means the cervix of the uterus has opened a little, and he will prefer to have you in the hospital where you can be watched more closely.

If you believe—or know—that you are in labor but for some reason cannot get your doctor on the phone, go to the hospital anyway. Another doctor will check you and get in touch with your doctor.

If you have been attending the outpatient maternity clinic, call your hospital before going. But if you cannot get to a phone or do not have time to call, go to the hospital anyway. Patients in labor are not turned away, even those who have had no prenatal care and have not registered ahead of time.

But in a first pregnancy there is usually plenty of time to get to the hospital, for the uterine muscles take longer to open the cervix the first time. The event of giving birth is the greatest experience in a woman's life. You will certainly be excited when you go to the hospital, so try to find out what to do beforehand, such as which door to use at the hospital and where to go after entering.

After you are admitted and taken to your room, you will be examined, your blood pressure taken, and the baby's heartbeat listened to. Hospital practices differ concerning shaving pubic hair. In many maternity departments all the pubic hair is shaven off; in others only the hair around the vagina; in some hospitals, shaving of pubic hair is omitted entirely. You may or may not be given an enema. You will be examined at frequent intervals during the course of labor, and the baby's heartbeat recorded. You may stay in your room, or you may be taken to a room near the delivery room.

THE THREE STAGES OF LABOR

During the *first stage* of labor, the cervix dilates gradually until the opening becomes large enough for the baby to pass through. This dilatation is entirely involuntary; pushing down will have no effect and only serves to exhaust you. Save your strength for later. Learning to relax the body during contractions, and resting between them, will make this stage more comfortable.

The *second stage* has its beginning after the cervix has become fully dilated and the top of the baby's head can be seen at the cervical opening during a contraction. At this point you are taken to the delivery room and placed on the delivery table in the position you have learned to assume for pelvic examinations. Now you will be asked to push down with each contraction; in fact, you will find it very hard not to push. The baby's head slowly emerges, followed by the rest of his body. The second stage is over; the baby has been born. (Not all babies come head first; some come buttocks first, called a breech delivery; some feet first.)

After the baby is born, his connecting cord is cut and you have a short period of rest. This is followed by the start of painless contractions as the afterbirth (the placenta and membranes which nourished the fetus) is expelled through the birth canal. During this, the *third stage*, a certain amount of bleeding occurs as the placenta separates itself from the lining of the uterus.

Use of forceps

The idea of forceps is frightening to many people, but it shouldn't be, for the modern use of forceps is far different from what it once was.

Many obstetricians now believe in the practice of prophylactic forceps. When your baby's head has descended to the outlet of the vagina, they use forceps to spare his head prolonged pressure against your perineum. It is thus a protective measure for your baby. After one or more births, the outlet may become more flexible and roomy, and then forceps probably will not be used.

Occasionally forceps are used earlier in delivery, if the uterus is fully dilated, the baby's head is descending, and the mother has a medical condition that makes it wise to shorten her labor —especially if the second stage of labor has gone on longer than usual and the mother is tiring. Or forceps may be used if the baby shows signs that his oxygen supply is getting low. Again, though, the use of forceps today is a simple affair which makes the delivery easier and safer for both mother and infant.

The episiotomy

As the baby's head emerges from the vagina, it is likely to tear the perineum around the vaginal outlet. To prevent this, it is customary to make a small surgical cut, called an *episiotomy*, after the patient's perineum is anesthetized. The idea is that a clean cut will heal better than a tear. After the birth is completed, the cut is sewn up. The stitches dissolve and will not need to be removed.

Cesarian section

Sometimes the natural process of birth may involve risks for the infant or mother—or both—because of the baby's position or his size or some condition that would make the stress of the birth process too exhausting for him, or because the mother has a small pelvis or a medical condition that might make going through labor too exhausting for her.

In such cases, the obstetrician decides to deliver the baby by Cesarian section, sometimes called simply *section*. The surgeon makes an incision down the middle of the abdomen, opens the uterus, and lifts the baby out. It is safe for both mother and child, and there is no reason why it cannot be performed during succeeding pregnancies if necessary. Because there is an incision to heal, the hospital stay is usually longer than for a vaginal birth —from 5 to 10 days.

WHAT HAPPENS RIGHT AFTER BIRTH?

As soon as the baby's head is delivered, mucus is sucked out of his nose and throat. After birth he is held upside down for a moment to allow fluid to run out of his mouth and nose. Remember, he has lived all his 9 months floating in fluid; no air has entered his lungs. Next he takes his first gasping breath, crying vigorously as he does so—and now he is really on his own as far as his body functions are concerned. The umbilical cord he no longer needs is clamped and cut off a few inches from his navel.

If you are awake and the baby is breathing properly, he will be shown to you and placed in your arms for a moment. He will then be wrapped warmly and put in a heated bassinet. Identification tags or bracelets will be put on his and your wrists, his footprints may be taken, his eyes will be treated to avoid infection, and off he will go to the nursery for a long rest. He needs a rest period after the strenuous experience of being born.

You will be watched rather carefully for the first hour, probably still in the delivery room. Your uterus, which had expanded to 30 times its normal size, needs to harden its muscles and contract. Blood clots and bits of tissue remaining in the uterus will be expelled, and the contracting muscles will clamp down on the blood vessels left open as the placenta peeled away from the lining of the uterus. Having been stretched for so long a time, these muscles tend to relax after birth, so the nurse may gently massage your abdomen with a kneading motion directly over the uterus. After the muscles have regained their firmness, you will be moved to the recovery room (if there is one) or to your own bed. You will be washed off, given some liquids to drink (if you are ready for them), and made comfortable for a long rest. If your husband has not seen you, he will be brought to your bedside for a few minutes before you go to sleep, and he will be taken to see his newborn child.

STILL IN THE HOSPITAL

After you have rested sufficiently, you will probably feel hungry and you will be allowed to eat as soon as you are ready. If you have had a general anesthetic, you probably will start a little slowly until your stomach is settled.

When you are rested and feel ready, you will be allowed to go to the bathroom, although the first time you will need someone to go with you. You may not be quite as strong as you thought you were. You may also feel considerable soreness in the perineal area, particularly if this is your first delivery.

You will be given supplies for attending to your own personal hygiene. These will include a sanitary belt and sanitary pads. You will have a flow which resembles menstruation but isn't, during the time the uterus gradually shrinks to nonpregnant size. For the first few days this discharge, called *lochia*, is red and contains small blood clots; later it becomes a deeper red or brown, finally becoming nearly colorless. It stops altogether in 3 to 4 weeks. The uterus regains its normal size about 6 weeks after the baby is born. Some doctors prefer that you rinse yourself off with sterile water, after urinating or having a bowel movement, and pat yourself dry with soft tissues, always cleansing from front to back. Others prefer that you use soap and water and disposable washcloths. Whichever method you use, you will be advised to continue for a few days after going home. Disposable washcloths are available in drugstores.

If stitches have been taken around the vaginal outlet at the time of the baby's birth, you will be shown how to use a heat lamp while in the hospital for keeping them dry and for relieving soreness.

Your doctor will indicate how soon you may walk around as much as you please. You need to keep in mind that you have just completed a very hard job of work, and your body needs plenty of rest. It is exciting to walk to the nursery window to watch activities there. It is also very satisfying to be able to use the toilet, take a shower, and generally take care of your own personal needs.

You will soon find that between caring for the baby, resting, eating, and attending to your own needs, there is no time to be bored in the hospital.

ROOMING-IN

If you have decided to room-in with your baby, to have him in a crib at your bedside, he will be there after the first 24 hours.

Hospitals differ in the way this system is set up. Many maternity departments have rooming-in available for patients in private or semiprivate rooms. Much depends on whether the hospital was built before the idea of rooming-in was common or whether it was built with provisions for rooming-in. In the United States this is a relatively new idea, though it has been in use in other countries for a long time.

In one plan, your baby goes back to the nursery at night, to ensure that you get a good night's rest, and comes to you in the morning after you have bathed and had breakfast. Under this plan, your baby is also taken to the nursery during visiting hours and during your daytime rest period.

Another interesting plan provides a small nursery with room for four babies, situated between two two-bed rooms. The mothers can go into the nursery, and the babies can come out. One nurse takes care of both you and your baby, as is true in any rooming-in plan. When it is not practical to provide this specialized service at night, the babies are taken into the big general nursery and brought back in the morning.

A few maternity departments allow the baby to stay at your bedside the entire time.

If you are practicing demand feeding, you will have to have your baby room-in. But even if you are not, the system has advantages. Rooming-in means that you as a first-time mother can become familiar with caring for your baby and develop confidence when handling him while still under supervision. You will be shown how to bathe, diaper, hold, and feed him and will have an opportunity to practice these skills while there is someone near to help. When you go home, you will find the new setup tiring enough; you will be much more relaxed and able to handle the situation if you and the baby have become accustomed to each other.

Your husband also can learn to care for his baby right in the hospital; he washes his hands, puts on a special gown, and practices being a father.

Some new mothers feel this experience would be overwhelming so soon after the birth. You certainly should not feel you have to choose rooming-in; it is in no way your duty. If you already have children at home, you will probably welcome the idea of a few days of rest in the hospital while a competent person takes care of your baby.

VISITING HOURS

With rooming-in, your visitors may be restricted to father and grandmother, or else the baby may be taken back to the nursery so that other visitors can be present.

Even without rooming-in, some hospitals restrict visitors to two members of the family, with no visitors in the room while the baby is with his mother for feeding, but sometimes allow the father to stay for an hour after visiting hours in the evening. Then the baby is brought to the bedside, the family has the hour alone together, and the father can, if he wishes, help care for his baby—and no longer be a stranger in a woman's world.

TO BREAST-FEED OR NOT TO BREAST-FEED

The merits of breast feeding versus formula feeding have been debated forever, it seems. We all know healthy, well-adjusted

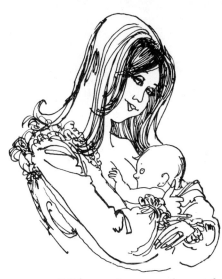

children who were breast-fed—and we also know healthy, well-adjusted children who managed very well with formula feeding. So the decision as to whether to offer breast or bottle would seem to be a matter of convenience and preference on the part of the mother unless a question of health is involved. This is, after all, your child and your life. But before you decide, look into the advantages of each method. (The actual techniques of both are discussed later in this chapter.)

The case for breast feeding

CONVENIENCE.   Breast feeding eliminates the work of sterilizing bottles and nipples and preparing formulas. Breast milk requires no mixing or diluting, is always ready, and does not have to be put in bottles and kept refrigerated. You can travel with your baby without packing nursing supplies. And if you are feeding your baby on demand, it is certainly easier to offer a breast than to prepare a bottle at a moment's notice. Finally, it's cheaper.

YOUR HEALTH.   Breast feeding will help your uterus shrink to normal size more quickly. And it will not spoil your figure. Your breasts will stay larger while you nurse the baby but will then return to normal size. Wearing a supportive bra will prevent stretching of the skin and breast tissues.

It really doesn't matter whether you have large or small breasts when it comes to producing milk for your baby. Nor should breast feeding tire you, as some people believe.

No special care of your breasts or nipples is needed. You should, of course, wash your hands before handling your nipples, just as you would before handling the baby. If your nipples are inverted, your baby will probably draw them out as he sucks. If they become sore, make sure that he is not clamping down on the nipple itself but is drawing the entire area around the nipple, the dark area called the areola, into his mouth. When bathing, just wash and dry your breasts and nipples as you do the rest of your body. If you have a seeping of milk between nursing periods, put a soft cloth inside your brassiere to prevent leakage onto your clothing.

YOUR EMOTIONAL NEEDS. Many mothers derive much emotional satisfaction from breast-feeding their infants. To them this is the ultimate fulfillment of their motherhood. They can feel the chlid's closeness and can give him something of themselves. It is when a woman starts taking care of her child that she gets the real feeling of motherhood, and there can be no closer relationship than that of feeding him.

THE BABY'S HEALTH. Babies rarely have allergic reactions to breast milk. The young infant is thought to receive some immunity to certain childhood infectious diseases through substances his mother passes on to him in her breast milk, but this cannot be relied on. What is sure, though, is that the milk is pure.

Your baby gets the kind of nourishment intended for him when he breast-feeds, though he will need supplements of vitamins C and D. And, if you breast-feed for more than a few weeks, the baby will also need some source of iron to prevent anemia.

THE BABY'S EMOTIONAL NEEDS. The young infant's need for security is as great as his need for food and physical warmth. He especially needs to be held close in an emotionally warm, loving manner. Breast feeding, when accompanied by a mother's love and acceptance, helps to give him this security and starts him on the road to a healthy, self-confident personality. But this start is brought about by his mother's attitude toward him; breast feeding in itself does not meet a baby's emotional needs.

THE BABY'S SUCKING NEEDS. Babies also have a definite need to suck, a need that is something more than the mere satisfaction of hunger. A breast-fed baby can suck for as long as he desires—within reasonable limits, of course—without taking in air bubbles to give him stomach distress.

THE WORKING MOTHER. A working mother in most cases will be obliged to put her baby on a formula. A baby may be breast-fed for the weeks the mother is home and then changed to a formula. Some young breast-fed babies, however, refuse to switch to the strange feel of a rubber nipple, and considerable difficulty arises. (Other babies become accustomed to the nipple and formula very quickly and refuse to go back to the breast.) Giving a baby water or juice by bottle, and perhaps an occasional formula feeding before he is expected to take all his nourishment that way, should accustom him to taking the bottle when the time comes.

Advantages of formula feeding

Commercially prepared formulas are ready for use and thus do away with lengthy preparation. Disposable "nursers," fitting into plastic holders, cut down markedly on preparation time. If you are a working mother, these preparations may well be worth the moderate extra cost in terms of convenience and timesaving.

HEALTH BENEFITS. Modern formulas, whether commercially prepared or mixed at home, closely approximate breast milk. Except for those who are allergic to cow's milk, most babies thrive equally well on them. (Special formulas are available for allergic babies, but whether they are needed should be the doctor's decision.)

THE BABY'S EMOTIONAL NEEDS. Your baby's fundamental need for love and security can be supplied by you as you hold him closely and lovingly while he takes his bottle. Bottle propping has *no* place in a baby's feeding routine. The young infant loses the nipple easily and becomes extremely frustrated. He also spits up easily and is apt to choke if you are not right there to help him.

THE BABY'S SUCKING NEEDS. If your baby is a robust, eager feeder, finishing his bottle in record time, a small-holed nipple will give him the extra sucking time he needs. It also tends to prevent his choking from drawing too fast, too eagerly. He also needs a stiff nipple to exercise his jaws; not one made soft through frequent boiling.

Your decision

Probably you started deciding as to whether you wanted to breast-feed long before your baby arrived. If you studied the matter, you discovered a wealth of printed material on the subject. You no doubt found some of the material absolutely crusading in its fervor for breast feeding. Reading it you may have felt you would be dehumanized if you dared to think about *not* breast feeding. Some of the pamphlets seem to imply that there is a sinister coalition in the medical and nursing profession to deny this birthright to infants.

Nonsense!

After more than twenty years' experience we think we've heard all the arguments. We agree that mother's milk is the *natural* food for young babies. But it is certainly not the *only* good food for babies.

Having worked with large numbers of both breast- and bottle-fed babies, we do not see any difference in results, but we admit the element of pleasure and satisfaction some mothers find in successfully breast-feeding their babies.

If you want to breast-feed your baby, do so. If you don't want to, forget it and don't feel a moment's guilt. There is no real evidence that breast feeding in itself is essential for a baby's emotional health, or that a formula-fed baby is shortchanged because he gets his nourishment from a bottle. If he is held and loved while nursing just as a breast-fed baby is, he will benefit the same way. So cuddle as you bottle-feed and turn a deaf ear to those who would make you feel inadequate. They have absolutely no right to condemn you, for they do so without really relevant facts.

WHEN THE MILK "COMES IN"

About the second or third day after giving birth, your breasts will become hard, tense, and rather uncomfortable. You need a firm, well-fitting brassiere to support them and help to relieve the discomfort. It is well to wear such a brassiere day and night until your breasts soften, whether you plan to breast-feed your baby or not.

This full feeling does not mean that your breasts are full to bursting with milk. Indeed, it will be another day or two before this swelling subsides and the breasts begin to secrete milk in any real quantity. The swelling comes before the production of milk, while the breasts are getting ready to fulfill their primary function of feeding your hungry baby. When the milk does "come in" on the third or fourth day, feeding your baby will help to relieve the discomfort, for your baby starts becoming really hungry at about the same time the milk arrives. In a few days your breasts become soft.

If you decide not to breast-feed, you will be given an inhibiting medication, one that helps prevent milk from forming. This medicine has the same composition as certain natural secretions in the body and therefore is not harmful. You may experience some breast tenderness, just as does the mother who breast-feeds.

LENGTH OF HOSPITAL STAY

In the United States, the customary length of hospital stay after childbirth is 5 days, although it may be as short as 3 days. If you are a new mother with your first baby, you will probably be encouraged to stay the full 5 days.

Before the advent of World War II, maternity patients were hospitalized for 10 to 14 days, with most of this time spent in bed. Naturally, by the time they got out of bed they were very weak because of unused muscles, but they were thought to be "recovering" from the ordeal of giving birth.

During the war, hospital beds were scarce and nurses even more so. Out of necessity patients went home earlier and therefore were allowed out of bed to gain strength to go home. Then it was discovered that early use of body muscles by walking, sitting up, and doing for oneself strengthened and hastened recovery. This of course must be within sensible limits. Too much

76

and too hard work before the body fully recovers is as harmful as too little.

THE NEWBORN—HIS FIRST WEEK OF LIFE

A newborn baby's appearance is quite a surprise to those who have never seen a person so young, for his development is not a finished thing, though he is anatomically complete. Before birth the upper portions of a baby's body are somewhat more advanced in development than the lower. His head seems large and his legs rather small and puny by comparison. These disproportions do not seem to concern mothers at all. If the baby is whole and healthy, they tend to see him, and rightly so, as a worthy result of their hard work. Fathers, on the other hand, may have a few questions and are apt to say, "Gee, Doc, he looks all out of proportion!"

Before birth, your baby needed extra quantities of red blood cells to transfer oxygen from your system to his own blood. This was because the placenta is not as efficient in supplying oxygen as his own lungs are after birth. Therefore, when you first see him, his color is usually quite red. It may become even deeper when he cries. (On the other hand, some newborn babies are temporarily quite pale or even blue-tinged and are still entirely normal.)

His skin has a protective covering of a white, cheesy material called *vernix*. Some babies are pretty well covered with this; on others it may be thick in the creases and thin otherwise. Before birth his body was more or less covered with fine hair; if he is born somewhat early, some of this prenatal hair is still present.

As we said, his head is large in proportion to his body, his legs and feet small. The bones of his head are flexible and not yet united into one solid single brain covering. This flexibility allows the head to slip through the birth canal easily; the bones can compress and overlap without injury. The spaces between the bones close shortly after birth, leaving only one opening on the top of his head, the fontanel. His head may be pulled somewhat out of shape during this molding process but goes back into proper shape in a few days.

The newborn's upper jaw is well developed, but not so his lower jaw. This does not mean he will grow up with a receding chin (unless it is a family pattern); it does mean that his jaws are ideally shaped for sucking, his major occupation for some time to come.

He does not coordinate the movements of his arms and legs. He can distinguish light and dark but cannot coordinate his eye movements, and so he has a cross-eyed look at times for the first few weeks.

His hearing is well established. Babies still in the delivery room have been known to quiet when spoken to in soft, soothing tones or to startle at loud, sudden noises.

Normal babies are born with a sucking reflex, although they have to learn how to grasp a nipple properly. One is sometimes startled to hear loud sucking sounds coming from the crib in the delivery room as the newborn finds his mouth and fingers.

Full-term healthy babies weigh somewhere between 5½ and 10 pounds. The "average" newborn is said to be 7 to 8 pounds in weight and 19 to 22 inches tall.

During the first few days of life, the newborn infant loses weight, sometimes as much as ¾ pound. This is to be expected, partly because he is not yet sufficiently interested in eating but mainly because of normal loss of fluid and bowel contents. He makes the weight loss up within the first 10 days and thereafter gains as much as 6 to 8 ounces a week, and sometimes more.

FIRST FEEDINGS

Your baby's need for rest is greater than his need for food during the first hours of life. If you have taken a childbirth education course, learning natural childbirth or Lamaze methods, you will probably expect to put your baby to your breast for a few minutes directly after he is born, while you are still in the delivery room. Otherwise, this is not a general practice. Your baby will be allowed a rest period of from 6 to 12 hours after birth before he is brought to you to be fed and admired.

Babies are born knowing how to suck, but they have to learn

how to grasp a nipple properly to obtain food. A baby given a formula in a nursing bottle has little difficulty learning. The nurse or mother opens his mouth, puts the nipple in, and the baby starts to suck. Not so the breast-fed baby; he has to find the nipple for himself.

Breast-feeding the newborn

If you plan to breast-feed your baby, you will probably find the first feeding goes easier if you lie on your side in a half-sitting position. Hold your baby in your arm, and brush your breast gently across his mouth.

The area around a baby's mouth is extremely sensitive to touch. When any object, even his own fist, brushes against his cheek or at the side of his mouth, he immediately turns his head in that direction and starts seeking a source of nourishment. This is called the *rooting reflex* and is instinctive in the newborn child. If you try to turn his head toward the breast by pushing on his cheek, he will turn toward the pushing hand rather than toward the breast. And if you hold his head firmly or squeeze his cheeks to make him open his mouth, you will only make him angry.

When your baby has grasped the nipple, it is important that he draw the entire dark area around the nipple—the areola—into his mouth. If he clamps his jaws down on the nipple itself, it will soon become sore and cause considerable discomfort. You can open his mouth by pushing gently down on his lower jaw and help him get the whole area into his mouth. This allows him to press the milk into the back of his mouth, ready for swallowing. Hold the top of your breast away from his nose with your finger to allow him to breathe.

As we said, milk is not secreted by the breast in any quantity until the third or fourth day after birth. Colostrum, a pre-milk secretion, does appear. This fluid is high in protein. Babies should nurse only 2 or 3 minutes at each breast before the milk comes in. After that, alternate the breasts for feeding, letting the baby feed for a period up to about 15 minutes. Later, when your nipples are no longer tender, he may be permitted to nurse as long as he wishes.

Few babies will refuse the breast unless forced to suck when they are not hungry. For the first few days after birth, babies are quite sleepy and not usually eager suckers. They waken after the mother's milk comes in. If you become tense and nervous over breast feeding, worried that you are not doing it right or determined that your child *must* nurse this time, you will be defeating your own purpose. Tenseness may actually keep your breast milk from flowing. If you can learn to relax when your baby wants to nurse there should be no difficulty.

If you have flat or retracted nipples, you may have difficulty getting your baby started. A very hungry, eager baby may become angry when he cannot immediately grasp the nipple, while a less aggressive baby may just give up and go back to sleep. If your baby starts crying and seems frustrated, just hold him close and comfort him. Then try again, getting the whole area around the nipple into his mouth. If your baby gives up and goes to sleep, he will waken later and you can try again. Few babies will give up trying altogether. But if you cannot seem to satisfy your baby's hunger, you may need to give him a supplementary bottle of formula. Keep in mind, though, that babies who are given supplementary bottle feedings are often reluctant to go back to the breast. So if you give a supplementary feeding, allow your child to breast-feed first, *before* the formula.

Frequency of feeding

A baby who is hungry and sucks vigorously gets nearly all he wants in the first 5 to 8 minutes. This is, of course, provided you have enough milk to satisfy him. When such a baby drops the nipple from his mouth with an expression of perfect satisfaction on his face as he drops off to sleep, there is no need to coax him to take more. Other babies are more leisurely feeders. While in the hospital the baby is still getting adjusted to the business of feeding. His desire for food is apt to be more unevenly timed than it will be later. Let him follow his own pattern at this early age. If he falls sound asleep after taking only a small amount, let him sleep. He has not yet adjusted to the rhythm of living outside the uterus. Waking him and coaxing will be useless—and take too much of your time and patience.

It will be simpler to feed him again when he wakens hungry in an hour or so. There is little point in trying to maintain a schedule now; he will make new adjustments.

Even newborn babies differ in personality. Some are alert, hungry, and vigorous from the start; others are inclined to dawdle over their feedings, catching quick naps, waking, and feeding again. Some may sleep throughout the entire nursing period, only to waken screaming with hunger when put back in the crib. But in time, all healthy babies discover the pleasure of eating. If your baby is allowed to nurse or to have his bottle when he seems genuinely hungry, and then sleep until his stomach signals its need again, he will very soon develop a rhythmic pattern. Three to 4 hours is the time it takes for an infant of normal size to empty his stomach. A premature or small baby may need feeding more frequently.

OTHER CARE OF THE NEWBORN

BOWEL MOVEMENT. For the first day or two of life, the baby's bowel movements are greenish black in color, usually quite large, and are smooth and sticky. This material is called *meconium*. It is composed of an accumulation of waste that has collected in the intestines before birth, before food enters the digestive tract.

After the meconium has been expelled, the baby's bowel movements vary in color when he is formula-fed and are usually yellowish when he is breast-fed.

THE UMBILICAL CORD STUMP. After the umbilical cord has been clamped and cut in the delivery room, a stump of cord remains. The stump will shrivel and dry and eventually fall off, leaving a moist area that heals quickly. This happens within 1 to 2 weeks after birth. No special care is needed except to keep the area as clean and dry as possible.

For a few days, there may be a little brownish spotting from this area. This is not abnormal. You can apply rubbing alcohol at each diaper change to help speed the drying process. The alcohol will not sting or hurt because there are no sensory nerves in the cord stump.

The cuff of skin around the area turns in to form the navel.

CIRCUMCISION. Circumcision is a minor operation consisting of the removal of most of the movable fold of skin, called the *foreskin,* surrounding the tip of the penis. Removal of the foreskin makes it easier to keep the area clean. If you do not have your child circumcised, you need do nothing until he is older, when he must learn proper cleansing.

Circumcision is performed on most boy babies in the United States, though not all doctors are in agreement as to its necessity. It is actually a socioreligious heritage and not a medical necessity, in most cases. It is usually done the first week of life, right in the hospital. If it is being done as a ritual rite, circumcision will take place on the seventh day of life of a full-term baby.

Bleeding following circumcision practically never occurs. But if the circumcision has been done at home, the baby should be checked occasionally for a few hours. If anything more than slight spotting of blood does occur, the doctor should be notified. Petroleum jelly and a strip of gauze is generally wrapped around the penis following the operation. The gauze falls off soon and need not be replaced. No special care is needed.

One argument in favor of circumcision during the newborn period, apart from ritualistic significance, is that it is a very painful procedure if needed later on. After the newborn period it should be avoided during early childhood, for at that time it may be the cause of psychological problems. The boy may subconsciously fear the loss of his penis as a form of punishment.

COMMON QUESTIONS ABOUT NEWBORN BABIES

Any questions you have about that new child of yours are in order. Your doctor will not think you ignorant or overanxious. But maybe we can anticipate some of your questions. You have read some of the answers already in this chapter, but let's put them all together.

Is my baby all right?

This is your first question, whether it is your first baby or your tenth. Obviously, only the doctor can answer it, but often even his assurance does not convince you. Nine months of pregnancy gives you plenty of time to worry. "Could something I did—or didn't do—have affected my baby in some way?"

Keep one thing in mind: It would be a rare doctor indeed who would assure you that your baby is healthy and normal if this were not so.

Within a minute after birth, your doctor or one of the hospital staff doctors has checked your baby against a routine list (called the Apgar Scoring System) for normal heart rate, breathing, muscle tone, reflexes, and color and has looked him over for any abnormalities. Later, the baby will be observed again at a more leisurely rate. So trust your doctor.

Nevertheless, look for yourself too. Don't be shy about examining your baby. When the nurse brings him to you, unwrap him. Turn up his shirt, unpin his diaper. Remember that his feet will seem small and inadequate for his body, but this is as it should be. They will have plenty of time to grow before they are called upon to support him.

My daughter has no hair—she's bald!

Well, not really. A mother is usually distressed when her baby girl's blond hair is so fine and soft it hardly shows. And some parents are embarrassed when their new baby boy shows a head of long black hair. "He needs a haircut already!"

The newborn baby's hair often changes considerably as he grows older and sometimes is replaced by a quite different type. So don't worry about what it looks like now.

Why is his head out of shape?

As your baby came through the bony part of your pelvis at birth, the soft, pliable bones of his skull overlapped to allow his head to pass through more easily and protect his brain from injury. Frequently this pulls the soft tissues of the baby's skull out of shape. But it will take only a few days for his head to round out.

The soft spot on his head is larger (or smaller)
than I supposed it would be. Is this normal?

As we saw, the newborn's skull is not the solid brain case it will become later. At the juncture of the frontal and side skull bones, there is a triangular space called the *anterior fontanel* or "soft spot." The size varies. If it is small, it is likely to become somewhat larger as the head grows. The fontanel closes sometime between the ages of 10 and 18 months.

The brain itself is covered by a very tough membrane; therefore, ordinary handling can cause no harm. Incidentally, there is another, much smaller fontanel at the back of the skull for the first 3 to 5 weeks of life. Because this spot is small and covered with hair, it is usually not noticed by parents.

Why is he so tense?
Even when he is asleep, his muscles are tight.

This is the normal state for a healthy, full-term newborn. Normally a newborn baby lies with his legs drawn up and his fists clenched, as though ready for action. He exercises frequently, waving arms and legs at random, just as he did before he was born.

My baby jumped when the nurse put him in my bed this morning. He did it again when someone dropped something on the floor. What's wrong with his nerves?

This is a normal reflex action for the newborn, called the *startle reflex*—much the same reaction you have to an unexpected noise or action. If your baby seems to jump and cry out frequently, ask your doctor about it.

Other normal reflexes of the newborn include:

The sucking and seeking or rooting reflex. The baby instinctively sucks on anything coming near his mouth. He actively seeks the source of nourishment, turning his face toward any object touching it.

The grasp reflex. Place your finger in the palm of your very young baby and he will grasp it tightly. This reflex fades after the first few weeks. He will not hold on to an object again for any length of time until he is old enough to do it voluntarily.

What are those white spots on his nose?

The tiny white spots appearing on many babies' faces, on or near the nose, are called *milia*. They are plugged sweat glands that open naturally within the first few weeks. They are normal and require no treatment.

My baby stares at me, though they say newborn babies can't see. Is this true?
The newborn baby is able to distinguish light from dark. Whatever image appears on his brain through his eyes has as yet no meaning for him. In a week or two he will follow an object briefly if it is held close before his eyes, but he will not turn his head when it goes out of his line of vision.

How long will he be cross-eyed?
In most cases the eyes become steady and straight as the baby grows older, though the time needed for a baby to learn to coordinate his eyes varies. If your baby still turns one or both eyes in—or out—after 3 months of age, tell your pediatrician and let him decide whether this has any significance.

My baby hiccups a great deal.
Does that mean I am not feeding him right?
Babies hiccup quite frequently during the first weeks of life. In fact, they are known to hiccup before they are born. Hiccups in the newborn seem to have no significance. Try holding him up on your shoulder for a few minutes and rubbing his back gently. This will bring up any air he has swallowed. If the hiccups persist, offer him a little water from a nursing bottle or let him nurse for another minute. But even without more food, they will soon stop.

My baby is nearly three days old, and he is still not interested in any food. Isn't it important for him to have some nourishment or at least some water?
Babies come into the world with ample stores of water to last them for 3 or even 4 days. So it does not matter whether or not he takes any fluids for the first few days. Offer him water; if he *is* thirsty, he will drink. Otherwise, don't force him.

This is my third (or fourth) day since delivery.
My breasts feel hard and full,
but my baby doesn't seem to be getting much.

The breasts usually feel firm, tense, and rather painful just *before* the milk starts to come in. Be sure to wear a well-fitting brassiere, night and day, whether you plan to breast-feed or not. This will make your breasts more comfortable.

My baby sneezed three times this morning when I had him
with me. Do you think he is catching cold?

Sneezing is nature's way of cleaning out any excess mucus in the nose. In the small child it serves the purpose of blowing the nose. It is not any sign of infection or allergy in the newborn.

Sometimes my baby's chin trembles. Sometimes one of his
arms or legs trembles. What does this mean?

The nervous system of the newborn baby is in the process of adjustment to independent living. The baby may occasionally twitch or tremble for no apparent reason. If you feel concerned about his twitching, talk to your doctor about it. But sneezing, yawning, hiccupping, and a certain amount of trembling are all normal signs of adjustment.

I have heard that baby girls sometimes have swollen breasts
from which a milky fluid oozes. My grandmother called this
"witch's milk." But my baby has this, and he is a boy.
What does that mean?

It is entirely normal for *both* boy and girl babies to have swollen breasts containing a little liquid. This is caused by glandular changes in the mother just before the baby is born and has nothing to do with the baby's sex. It is important not to squeeze or massage the swollen breasts. The swelling disappears spontaneously after a few days.

Why did my baby girl have a few drops of blood on her diaper?
It seemed to be coming from her genital area.

This too is normal and due to glandular changes in the mother before the baby is born. The spotting disappears in a few days.

Why is my son's scrotum bruised and swollen?

Babies who were born buttocks first—instead of head first—frequently show swelling and discoloration of the genitals. This happens during the labor process. The swelling and discoloration may persist for a time but will eventually disappear without damage.

THE PREMATURE BABY

A baby weighing under 5½ pounds at birth is classed as a *premature,* meaning one who is born before the end of the normal nine months of pregnancy. The term is not always accurate, since your baby may weigh less than 5½ pounds at birth and still be a full-term baby. The World Health Organization prefers the term *"low birth-weight"* for those full-term babies who still do not make the desired 5½ pounds.

The small full-term baby. In some hospitals all babies with a birth weight under 5½ pounds are admitted to the premature nursery. These larger "prematures," if healthy and sturdy, are usually put in heated cribs rather than in incubators. If your baby is one of these, he may be able to come out to you for feedings and will probably be ready to go home as soon as his initial normal weight loss has been made up.

The small premature baby. When a small premature baby is born at home, as occasionally happens, it is vital that he be transferred to a hospital as soon as possible. These tiny babies are not yet equipped to cope with life without specialized help. The premature unit of a hospital has everything needed to give them the best possible care.

Babies weighing as little as 2 pounds have survived, but a hospital nursery set up especially for their care is essential. The doctor or visiting nurse will arrange for the small baby to be taken to the hospital in a traveling incubator. This is a heated boxlike affair, equipped with means for giving him oxygen and any other first aid needed.

While still at home the baby should be handled as little as possible. He will not need feeding for several hours after birth. He will need to be kept warm, wrapped in a light blanket. Hot-water bottles filled with *warm*—not hot—water placed *under* his crib mattress will be helpful if they are readily available.

In the hospital the small premature will be put in a preheated incubator, and the incubator will be adjusted to supply warmth, humidity, and oxygen according to his need. Small prematures use up energy by simply being handled; therefore they are not dressed or disturbed any more than is necessary. Modern incubators, such as the Isolette, are very finely adjusted to care for these tiny beings and have been the means of saving many lives.

While in the hospital the small premature will be fed in his incubator until he can tolerate coming out for feeding periods. If he is not strong enough to suck on a nipple, he will be fed with a medicine dropper or a tiny soft plastic stomach tube. Special commercial formulas, or hospital-prepared formulas especially modified for the premature, are available. These have been highly successful in meeting the tiny infant's needs.

Some maternity departments have set up their premature nurseries so that the baby's mother may come in and see her baby and put her hand in his incubator to touch him. If this is not possible, the incubator will be brought to the nursery window.

The period of waiting for your premature infant to come home is a very difficult one for any parent. The anxiety you feel about the child himself, the disappointment over having no baby to take home, and the additional financial burden involved make this a trying time indeed.

But as the parent of a premature baby, you will be welcome —indeed, encouraged—to go to the hospital frequently to see him. Find out whether special hours are set for showing such babies to their parents. If you are not able to come at the specified times, ask about making special arrangements for a time when you can come.

If the department holds classes for waiting parents, attend them. You will see small babies being bathed, fed, and clothed, and will have an opportunity to practice these skills yourself, using a doll rather than a squirming baby. The anxious waiting period, followed by the bringing home of a still pretty small baby, is likely to make you feel somewhat insecure and fearful. Any practice you can have before he comes home will help greatly.

If the maternity department does not provide for this kind of observation and practice, ask for an opportunity to bathe, dress, and perhaps feed your baby a day or two before you take him home. In this way you will have the nurse's help and advice before you assume complete responsibility for your baby at home.

Nursery personnel are not surprised to receive phone calls from parents during the first few days a premature baby is at home. They understand and are willing to help. Be aware, though, that they are busy people, and limit your calls to those that seem really important.

A visiting nurse can be of great help. Get in touch with one before your baby comes home. The welfare of premature babies is an area of special concern to public health and visiting nurses.

Remember one thing: Your doctor will not send your baby home if he has not reached the stage where he can stand the stress of living as well as any full-term baby.

BABIES OF DIABETIC MOTHERS

If you are diabetic but have kept your diabetes under good control, you are not likely to have difficulties during pregnancy. The baby you are carrying tends to grow rapidly, however, and is usually quite large at birth. But after he is born, his body processes take longer to settle into a normal pattern than those of other babies. He has had access to an unusually rich supply of sugar before birth; once this is cut off he tends to suffer temporarily from a *low* supply of blood sugar. He needs careful watching during his first 48 hours and possibly some treatment to help him adjust to his new environment.

For this reason babies of diabetic mothers, big as they are, are usually kept in the premature or intensive care nursery while in the hospital. There they can be watched and given special care when needed. After they have weathered the initial period of adjustment, they need no more special care than any other newborn infants.

THE BABY WITH A VISIBLE DEFECT

A young mother-to-be is naturally excited over the prospect

of bringing home her first baby. Relatives and friends are looking forward to the new arrival. There has been much preparation in anticipation of the homecoming.

When, under these circumstances, a baby is born with a defect of some sort, it comes as a great shock. If the defect is external, such as a split lip, extra fingers or toes, or a twisted foot, it may seem doubly difficult, for the new mother tends to dread her friends' reactions and sympathy.

These surface defects are, in most cases, correctable, as the doctor will explain. Still, it will take a while for the importance of that fact to sink in. The thought of taking the baby home may be a difficult instead of a joyous one. And hospital personnel, knowing that these flaws can be repaired, may not give the new mother the concern and understanding she expects.

The important thing for parents to realize is that their baby is essentially sound and these worrisome defects can be corrected.

CLEFT LIP. Cleft lip is the result of imperfect closure of the upper jaw early in fetal life. Nothing the mother did or did not do during pregnancy caused this defect, so she has no reason to feel guilty.

If the baby weighs 7 pounds or more at birth and is healthy, the lip can be sewn together sometime during the first weeks of life. As soon as the stitches are removed the baby goes home, able to suck and to receive the normal care of any baby. Repairs today leave very little scarring.

Occasionally, though, the gap in the upper lip is quite wide. Then it is often better to wait until the baby has grown larger and has more tissue to use in correcting the defect.

If the roof of the mouth (cleft palate) is involved as well, it may have to be fixed in two or more stages over a period of time, but the result is excellent.

CLUBFOOT. Everyone has heard tales of people crippled because of clubfoot, a condition in which the infant is born with his foot or feet twisted out of shape. In the most common type, the child's foot is turned inward, causing the child to walk on the toes and side of the foot. (See also Clubfoot in Chapter 9.)

3
Growth and Development the First Year

THE HOMECOMING

Bringing a first baby home from the hospital is an exciting experience, filled with feelings of pride and joy, mixed with a new sense of responsibility. But after the excitement and fanfare have died down, you may suddenly realize that *you* are solely responsible for the health, the well-being, the very life of this tiny, helpless baby. At that moment you are quite likely to develop a sense of insecurity, regardless of any preparations you have made earlier.

Take heart and relax. Babies are meant to be enjoyed. Healthy babies are pretty husky, not nearly as helpless as they appear. Sure, you will make mistakes—you can count on it. But you will learn quickly enough, and your baby will be fine in the mean-time, just as long as he receives the essentials.

What are these essentials? Food, shelter, and physical care, of course, but most of all a sense of security. Your baby needs to be able to put absolute trust in those responsible for him before he will feel safe and assured that all is well.

For 9 months he has lived in a small, quiet world where all his needs were supplied. Indeed, he was not even aware that he

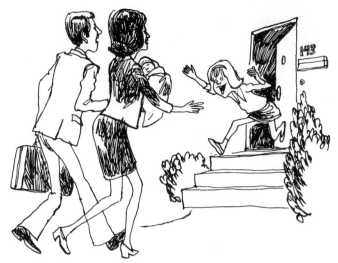

had any needs. He slept and wakened, moved about at his pleasure. He was soothed and comforted by the gentle rocking of your movements and the rhythmic sound of your heartbeat. Suddenly he was forced into a larger world with an overwhelming confusion of sights and sounds. No wonder he needs security.

There is only one way he can achieve it: through immediate attention to his physical needs. Experience cannot tell him, "Mother is busy for a few minutes, but I know she has always fed me when I am hungry. I can wait." Only when he has been fed, clothed, comforted, and loved over and over again will he learn to trust. Then, and only then, when he knows that he *will* be cared for, can he take the next step—of enduring a temporary frustration for a greater good to follow.

This is not to say that you must jump to respond to his every whim. You and your baby both have rights; respect is a two-way street. In a very short time you will each learn to understand the other. Just remember this experience is new to your baby. He has so much to learn. You can count on one thing: He starts learning from the moment of his first cry. All you need do is to try not to stand in his way.

OLDER CHILDREN IN THE HOME

As we said, homecoming takes on a different aspect when there are older children to be considered. To each of them it will mean a further sharing of his parents' love and attention.

Your toddler who, up until now, has been the baby himself, no doubt will be thrilled to see the new "doll." When he discovers it is not his to play with, and furthermore that this new member of the family is getting—in his opinion—more than his share of attention, the story becomes quite different. You must be prepared to accept some resentment and jealousy for a time from the displaced baby. Your greatest care must be to do nothing to make his resentment greater. This applies to older children as well.

There are ways for helping children through this period. These will be discussed in detail in the chapters concerned with the various age groups. It should be mentioned here, however, that it is not good practice to leave a toddler or small child alone with a tiny baby. The small child is not yet mature enough to control his feelings, nor can he visualize the results of his actions. He may not even consciously realize any harmful intent.

VISITING HOURS

Your baby can be gazed at, cooed over, and admired without being disturbed in the least. But he tires easily when handled; the word is "Look, don't touch." And you will have to be stern with the visitor who is sniffly, even though you are assured that it is just "hay fever." Most people who are not feeling well will stay away from the baby of their own accord. If not, be firm and ask them to come back another time.

It is very difficult to refuse to see visitors, especially when you are brimming with pride and anxious to show your new baby. But you must be realistic and if necessary selfish. When you have a visitor and begin to feel tired, say so. Don't let your friends stay on and on. It is easy to get overtired in the first few days after coming home, and you should avoid it. Your short stay in the hospital did not give you enough time to return to your usual strength and vitality. In addition, you will be facing a completely new home situation with new responsibilities. This in itself will tax you considerably.

But the main thing is your own reaction. If you like being with others, you will welcome having friends and neighbors drop in— within reasonable limits. But if you prefer to be alone, you probably will find yourself tiring much more quickly.

Either way, learn to respect your limits. It is especially important if you are breast-feeding. Don't be afraid to say, "I love having you here, but I get so tired these days that I can't ask you to stay long. Will you come back soon?"

Your husband, too, needs to consider the strain that too many visitors may put on you. He should always check with you before inviting friends or associates in to see the baby. He can help by suggesting a slowdown when he considers you are becoming over-tired. He may even take a hand in spreading the word: "Mary has had a lot of visitors and I think she is getting pretty tired. Will you ask everybody to take it easy for a while?"

Relative peace and quiet are best for both you and your husband at this time. Parties can come a little later.

COPING WITH THE HOUSEHOLD

If you were employed before the baby came, you have already learned to handle two jobs reasonably well. You and your husband probably work as a team around the house. Nevertheless, you will have your hands full caring for a tiny baby so soon after giving birth.

If relatives, neighbors, or friends can come in to take care of the housework, it will be a great help, of course, for it will leave you free to look after the baby and to get needed rest. But in present-day society this does not always work out. Families are scattered; friends and neighbors quite likely are working and cannot help. This means that young parents need to work out come sort of arrangement to ease the load for a week or two.

If you can afford to have someone come in and do the heavy work, this is ideal. But many young couples cannot afford this. Just remember that kitchen floors, rugs, and furniture will not deteriorate if they get dustier than usual. If your husband wants to feel part of the total scene, he can help with cooking, washing dishes, even running clothes through the washer.

If you can't afford diaper service for a long period, try to have it for the first few weeks. It will save a great deal of work. Otherwise, try some of the newer brands of diapers.

There are all kinds of housekeeping shortcuts available, from disposable bottles to TV dinners. But they are expensive too.

Do what you can to save your strength, and don't worry about what you can't get done.

There is a time shortly after coming home when many a new mother is apt to feel let down and depressed. The baby cries at night, for no reason anyone can determine. The house looks dismal. Nothing seems to go right. You suspect your husband is discouraged too. This is a trying time, even more so if you did not expect it.

But things *will* get better, a healthy baby *will* learn to sleep at night, and you *will* start feeling stronger. This is as temporary as it is common. Again, don't worry more than you have to about routines. Shut that pile of dirty dishes out of your mind and catch that much-needed nap while your baby is taking his. Ignore the phone, or take the receiver off the hook for an hour. Try to relax. Whatever you do, don't be concerned about what your friends will think. They have probably gone through the same experience.

THE ESSENTIALS OF BABY CARE

It will probably be a few days before your baby settles down into some sort of schedule. A little patience, tolerance, and understanding is needed. Soon the hectic days are over and everyone can relax.

SLEEPING

For about the first 2 weeks most new babies spend the greater part of their time sleeping. And, much as we might prefer it, they do not necessarily confine their waking periods to the daytime.

If your baby wakes and cries the first few nights he is at home, pick him up and rock him for a few minutes. You won't spoil him. But don't take him into your bed; the danger of your rolling over on him in your sleep is too real.

The very young baby wakens primarily when he is hungry. But after the first 2 or 3 weeks he stays awake for longer periods and begins to show some interest in kicking and waving his arms about. When his hand accidentally touches his mouth, he starts sucking his finger or thumb. Sucking in itself gives him pleasure.

Individual babies differ in the amount of time they sleep, just as they differ in other aspects of adjustment. Some sleep 18 to 20 hours a day. Some healthy babies sleep much less, seeming not to need as much sleep. You can safely let your young baby set his own pattern.

The sleep requirement is an inborn trait and there's not too much you can do about it. Babies have no sleep button you can turn on and off.

How do you know when a baby's sleep patterns are beyond the range of normal? If your baby sleeps a lot but is happy, alert, and pleasant when awake, don't worry about how much sleep he wants. If your baby sleeps poorly and not very much but is still pleasant and happy when awake, you'll know that he is one of those who just doesn't need more sleep. But if your baby sleeps poorly and not very much and is unhappy and irritable when awake, ask your doctor about it.

Where should the baby sleep?

Many mothers worry less if the baby sleeps in the same room with them for the first few weeks. But after that it will be much better if the baby can sleep in a separate room.

As your baby grows a little older, his sleeping habits change. He stays awake longer in the day and sleeps through longer periods at night. But he also wakens more easily. He should be sleeping in a separate room from his parents by the time he is 7 or 8 months old. If no separate room is available he should at least be separated by some sort of screen. Or perhaps his crib can be rolled into the living room at night and back into the bedroom during the day. At this age even your softest talk may wake him, and he is likely to drop off to sleep again only if there is nothing to attract his attention. Studies have shown that babies do not sleep soundly at night for 8 to 12 hours; instead, they have little wakeful periods and then drop off to sleep again *if* there is nothing to attract their attention: no sound, movement, music, voices, snoring, or other activity. But if he's in a room to himself, you do not have to keep the rest of the household overly quiet. Ordinary household sounds should not disturb him at all.

Right now you are setting up your child's nighttime sleep patterns for a long while to come. You may as well make it easy for yourself later by making it easy for him to sleep at night now.

What's the best sleeping position?

Some young babies sleep contentedly in whatever position they are placed. Others show a definite preference for lying on their abdomens with their legs drawn up under them and will fuss until they are in this position. There appears to be no reason why a newborn baby should not lie this way if he wishes. A healthy, vigorous baby will turn his head to one side for breathing. Just make sure he has a firm mattress or pad under him, so he *can* turn his head to breathe.

Some young babies will stay lying on one side or the other if placed in that position, with a rolled blanket or pad at their back. Don't be surprised, though, if even the youngest squirms away from this support and rolls onto his back.

If your baby insists on sleeping on his back, raise the head of his crib by placing a folded blanket under the mattress. Young babies are quite likely to spit up a mouthful or two of milk after a feeding, and a back-sleeping baby may choke on it. If you raise his head, the spit-up milk will flow out of his mouth instead.

The baby who insists on sleeping on one side only, or on his back, may flatten his head. This will correct itself eventually, but in the meantime you can encourage him to be willing to sleep in different positions by placing him alternately on one side and then the other. Babies usually tend to lie with their faces turned toward the light. Turning the baby or the crib around may be all that's needed.

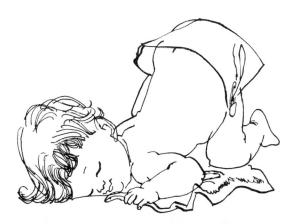

HOW TO PICK UP YOUR BABY

It's a bit of a trick to pick up your young baby, because he has not developed his neck muscles enough to hold his head upright for more than a brief minute. The best he can do is raise it momentarily, when he lies on his abdomen on a flat surface.

To pick him up, turn him over on his back and slide your hand up his back toward his head, supporting his body on your arm. Raise him up with your arm still under him and with your hand firmly but gently supporting his head. You can then easily place him in your other arm for carrying.

CARE OF THE NAVEL AND CIRCUMCISION

Your baby should be given only sponge baths until his navel has healed. No special care of the navel is needed except to keep the area clean and dry. The stump of the umbilical cord usually drops off 5 to 8 days after birth, although occasionally it may stay connected as long as 12 to 14 days. If any inflammation or bleeding should appear, notify your physician.

If your baby was circumcised in the hospital, he will probably have a strip of gauze that has been saturated with petroleum jelly wound around the site of operation, at the end of his penis. When this dressing drops off, it does not need to be replaced. The area should be gently cleansed with cotton balls moistened in warm water daily, or more often if the infant has had a bowel movement. Don't give him a tub bath until the penis has healed.

BATHING

You may think your baby needs to be bathed daily, but it is doubtful whether he cares at all. A daily bath will make him smell sweet, but it is far from essential, especially if his skin is dry.

Just wash his face and hands and the diaper area as often as necessary. Wash after bowel movements and occasionally after your baby has been lying in a wet diaper for a long time. Give him a complete sponge or tub bath 2 or 3 times a week to keep his skin in good condition.

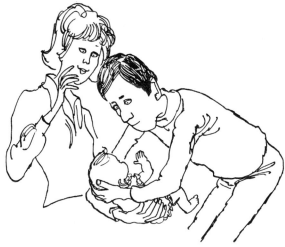

There is no sacred time of day for bathing a baby. However, it is not practical to bathe him directly after he has been fed. He is more likely to spit up some or all of his meal if handled too much at that time.

Before you start, have the following items ready:

A baby bathtub (or a basin of water for a sponge bath)

A cake of mild soap

Washcloth, small towel for drying, and a large soft towel or cotton blanket to wrap the baby in when you lift him from the tub

A small jar of cotton

A small jar of mineral oil

Clean diaper, shirt, and gown or sleeper

A table covered with a folded towel, blanket, or pad on which to place baby, tub, and supplies (the padding will protect the table and keep the baby from rolling)

For a sponge bath, start with the baby on his back on the padded table and then turn him over. Follow the washing procedure given below for the tub bath; just don't put the baby in the tub.

For a regular bath, the molded plastic baby tub seems the most practical. It is oval in shape and comes with a canvas hammock on which to rest the baby. (Note that even with the hammock you will still need to hold the baby firmly.)

Now for the procedure:

1. Place the tub or basin at one end of the padded table.

2. Fill the tub *less* than half full with warm water. (Use only a little water at first, until you get used to holding a wet

baby.) Dip your elbow in the water; it should feel pleasantly warm. If you have a bath thermometer, check that the temperature is not over 100 degrees F. (A bath thermometer is nice but not necessary; your elbow will do fine.)

3. Lay your baby, still dressed, on the padded table next to the tub. Wash his face with a washcloth wrung out of *clear* water. Babies do not like to have their faces washed, so wring the washcloth quite dry so it does not drip.

Still using clear water, wash carefully behind his ears and in the folds of his ears with the washcloth. As the old saying goes, "Use nothing smaller than your elbow to clean in the ear canal"; a small baby is not going to lie quietly while you poke in his ear, and it is all too easy to damage the delicate membranes if you go into the canal. Just clean the entrance. Ear wax belongs in the ear; if it appears excessive, do *not* try to remove it but mention it to your doctor the next time you take your baby to see him. Your baby's hearing is one of his most important assets, so do nothing that might impair it. *Don't go in the ear canal at all, not even with cotton tips.*

Wash around his eyes with water. You don't need any medicine around or in the baby's eyes, unless he has a special condition—and then your doctor will prescribe the right kind of drops or ointment.

Boric acid is no longer considered safe for use.

Wipe away any mucus at the entrance of his nose with the wet washcloth. Do *not* poke into his nose. The mucous lining is delicate and easily injured. If a small ball of mucus just inside his nostril annoys you, roll a wisp of wet cotton around just inside the nostril with your fingers. This will probably make him sneeze the mucus out.

Wash in the crease under the baby's chin and dry his face.

4. About once or twice a week, wash the baby's head with soap. Lather your hand or washcloth with soap and wash his scalp. Be sure to wash over the soft spot as well. Next, pick the baby up by running your arm up his back with your hand holding his head. Hold his head over the tub and rinse it thoroughly. He will not like it if you splash in his eyes, so do it carefully. Lay him down on the table and dry his head.

5. *Now* undress the baby. You may prefer to remove all clothes except the diaper before starting the bath, but a clothed baby is easier to pick up than an unclothed one. And it does not matter if his shirt or gown gets wet: you will be changing it anyway.

If the baby's diaper area is soiled with bowel movement, dip a piece of clean cotton in the water and wash him off, working from the front to the buttocks. Use more than one piece of cotton if necessary; do not dip the soiled cotton back into the bath water.

6. To wash your baby's body, use either of the following methods, whichever seems easier. The second is suggested in case you find a soapy baby too slippery to handle.

Soap his body all over, paying attention to creases under the arms and in the thighs. Lifting your baby as before, let him down gently into the water, keeping your arm and hand in position. Rinse him off with your other hand, lift him out into the soft cotton blanket, and *pat* him dry.

Or put him in the tub first, holding him the same way. Then soap and rinse him with your other hand or with the washcloth. After taking him out of the water, check his creases to be sure they are clean.

Young babies do not always need soaping. If your baby's skin is dry, omit the soap and just use mineral oil to cleanse the soiled diaper area.

A freshly bathed baby has a sweet, clean smell of his own that does not need to be enhanced by any other fragrance. Powders tend to cake in the body creases and cause irritation, especially in warm weather. If your baby has a tendency toward heat or diaper rash, first try to remove the cause. Perhaps he is dressed too warmly, or his diapers are not changed often enough, or his skin is delicate. Cornstarch dusted lightly over his skin will be protective and soothing.

Baby lotions are not a "must" for the baby's skin either; some babies develop a rash from the ingredients in commercial lotions. If your baby's skin is dry, use a bland, unperfumed cream or lotion. For a severe diaper rash see Chapter 10.

DRESSING

The young baby does not need to wear many clothes. Many babies are dressed far too warmly. But it is also true that so many mothers have been cautioned against overdressing their babies that some have erred in the opposite direction. Feel your baby's arms, legs, and body to find out whether he is cold. You can't judge by hands and feet, since they may feel cool even when the baby is comfortably warm.

Much, of course, depends on the climate and the time of year. The sensible course is to remember that your baby feels the heat or cold just as you do. It is distressing on a hot day to see a mother carrying a bundle of blankets, inside of which, presumably, is a small baby. The mother, meanwhile, is smart enough to wear a minimum of clothing.

How much does he need? In very hot weather even the newborn baby needs nothing more than a diaper. When the temperature becomes cooler, he will probably be comfortable in a shirt and diaper, with a light cotton blanket over him as he sleeps.

As your baby gets a few weeks older and becomes more active he is not likely to stay under a blanket. You do not want to restrain him by tucking the blankets too tightly over him; he needs to exercise. (Even if you try, you will have little success; he will manage to wriggle out from under.)

A knit cotton gown, sleepers, or sleeping gown* will keep him warm in cold weather even when he becomes uncovered. When you take him outside, see how much extra clothing you need and use that as a guide for clothing him.

It isn't easy to dress a young baby who really isn't interested anyway. But if you use a little know-how and easy clothes, you will soon master the art. Let's start with the part that you will be doing most often: putting on a diaper.

Diapers

For disposable diapers, follow the directions on the package.

* A description of these and other kinds of clothing is given in the first chapter under What to Buy for the Baby.

Some brands caution against disposing in the toilet; others can be flushed away. Some use an outer pant to hold them in place; others have their own waterproof backing. Some require the use of safety pins; others are self-fastening.

Cloth diapers may be of layered gauze or bird's-eye cotton—oblong, square, or ready-shaped. Here's how to deal with each:

THE OBLONG-SHAPED DIAPER. Fold both sides in to overlap and make a 3-fold thickness. Fold up one end about ⅓ of the way. Place the folded end under the baby's buttocks if a girl, or in front if a boy. Bring the other end of the diaper up between the baby's legs and pin front and back together over each hip. Safety pins at the leg opening are useful for keeping the bowel movements inside the diaper. As your baby grows larger, the folds can be smaller to make a larger-sized diaper.

THE SQUARE DIAPER. A popular way to fold this diaper is in "kite" fashion. Place the diaper on the table with a corner pointing straight up. Fold the two sides to make a long kite-shaped V. Fold the top down to form a triangle, and bring the point of the V up, envelope style. Lay the baby down with his buttocks over the folded diaper and bring the front up over the baby's abdomen. Pin at the hips and leg openings.

THE READY-SHAPED DIAPER. These save the time spent on folding stacks of diapers, but they have one disadvantage: they cannot be made larger or smaller unless they are made of a stretch fabric. The wider end of the diaper goes under the baby's buttocks; the narrower end is brought up and pinned in the usual manner.

SOME PRECAUTIONS. Be sure when putting on a diaper that it is not so tight as to restrict circulation. When pinning the diaper, place your finger between your baby's body and the diaper material. In this way you will avoid sticking the baby, should he kick or should you misjudge the thickness of the material. It is also a good idea to place the open end of the safety pin *away* from the baby's body. If the pin should accidentally open, the point is much less likely to stick into the baby.

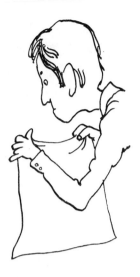
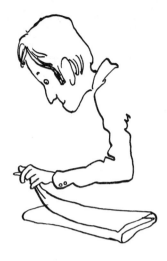

How Often Should Diapers Be Changed?   It is not necessary to grab a clean diaper every time your small baby becomes wet. If he is changed before and after feedings (if needed), after a bowel movement, and when he seems fretful or uncomfortable, this is usually enough. If his skin is unusually sensitive or he develops diaper rash, he will need to be changed more frequently.

After a bowel movement, cleanse the diaper area with soap and water or with mineral oil.

Remember that if you keep waterproof pants on your baby all the time, he will need to be changed just as frequently as without them, for the moisture kept in the diaper may cause diaper rash.

Shirts

As we said, babies hate to have things pulled on over their heads and will usually resist quite vigorously. If you have chosen—or received—the pullover type of shirt, make sure the head opening is large and can be stretched when pulled on.

The doublebreasted kind with snap fasteners or ties may be easier to put on. Hold the shirt by one shoulder and run your fingers up inside the sleeve from the wrist opening. Grasp the baby's hand and pull it gently down through the sleeve. Place the back of the shirt under him and pull the other sleeve on in the same manner. Fasten the front with the snaps or ties.

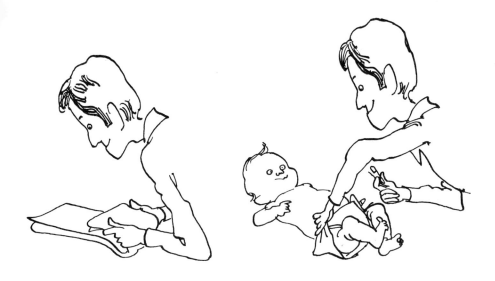

Whether you use long- or short-sleeved shirts, or shirts with no sleeves, depends on the climate and the temperature.

Dresses, gowns, sleepers

It is fun to dress up your baby, but fancy dresses and suits make a great deal of extra work; you cannot tell your young baby to be careful with his good clothes. So look for gowns that are both practical and attractive, and don't overlook the dress-up set of knit cotton sacque with diaper cover to match.

CARE OF THE BABY'S CLOTHES

If you are not using a diaper service, keep a covered pail partially filled with soapy water for wet or soiled diapers. Rinse soiled diapers in the toilet bowl before putting them in the pail.

When washing diapers in an automatic washer, use hot water and any detergent or soap recommended for baby clothes. An automatic dryer will make the diapers come out soft and fluffy.

If your washing machine is not automatic, rinse the diapers until the water is clear. If you don't have a machine and are washing by hand, you may find it is easier to remove stains by boiling the diapers in soapy water and then rinsing them thoroughly. If it is possible, hang the diapers in the sunshine, for this helps to remove stains, destroy bacteria, and keep the diapers soft. It is important that all soap be rinsed out before drying, especially if the baby has a diaper rash.

Other baby clothes can usually be washed in an automatic washing machine with a mild detergent or soap. Always make sure that all soap or detergent is rinsed out. When plastic pants or protectors are used, check the manufacturer's suggestions for laundering.

FEEDING

Babies are sensitive to change. They take a while to settle down at home, and their feeding habits reflect that. They may be fretful and fussy the first few weeks. As in the hospital, your child may wake up and act hungry as often as every hour at the beginning or may go to sleep in the middle of a feeding and then wake up hungry in a couple of hours.

If your baby eats only a little at a time but wakens and cries frequently, try waiting a few minutes before feeding him. But don't let him "cry it out"; there is nothing to be gained by that at this age.

If he habitually wakens and cries within a few minutes or a half hour after a feeding, he may not be getting enough, or he may have indigestion from swallowing air. It is difficult to tell which is the trouble from his cry. Try burping him or offering him a little warm water. If he still cries, check with the well-baby clinic or your doctor to see if he is getting enough to eat.

To burp him, either hold him up on your shoulder and gently rub his back—don't slap or pat hard or you may get back more than air—or else sit him upright on your lap and support his head and neck with one hand while you rub his back with the other. Don't be upset if he doesn't bring up any air. Some babies never do. If no air is swallowed, there will be no burp.

Don't interrupt his feeding to burp him; he may resent being stopped. Burp him only if he stops of his own accord.

Breast-fed babies do not usually swallow so much air, and so they may never need burping. But it is a good idea to try after a feeding.

If your baby nurses well but still has trouble settling down, try wrapping him rather snugly in a light blanket. This seems to soothe an infant; perhaps it reminds him of his snug uterine home. Or rock him for a short time.

Some babies are normally somewhat fussy. They suck their thumbs and whimper for a few minutes before going back to sleep. Other babies stay awake for quite a while after feeding, waving their arms about. If your child is gaining weight and is healthy, there is no need to worry.

Schedules?

Most babies adjust to a 3- or 4-hour schedule after the first or second week, because, as we said, that is about the length of time it takes their stomachs to empty. So it is *not* a question of imposing a schedule on your child—of forcing him to eat if the clock says it is time, or of making him cry himself hungrily back to sleep if the clock says the time is not right—the way it used to be done. It is simply a matter of encouraging him to do what comes naturally.

Nevertheless, when your baby arrived home, he became part of the family. His feeding should not be allowed to disrupt the entire household. After all, living in a family is a shared experience, and even a baby must make some adjustments.

If he has nursed well and fallen off to sleep, don't run to pick him up to feed him again the moment he stirs. He may wave his arms around a bit, even whimper, but if you wait a while he will probably fall back to sleep. If he does wake up completely and start protesting, check his diaper and turn him on his other side. If he is really hungry, he will continue crying; feed him then, even if it is only 2 hours since his last meal.

For the first 3 or 4 weeks, your baby will probably need a feeding between 10 P.M. and 6 A.M.—usually at 2 A.M. If you feed him late in the evening, it may help him to sleep longer at night, though you will probably have to give him an early morning feeding. In any event, after the first few weeks he will start to sleep later and soon will sleep through the night. The bigger he is, the more he will take at a feeding, and the longer he will take to get hungry. Remember, though, that if your baby does wake at night, he shouldn't be made to cry it out. That will teach him nothing except that his needs for loving are not being met.

There is no harm in waking him after he has had 3 or 4 hours' sleep. As soon as he is fully awake, he will realize that he is

107

ravenously hungry. And, on the other hand, it won't do him any harm to sleep longer than 4 hours if he wants to, except that it may take him longer to set up his own schedule.

For the working mother: a semidemand schedule. If you are going back to an outside job within a few weeks after your baby's birth, you will have to schedule his feedings more precisely. Your infant will adapt quite easily if you work toward this goal from the start—and if you are prepared to bend a little on occasion.

Set your own schedule ahead of time, and try to adapt your baby to it before you go back to work. If you have to be at work early, wake your baby early to feed him before you leave. It will not bother him at all; he will fall back to sleep when his stomach is full. He should settle quite comfortably into a relatively scheduled pattern of 6 A.M., 10 A.M., 2 P.M., 6 P.M., 10 P.M.—and another feeding at 2 A.M. if he awakens.

If your job starts later or if you work at night, help your baby adjust to a later waking. Gradually push the evening feeding to a later time by letting him sleep until 11 P.M. or so. This will postpone his middle-of-the-night feeding and may cause him to sleep later in the morning. If he still wakes up early for a few mornings, wait 5 or 10 minutes before giving him his feeding. He may drop back to sleep.

Leave instructions with your baby-sitter about the feeding hours, but make it clear that if your child wakes an hour or so early and acts hungry, he should be fed, and that if he sleeps a half hour later he should be allowed to. Have a couple of extra bottles in the refrigerator for the sitter's use if needed, but be sure to tell her not to save a partly empty bottle for later use, because bacteria multiply in milk that has been exposed to the air. And remind your sitter that if your child fusses a short time after he has nursed well, a good burping rather than more food may be in order.

Breast feeding

If you are breast-feeding, make sure that your diet is adequate for yourself and your baby. You should be following the balanced diet of your pregnancy, with plenty of fluids and protein. Milk in any form—as a beverage or in soups, custards, or yogurt—fruit juices, and water are all good for you. Any foods that you tolerate and can digest are not likely to upset your baby, but if he is distressed and you know you have eaten something different, try leaving it out of your diet and see whether his discomfort ends.

Certain drugs are excreted into the breast milk and may affect your baby, so check with your doctor about any medicine you wish to take.

Remember that worry, overtiredness, or a general state of tension will affect your milk supply, so make sure you get enough rest. Try to take a nap every day while your baby is sleeping—even if it means turning away visitors or letting the kitchen floor stay dirty.

The average baby gains about 6 to 8 ounces a week during the first 3 months. If your baby is healthy and satisfied yet gains less, don't worry about it. He is probably just a slow gainer. But if he seems hungry after feedings, weigh him before and after each feeding for 24 hours and let the results help your doctor decide whether your child needs more food.

Techniques of breast feeding. Once your breast milk has become well established, you will have to decide whether to offer one or both breasts at a feeding. If you are to stimulate the secretion of the maximum amount of milk, your breasts need to be completely emptied. If your baby empties one breast and is satisfied, leave it at that and have him nurse the other breast at the next feeding.

But if you prefer to use both breasts at each feeding, nurse your baby on one breast for 10 to 15 minutes and then transfer him to the other breast and let him continue there until he seems satisfied. At the next feeding, start with the breast you used last to make sure each breast is emptied at least every 8 hours. Tie a ribbon on your bra strap so you'll remember which side to use next.

You can make sure both breasts are emptied by using either a breast pump or your own hands. In manual pumping, wash your hands, then place your thumb and forefinger on opposite sides, about an inch from the nipple, so that your fingers are outside the areola. Press your fingers deeply into the breast and squeeze them together to push the milk out of the milk sacs. Continue as long as the milk flows freely.

Can the working mother continue to breast-feed? It is usually difficult for two reasons—one yours, one your child's. First, if your baby is given a bottle during your working hours, your breasts will lack the necessary stimulation and may dry up. Second, as we noted earlier, many—even most—babies do not change easily from breast to bottle and may not go back to the breast after having been given a bottle.

So unless yours is part-time work—or unless your job is so close to your home that you don't have to miss any feedings—you should probably not breast-feed once you have gone back to work.

Remember, though, that you are not depriving your child by not nursing him. He will be well taken care of by a bottle, as long as he gets affection along with the formula.

Formula feeding

Let's repeat the most important thing: Hold your baby while you are feeding him. When he gets older, he will want to hold his own bottle and will enjoy having it in his crib; he will put himself to sleep with it. But now he needs the comfort of being held closely. Furthermore, there is the very real chance that he will choke if left alone with a propped bottle—or that he will lose the nipple and become angry and frustrated. So don't prop your baby's bottle until the day comes that he brushes your hand away and insists on holding it himself.

And when you are feeding him the bottle, make sure that milk fills the neck and nipple so that he is not sucking air with his formula.

When you are making up the formula, prepare an extra bottle or two, in case he doesn't take enough at one feeding to hold him for 3 or 4 hours. But remember, if he doesn't finish his bottle, *don't save the leftover formula;* bacteria multiply rapidly in milk that has been warmed or kept at room temperature.

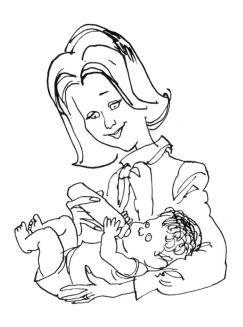

Prepared formulas. Your doctor will advise you on the amount and strength of the formula needed for your baby's age and weight. He will also suggest the kind of formula best for him. If you are particularly interested in the commercially prepared formulas, ask your doctor about them. There are several on the market that closely resemble breast milk. These commercial formulas are often a great help to the mother who plans to return to work. They cost more than a home-prepared formula, but they are more convenient. They can be purchased in powdered or concentrated liquid form, or ready to use. The powdered or concentrated preparations need to be diluted according to directions. The ready-to-use is poured directly from the can into a nursing bottle.

All three commercial forms contain approximately the same amount of nutrients and supply the same number of calories per ounce. All are reinforced with the daily requirement of vitamins.

Several companies have added an additional service. Ready-to-use formula is prepared in 4,- 6-, or 8-ounce nursing bottles. All you need do is remove the cap and replace it with a nipple. The bottle does not need to be stored in the refrigerator before being opened and can be discarded after use. These ready-to-use nursing bottles are more expensive but are very convenient when traveling or when an inexperienced person is caring for your baby. The chief advantages of all the commercially prepared formulas are their convenience and timesaving.

Warm or cold bottles? There is one way you can save time no matter what formula you use: you do not have to warm it. For ages, parents thought that a formula had to be warmed to be properly digested, but it just isn't so. Milk given straight from the refrigerator or at room temperature has not been proved to cause indigestion. Warm milk may be more soothing to your baby's taste and may be more readily accepted by him, but there is no law that says formulas must be warmed.

Kinds of milk. Cow's milk is used for formulas, but it has to be specially prepared to make it right for human babies. An occasional baby cannot tolerate milk and needs a special formula, but this is for the doctor to decide. Most babies tolerate cow's milk diluted with water, with some form of sugar or syrup.

Of the various kinds of milk from which you can make formulas at home, *evaporated milk* (canned milk with half the water removed) is the most widely used, and for good reason. It is the least expensive (a formula made with evaporated milk, water, and sugar or corn syrup can be as much as 11 cents a day cheaper than a commercial formula), it is readily available, it compares well with commercial formulas in nutrients and calorie contents, and it is safe and easy to use. Evaporated milk is sterile, uniform in composition (the milk and cream are completely mixed), and convenient; as long as the can is unopened, it can be kept indefinitely without refrigeration (though after it is opened, it must be refrigerated like fresh milk).

If *whole milk* is used it should be pasteurized to kill bacteria. Most milk sold in bottles in the United States is pasteurized. But in some areas there is "certified milk" which may not have been pasteurized; we do not believe it should be used for babies. If the milk you buy has been homogenized, the cream has been broken up into small particles and mixed throughout the milk so that it cannot rise to the top and does not need shaking or mixing.

Vitamin D is frequently added to whole milk and evaporated milk before you buy it. A quart of whole milk, fortified with

Vitamin D, contains a day's supply of this vitamin. But your baby would have to drink the entire quart in 24 hours to get sufficient Vitamin D from this source. As he will not be drinking as much as this, he will need an additional source.

Equipment for making the formula. Nursing bottles, as we have noted, come in glass or Pyrex, in plastic (that can be boiled), or in a disposable form. The wide-mouth kind of nursing bottle is most easily cleaned. These take a wide-based nipple.

Nipples should be firm enough to allow the baby to suck vigorously. Although a young baby needs a small-holed nipple, he should not have to work so hard as to leave him exhausted or frustrated.

The test of a proper hole size can be made by holding the milk-filled bottle upside down. The milk should run out through the nipple drop by drop without squeezing. It should not, however, run out in a stream.

Some nipples are "cross cut" instead of having small holes. A small cross had been cut in the tip of the nipple, and the cut edges stay together until the baby sucks. You might wish to try both kinds to find out which works better for your child.

If the hole needs to be enlarged, this can easily be done. Just heat a fine needle over a flame until it is red hot and then plunge it into the hole. You will need something to hold the needle, as it will be too hot to handle. Be careful not to spoil the nipple by making the hole too large. It may take a little practice.

If you can, use the utensils you need for preparing the formula for that purpose alone. You will need:

1. Eight or more bottles.

2. Eight or more nipples. Having enough bottles and nipples for a 24-hour supply is a considerable time-saver. Formulas can, however, be made up one bottle at a time, as shown later.

3. One large container with a lid for boiling the formula after it has been bottled. You can buy formula sterilizers complete with rack to hold the bottles. But if you do not want to spend the money to buy one, make your own from a kettle or Dutch oven with a tight-fitting lid, large enough to hold eight bottles but not so large that the bottles will bump together as the water

boils. (To be really economical, get a kettle high enough for 8-ounce bottles to stand upright. Your baby will be ready surprisingly soon for more formula than a 4-ounce bottle will hold.)

Put something between the bottles and the bottom of the sterilizing kettle. A folded towel or cloth will do. A pie pan, perforated with holes, can be set bottom side up in the kettle, or you can buy bottle racks that hold the bottles upright.

4. A quart measure marked in ounces. A Pyrex measure with a lip for pouring is best. Otherwise you can use a pitcher, saucepan, or any clean container that holds 1 quart, and do the measuring with a nursing bottle or a measuring cup marked in ounces.

5. A can opener if you are using canned milk.

6. A funnel for pouring into the nursing bottles. You can do without this if your pitcher or pan has a pouring lip or if you are using wide-mouthed bottles.

7. A tablespoon for stirring and a measuring spoon for the sugar or syrup to be added. Some preparations such as a dextrin-maltose sweetener supply a measuring spoon with the can.

8. Milk for the formula, water, and the sweetening you use.

Preparing the formula. Home-prepared formula must be sterilized, because germs grow and multiply quickly in milk, and you cannot always be certain that the water you used in the formula is not contaminated. Take comfort, though; you will not have to sterilize the dishes, spoons, and cups you use for his first foods. And when he is old enough to take straight pasteurized milk, either by bottle or cup, you will no longer need to boil his bottles or utensils.

But right now, you must sterilize—unless you use a commercially prepared formula and pour it into each bottle *at the time the baby takes it,* and keep the opened can refrigerated. Then all you will need to do is to wash the used bottle and nipple thoroughly with warm water and let them dry. But note: if you prepare several bottles of commercial formula in advance to store until used, sterilization of bottles and nipples is necessary.

Here is how to go about it:

Measure the amount of water called for in the formula and

add the specified amount of milk. If you use canned milk, wash the top of the can before opening. Add the sweetening and stir. Pour the formula into the nursing bottles and cap the bottles. If you use screw-on caps, do not tighten them until after the formula has been sterilized.

Place the bottles upright in the kettle you have prepared for sterilizing. Put 2 or 3 inches of water in the bottom of the kettle, and cover with a tight-fitting lid. Place over high heat and boil for 25 minutes. Then let bottles stand in the covered kettle until they have cooled. When you take them out of the kettle, tighten the caps and put bottles in the refrigerator.

Formulas made this way may be kept for as long as 48 hours refrigerated. Any milk you have left over after mixing the formula can be used in cooking or on the table. *But don't save milk in an opened milk bottle or can for tomorrow's formula.*

Some wide-mouthed nursing bottles have a ring-shaped cap through which the nipple is placed. If you use this kind, put the nipple on upside down before sterilizing the bottles of formula. Just before feeding your baby, turn the nipples up. Or else boil the nipples separately for 2 or 3 minutes and keep them in a dry covered jar that has been sterilized.

When using bottles that do not have caps, you can sterilize them with nipples in place if you wish, but this long boiling softens the nipples. Instead, when you take the bottles out of the kettle, cover the tops with clean wax paper. Don't put wax paper on before sterilizing or the paper will stick to the bottle.

Cleaning bottles and nipples. After the baby has finished his feeding, discard the remainder of the formula and rinse the bottle with cold water (unless you use a disposable bottle). If you do not plan to wash it right away, leave the bottle filled with water; it will be easier to get it clean.

Rinse the nipples right after use and squeeze cold water through the holes to prevent them from becoming clogged. It is better to keep rubber nipples in a dry container after cleaning; otherwise they will soften too quickly.

Most mothers find it convenient and timesaving to wash a day's supply of bottles and nipples at one time. Use a pan of warm, soapy water and a bottle brush to clean the bottles thoroughly. Wash the nipples and bottle caps in the same way. Rinse with hot water.

Other methods of formula preparation. If you are short of bottles or of refrigeration space, the sterilized formula can be kept in a boiled covered jar and one clean bottle at a time filled as needed. If the bottle is clean and does not have formula stored in it, there will be no need to boil the bottle before using it.

If only one bottle of formula is needed, you can boil the water and sugar or syrup, pour them into the clean bottle, and then add the evaporated or pasteurized milk directly from the can or milk bottle.

For the very young baby, use milk from a previously unopened can or bottle. If you have to use an opened bottle or can, boil the milk before adding it.

Sample formulas. For *the first month,* a basic rule to follow when starting formula feedings is this:

1 ounce of evaporated milk per pound of baby's weight
2 ounces of water per pound of baby's weight
3 tablespoonsful of corn syrup (Karo) for each 24 ounces of milk-and-water mixture

Thus the formula for a baby weighing 8 pounds would be: evaporated milk, 8 ounces; water, 16 ounces; and Karo syrup, 3 tablespoonsful. This makes up a 24-ounce formula for use over 24 hours. Divide it into feedings to fit your baby's pattern of eating. If you intend to feed him on a "demand schedule," you will find it most convenient to put the entire formula into a sterilized 2-quart jar and then pour out 2 or 3 ounces for each feeding until your baby has settled into a routine. Otherwise, try putting about 3½ ounces into each of seven bottles, or 3 ounces into eight bottles if you prefer. Remember to discard any portion of formula left in a bottle after a feeding.

At *2 to 4 months,* a somewhat stronger formula is needed. From now on, you can use half evaporated milk and half water.

13 ounces (one can) evaporated milk
13 ounces water
2 tablespoonsful Karo syrup

Divide according to the number of bottles your baby is taking. Some babies will want more than this amount. That's O.K.; just keep the proportions the same, 1 to 1 of evaporated milk and water.

At *4 or 5 months* babies can be switched to whole milk. Use fresh pasteurized milk and keep the bottle covered. The milk will not need to be boiled.

Many babies tend to become a little constipated when they first change from one of these formulas to whole milk. So it is a good plan to add 2 to 3 tablespoonsful of Karo syrup to each quart of whole milk at first. Gradually taper off by reducing the Karo by ½ tablespoonful every 2 weeks. If the baby's bowel movements become too frequent, reduce the Karo more rapidly.

Vitamins

Vitamins A, C, and D are needed by every baby. Commercially prepared formulas usually contain these vitamins. In the United States bottled or evaporated milk is usually fortified with vitamin D, but the young formula-fed baby may not get enough in the amount of milk he takes. Breast milk contains vitamin C, but whether enough for the baby depends on the amount of citrus fruits and vegetables the mother eats.

Because A, C, and D vitamins are so important for your baby's growth and health, doctors routinely advise giving him a vitamin preparation.* This can be dropped directly into your baby's mouth with the dropper that comes with the liquid vitamin preparation. But do *not* put the dropper itself in the baby's mouth and then back in the bottle. Empty any leftover drops in the sink and wash the dropper thoroughly. It is usually best to give the vitamin preparation just before a feeding, when the baby is hungry and most willing to swallow it.

Vitamin drops can be started during the second to fourth week of life. Draw the preparation up to the mark on the dropper for the young baby, unless your doctor prescribes a larger amount. This will fill his daily vitamin needs.

* With ready-prepared commercial formulas, fortified with vitamins, a baby will not need additional vitamins unless his doctor has a special reason for recommending them.

Orange juice for vitamin C and fish liver oil for vitamin D are generally not given at this early age. Some babies are allergic to orange juice, and most babies dislike cod liver oil and may choke on it. Vitamin drops are at least as inexpensive and are much easier to use.

Fluoride

Studies have shown that the baby who gets fluoride in his diet early in life develops teeth that are stronger and more resistant to decay. Fluoride helps to calcify the teeth while they are being formed.

In some areas fluoride is added to the water supply. If the water in your area does not contain fluoride, either naturally or by addition, your pediatrician or dentist can prescribe fluoride drops to give to your baby. These are generally started at around 1 month of age.

Combined fluoride-vitamin drops are available and are easy to give to your young baby.

What about water between feedings?

Most young babies resent being offered water to drink and will refuse it unless they are hot and thirsty. It does no harm to offer water to your baby, but if he refuses it don't worry. Your baby gets enough water in his formula or breast milk for his usual needs.

If your baby is fretful, or the weather is hot, a drink of water from a nursing bottle may be the answer.

If you are confident that your city water supply is pure, you can give it to your baby to drink without boiling it. If there is any doubt, or if you use well water, better play safe and boil it for 3 minutes. You can boil a couple of bottles of water along with the formula, or boil up a few ounces and keep in a covered boiled jar for use.

Your baby's weight gain

A young baby normally gains 5 to 8 ounces a week. You do not

118

need to weigh him every day; in fact, if you are taking him to the doctor regularly for checkups, you do not need to buy a scale at all.

When your child appears contented after feedings and is willing, most of the time, to wait at least 2 hours between feedings, he is getting enough to eat and will gain weight. If he is cross and appears hungry shortly after being fed, he may well need more milk or a stronger formula.

BOWEL MOVEMENTS

Breast-fed babies are quite apt to have several bowel movements a day during their first weeks of life, though after the first 2 or 3 weeks some will reverse the procedure and have a movement only every 2 or 3 days; they are still perfectly all right. A formula-fed baby usually has fewer movements, occasionally as few as one every 2 or 3 days. The normal movement is soft and pasty; there may be some soft, loose lumps in the formula-fed baby's movements.

Normally you will not have trouble with constipation or diarrhea in a baby at this age. But if you are nursing your baby and have taken certain laxatives, your baby may have a loose movement.

If your baby should start having several loose watery stools, call your doctor. It may be only a reaction to his feeding, which can be straightened out, but it could mean an infection and need prompt treatment.

SAFETY CONSIDERATIONS

While bathing

Does the water temperature feel just comfortable to your elbow? Or if you use a bath thermometer, does it register between 90 and 100 degrees?

Do you keep one hand on the baby at all times?

Do you let the doorbell or telephone ring and *never* leave the baby alone in the tub or on the bathing table, even if you are using some sort of harness or strap to hold him?

In bed

Do you remember *always* to keep the crib sides up, even though you never have seen your child roll over?

Are the side bars of his crib close enough together so he cannot get his head caught between them?

Are you aware that even a newborn baby can move about and that the only really safe place to leave him is his crib (or the floor, if you must—he can't fall off that)?

You never use a thin piece of plastic or a plastic bag in his crib, do you? He could smother.

For the same reason, do you use a firm mattress or folded blanket in his crib rather than a soft pillow for a mattress?

While feeding

If you prop his bottle "just this once," are you *sure* this will not be the time he will choke?

If he insists on lying on his back after a feeding, do you raise the head of his crib (by placing a folded blanket under the top of the mattress) to help prevent choking on spit-up milk?

THE FIRST FOUR MONTHS

Your baby is born out of a world that is nearly soundless into one of great noise and confusion. So he does the only sensible thing. He sleeps most of the time.

Around the second or third week you can expect to find him awake for much longer periods of time and beginning to take notice. Just hope he chooses the daytime hours. If he doesn't, have patience. He will soon set up a schedule that will fit into the routine of his home, given a little nudge from you.

PHYSICAL GROWTH

Your baby is in for an extremely busy growth time. During the first half of his first year, he will grow so fast he will double his birth weight. He will never grow at that rate again.

An average full-term baby (5½ to 7 pounds, 19 to 22 inches at birth) loses 5 to 10 ounces the first few days and then gains 1 to 2 pounds monthly and approximately 1 inch a month for the first 6 months of his life.

But remember that your baby is an individual. So use those figures only to tell you *about* where he will be in terms of growth during the first 6 months.

PERIODIC CHECKUPS

Every baby should have regular examinations. During early babyhood a monthly or 6-week checkup offers the best kind of insurance. (See Chapter 8 on choosing a doctor.)

If you are having a pediatrician or your family doctor care for your baby, he will probably have examined your baby shortly after birth.

Well-baby clinics or child health stations are for the express purpose of safeguarding the health of your baby. These facilities exist in most parts of the world, but there are not enough of them to be always easily accessible to everyone who needs to use them. If there is none in your locality, and you and your neighbors are very much in need of such help, why not get together and put in a petition to your health department? Perhaps you or your friends could find volunteers to help in such a clinic. If distance is the problem, how about making up a list of volunteer drivers?

Whether your baby gets his checkups in a doctor's office or in a clinic, he will be well served. At each visit he will be weighed, examined carefully, his feeding schedule checked, and his general daily behavior reviewed.

The first time you take him for a checkup, pull out that list of questions you have been making all month. Such as: "He still wakes up and cries for his two A.M. feeding. His brother slept right through from the start. My sister tells me to let him cry it out, but my husband says he can't sleep with the baby crying. What should I do?" Or: "I just cannot clear up that rash on his bottom. What can I do?" Or even: "How about starting baby foods? All my friends started earlier than this."

Don't be afraid to ask a question because you feel the doctor will think you should know the answer. He doesn't expect you to know as much about babies as he does.

The doctor will help you plan and will make recommendations for changes. His suggestions may differ from the routine your neighbor is using, because he's concerned with *your* baby, not your neighbor's.

The doctor will also check anything that does not seem to be exactly as it should in your baby's health and development. He may put your child on a "watch and wait" routine to prevent trouble from developing or to correct a condition that could become troublesome when the baby grows older.

Immunizations

It is easy enough to forget the importance of preventive inoculations. No longer do we hear of children dying of lockjaw. Gone are the devastating neighborhood epidemics of whooping cough. We do not have to face the horror of a child slowly suffocating with diphtheria. The youngster mentally and physically crippled by measles encephalitis is becoming a medical rarity. Soon there will be few, if any, newborn babies blinded or otherwise damaged because their mothers had German measles during pregnancy. Smallpox no longer kills by the hundreds of thousands; it is disappearing as a result of years of nearly worldwide vaccination. Polio, with its death and paralysis, is everywhere being defeated. *But only because of preventive measures*

If children are to be protected, they *must* have their immunizations very early in life. The cost is trivial compared to the protection. The materials used have been steadily improved until now even mild reactions to the vaccines are uncommon.*

NORMAL DEVELOPMENT

"Mrs. Jones says her baby knew she was his mother when he was two months old. My baby lets anyone pick him up and he smiles at them as much as at me. Is he 'normal'?"

You need not be entirely dependent on your doctor's exami-

* See the Basic Schedule of Immunizations in Chapter 9.

nation for an idea of your child's progress. You can have at least a general idea of what to expect at any particular age.

The following table gives you that general idea during this age period. Just remember that even though your baby may not fit all the categories, he may still grow up to be a genius. But if he is quite a bit away from the average range, mention it to your doctor, if only for your own peace of mind.

Development is an orderly process, continuing from the moment of birth until the person has reached the limit of his ability.

Motor Ability

At 1 month	At 4 months
Can raise head briefly when placed prone on a firm surface. Needs head supported when held upright.	Can raise head and shoulders when lying prone on firm surface. Holds head up and steady when held upright, though head may bob occasionally.
Keeps fist closed most of time. Will grasp object placed in his hand but only as reflex action; soon drops object.	Holds object placed in his hand, begins to look at it. Will soon let object fall. Reaches in direction of bright object held near him. Reaches with entire body, head, shoulders, arms. Not yet able to come in contact with object, except accidentally.

Vocal, Social, Visual Ability

At 1 month	At 4 months
Cries and makes small sounds in throat. Stops motor activity momentarily at sound of human voice speaking soothingly to him.	Cries, coos, gurgles. Laughs aloud on social stimulation. Responds to human contact with social smile. Is beginning to become excited when familiar routine signifies that bathing, dressing, or feeding is about to occur.
Enjoys being held closely and will soothe momentarily even when hungry. (The feeding had better be forthcoming immediately, though.)	Enjoys social activity around him. Likes having head elevated so he can look around.
Stares vacantly at large objects or at the human face when in his direct line of vision.	May show some recognition of familiar faces. May sober at sight of strange face (much to dismay of grandparents) but will show appreciation of anyone who attends to his needs.

At 1 month	At 4 months
Will follow an object with his eyes when held before him. *May* turn head to follow. Eyes focus momentarily, if at all. May stare at own hand when it comes accidentally into his line of vision.	Will follow object with interest and show signs of reaching out for it. Focuses eyes most of time when looking. Eye and hand coordination good. Will voluntarily bring hands into field of vision and look at them intently.
Waves hands around without conscious purpose.	Clasps hands together. Glances from hand or hands to bright object held before him. Will soon reach out for it.
Sucks own finger or hand when it brushes against his mouth.	Sucks finger or thumb by bringing hand to face for that purpose.

BABY FOODS

While your baby is in this fast-growing period, he will need plenty of nourishment. His formula may be strengthened and will be increased in amount to meet his growing needs and baby foods will be started.

There is no set time for starting a baby on solid food. An energetic, fast-growing baby probably will demand more food than a more placid infant of the same age and may therefore get an earlier introduction to solid food. In general, this will be when your baby is between 3 and 6 or 8 weeks old. Usually cereal is the first food offered; its bland, smooth character makes it more acceptable to an infant used to liquids.

Make the cereal quite thin until your baby gets used to it. Rice, barley, and wheat are all good starters, but if you cook them at home they will need to be strained. Commercially prepared baby cereals are ready cooked and need only to be mixed with a little formula or plain water. It may be better to use water so your baby will learn that not everything tastes like his milk or formula.

Learning how to eat

A young baby knows only one way to take food, and that is to push his tongue forward as if to suck. Try sucking on a straw, and you will see how differently you hold your mouth and tongue. Your child now has to learn a very complicated skill— how to transfer food from the front of his mouth to his throat for swallowing.

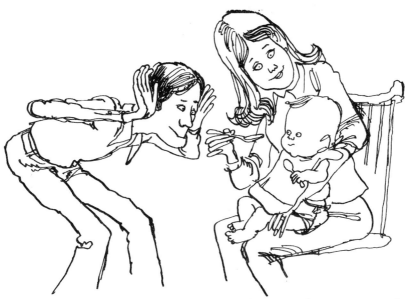

The eager, hungry baby is quite puzzled over this new turn of events and is apt to become frustrated and annoyed by it. "What's this all about, anyhow? Where's my bottle?" he is likely to protest in loud and clear terms. In fact, you will find it best to give the very hungry baby part of his formula or let him nurse for a few minutes before you introduce him to the new method of feeding.

Once you understand that the queer look your baby is giving you is one of astonishment, and that his pushing the food out with his tongue is habit, it will be easier to relax and be patient with him. Make up your mind right from the beginning, however, that you will never force him to eat. *Never.*

Offer him food, help him, but let him take only as much as he enjoys.

Your baby's clothing (and yours too) will need protection. A small spoon will fit his mouth better than a large one and will make it easier to put food further back on his tongue. Don't put it so far back that he gags. Put only a small amount on the spoon at a time. When he pushes it out with his tongue, catch it and offer it again. Be patient; your baby will soon learn how to manipulate the food and will come to enjoy this novel way of eating. Let him be the judge of how much he wants.

The choice of mealtime does not matter, although it is not good practice to try at first when he is ravenously hungry. He will be too impatient.

A food timetable

Strained fruits are usually added to the baby's diet after he has become accustomed to cereals. A few weeks later, strained vegetables and pureed meats, or meat-vegetable mixtures, are introduced. Mashed hard-boiled egg yolk may also be given. Whole eggs are not offered until much later. Many babies become allergic to the albumen in egg whites if started on them too early.

Pediatricians differ in the timing for starting babies on foods other than milk. Follow your doctor's schedule; he knows your baby.

The authors of this book find the following timetable useful. It works well for most babies.

At 3 to 6 weeks of age, start with cereal, very thin and smooth. Commercially prepared baby cereals come in dry precooked form. Pour a small amount into a bowl and mix with water to a thin paste. Later, after your baby has learned how to use his mouth for eating, he will enjoy having it thicker.

After he has become somewhat used to being fed, rotate the different kinds of cereal to get him accustomed to various flavors.

At 6 weeks to 2 months, add strained fruit. Babies usually enjoy the taste of fruit and accept it eagerly. Vary the kinds offered, but don't force him to take any he does not seem to like. Wait a while and try it again; if he still refuses, let it go and try another flavor. If you give prunes, try only a small portion the first time. For some babies, they are too laxative.

At 2 to 3 months (usually about 3), introduce various strained vegetables and pureed meats. Some babies prefer meat-vegetable mixtures. Mashed hard-boiled egg yolk may also be given.

Give him his food first and his bottle as dessert; whatever his reaction to the food, he won't give up his bottle at this age.

We do not specify the amount of food to offer; again, it is safe to let your baby be the judge. You will probably start him with less than a teaspoonful of cereal or fruit and work up until he is taking half a jar or more. The important thing is neither to coax him to take more than he wants nor to stop him if he wants more.

Do not force a baby or small child to take any food he does not like. Wait a few days and offer it again. If he repeatedly refuses, do not make an issue of it. There is always something else to give him the needed nutrients. There are plenty of varieties of fruits, vegetables, meats and cereals to meet his needs.

One of the very best ways known for making a child into a poor eater is to force him into eating something he does not want or to take more of a food than he wants at a particular time.

Preparation and storage of baby foods

Every kind of food a baby needs—and some he does not—can be bought ready to serve in small jars. These commercially prepared foods are great time and labor savers, and ideal for use when traveling or visiting, but more expensive than food prepared at home. You may decide to use the prepared foods and economize in other ways.

If you find the strain on your budget is too much, you can cook your own vegetables and fruits—often using the same foods you are serving the rest of the family—just as long as you strain them. A blender is a marvelous help—it will puree just about any kind of food and soon pay for itself—but if the initial cost is the stumbling block, an old-fashioned strainer will do the job.

If you use commercially prepared food, keep any opened jars in the refrigerator or else discard the unused portion.

If your baby is taking only a few spoonsful at a meal, pour some of the food out into a dish rather than dipping the spoon into the jar, and put the opened jar back in the refrigerator. In this way you can avoid contamination of the food and can use the unused portion at a later feeding.

A last word: Some mothers make a practice of mixing the young baby's foods into his formula and letting him take it from a bottle. This is not teaching him how to eat. The only time this is permissible is on the rare occasion that a sick, malnourished baby needs food quickly and is too weak to take it any other way.

SOCIAL DEVELOPMENT

There is an important fact about babies, even young babies, that has received little attention in the past: They can, and often do, get bored. It was once thought that babies were born with minds like blank slates. Now we know that every normal baby starts early in life to show an immense curiosity. As soon as he has had enough experience in any area to remember, he starts to learn.

Then, too, as soon as any object or experience has meaning for him, he uses that knowledge to build on for more learning. You do not have to teach him to do that; it is part of his natural development. For example:

Each normal baby is born with an instinct to suck, though he has to be guided to the nipple and perhaps taught how to grasp it. Once he has learned to grasp the nipple and has obtained milk from it, sucking becomes a pleasure for him. He soon begins to put together *sucking* and *food*. It will not be long before he *anticipates* food when he sees a nursing bottle or is picked up at feeding time. In other words, development comes by living.

A baby learns through experience and memory, but his every-day environment must provide the opportunities for experience. Without any such opportunities to learn, he will become dull.

Johnny, at 1 month of age, was staying awake several hours during the day. His conscientious mother fed him, bathed and dressed him, and put him in his favorite position in his crib in his own quiet room. Yet Johnny cried for no reason anyone could discover.

One day his mother in despair moved his crib out into the breakfast room where the rest of the family were gathered. Johnny's face brightened and his crying stopped. He plainly showed that he too was a social being and was becoming just plain tired of being alone in his room.

Your baby learns through all his senses

Babies really need to be touched and handled. (Obviously, you shouldn't overdo this or you will tire them.) You may have noticed how a fretful baby will soothe when his mother rocks him gently or his father walks the floor with him. We are not advocating that you walk your baby every night; fathers have rights too. But a baby's need to be handled is very real. He needs what is called "tactile stimulation" to grow and develop properly.

Babies who are left in their cribs and never held or played with become dull and listless, showing no interest in their surroundings. They need the physical stimulation of being held and of being handled. Rocking your baby, rubbing his back gently when he is fretful, handling him when bathing and dressing him —these are all stimulating to him.

Babies need to be talked to

The coos, gurgles, and babbles of your baby are the beginning of speech for him. Some parents have the mistaken idea that "baby talk" should never be used. But speech specialists tell us that a young baby *should* be babbled back to in the same way he is babbling.

So don't be afraid of baby talk. It is partly a social interaction; just watch how your baby enjoys it. But it is more than that. Your baby is learning to make sounds that he will use later in forming words. He is a great imitator—he watches your face intently as you make sounds—but he is not yet ready to learn the extremely complicated process of putting them into words.

Babies love "whistle talk." When you are relaxed and playing with your 2- or 3-month-old child, whistle to him softly. Almost all babies respond. It needn't be a tune, just a variety of soft little whistle sounds. A doctor who is skillful at this can usually get a wonderful smile this way from the soberest little patient. So can you.

Don't try to get your baby to say words that use combinations of sounds entirely beyond his ability. Being unable to imitate much of it, he is likely to become discouraged and quit trying. It is really the pleasant give-and-take that matters.

When your child is old enough to learn real words, that is the time to make sure he hears them spoken correctly. Don't keep up the baby talk past babyhood.

Toys for your baby

TOYS TO LOOK AT. Just as your newborn baby has to learn to

129

focus his eyes, he has to learn to recognize what he sees. To help him develop this important sense of sight, he needs to have something to look at.

There are many toys designed to aid babies and young children in their development, and they make fine gifts from proud aunts and grandparents. But playthings do not need to be expensive to be "educational." Your infant will be equally happy with those you make for him at little or no cost.

By the age of 2 or 3 months, he will enjoy looking at bright objects strung across his crib. *Cradle gyms* are very popular and can be bought cheaply in any infant department. These consist of a heavy cord strung from one side of the crib to the other, from which hang brightly colored balls, rings, or small bells. A cradle gym can easily be made at home. Painted spools, painted toilet paper rollers, plastic cups, bells, bracelets may be used. Get a piece of heavy cord long enough to string across the baby's crib from side to side. Tie 3 to 5 short lengths of cord to dangle from it. Tie large spools (painted bright colors), a rattle, a small bell, or other bright unbreakable objects to the ends of the short cords. After your baby has kicked at these objects a few times in his random movements, you will be surprised how soon he will kick at them deliberately and reach out toward them with his hands.

Mobiles can be bought in a wide variety of forms, ranging from simple to quite sophisticated. Mobiles are also great fun for parents and older brothers and sisters to make. The thin wire used for making artificial flower arrangements is good for making mobiles. Heavy nylon threads hanging down from the wires support paper or pipe-cleaner objects floating about gently. Hang the mobile high out of the baby's reach.

Wind chimes make a gentle tinkling sound that may capture your baby's attention.

MUSIC. Babies seem to be born with an appreciation of rhythm. Even a very young baby may be soothed by soft music on a record player or radio—but no record or radio can take the place of a mother or father gently rocking the baby while crooning a quiet lullaby. Be careful not to frighten him with loud, blaring music.

TOYS TO TOUCH. *Rattles* come in every possible shape and size. Be sure to get sturdy and durable ones. Check plastic rattles carefully for cracks and breaks.

Chains of brightly colored *plastic disks* make a pleasing sound when the baby shakes them. They seem to taste good too.

Babies like to manipulate strings of large, *plastic or wooden beads.* Make sure they are on heavy cord and are made of unbreakable material. The individual pieces should be too large to swallow.

General social experience

Years ago it was the custom in hospitals, institutions, and sometimes even in the home to keep babies carefully screened from any sort of contact with others. Crib sides were draped with white sheets, so the baby could see nothing around him.

This was at a time when infections were widespread and infant mortality was high. Keeping each baby carefully isolated certainly cut down the spread of infections, but nevertheless some babies refused food, sickened, and died. Eventually it was realized that a baby's need for social stimulation and a feeling of being loved is as vital as his need for physical care.

Your baby will enjoy having the head of his crib elevated when he is awake, so he can look around. You can use a blanket folded under the top of his mattress or a specially constructed infant carrier.

Babies around the age of 3 or 4 months also usually enjoy a playpen. In fact, they enjoy it more than they will later when their curiosity and independence cause them to view the playpen as a sort of prison. Of course you will not want to leave a 3-month-old in a playpen or infant seat after he clearly indicates that he is getting tired or bored.

The playpen also comes in handy as a safe place to put your baby while you are preparing his bath, mixing his bottle, or perhaps answering the phone or doorbell.

Learning to recognize faces

At about 4 months of age or very soon after, babies begin to show signs of recognizing familiar faces. Your baby will become excited, laugh, and coo when you lean over him. About the same time you will notice that he stays quiet when the face is that of a person he does not see very often. He is still too young to fear strangers; that will come later. At this age he will become sober, but just let the stranger smile and speak softly to him, and very soon he will be beaming and cooing in response.

MOTHER-BABY INTERACTION

When it was realized how very important it is for babies to have a strong relationship with another person, it was believed that the relationship had to be between the baby and his own mother. This was pretty rough on those mothers who went out and worked for a living.

After a time it was discovered that any person who gave a young baby attention, love, and care was perfectly acceptable to him, but it was still thought that this must be a one-to-one relationship, either between the baby and his natural mother or a "mother substitute."

We are now looking at this a little more closely. *Is* a baby who gets little or no emotional support in his own home really better off than a baby in a day care center or even an institution, if the latter is getting the emotional and social support he needs from many substitute mothers? Here is one example.

Sally, a 4-month-old baby, was brought to the children's hospital after she had been found alone and crying in an apartment. Sally did not smile, look at people, or show any interest in anything going on around her. She seemed totally withdrawn, and it was thought she was probably mentally retarded. It was decided that any nurse passing her crib would smile and speak to her, while her own nurse made a point of holding, rocking, and singing to her. Nurses do not work 24-hour shifts, and they do have days off, so Sally had a variety of nurses to care for her. In only a week or so, Sally rewarded her nurses with a broad smile. She started to play and to enjoy being put in a sitting position and showed every indication of being a normal baby.

This may be an extreme example, but babies in many homes get very little social attention. The point is not how much neglect Sally received but rather how fast she responded when cared for by several people who were interested in her.

Experiments in group care have been tried in several European countries in recent years. One notable example is in the Israeli kibbutz. There babies are nursed by their mothers, visited daily by their parents, but live in infant houses and are cared for by trained aides. From four to six babies share a room; an individual baby is never alone. Babies learn from each other.

Although only a very small number of Israeli children are raised in this manner, the kibbutzim have been of great interest to people concerned with child welfare. Bruno Bettelheim, after observing babies and children in kibbutzim for a time, wrote, "I suggest that the inner experience of the infant leading to trust is that of security, whatever the outer experience that creates such a feeling, and whether or not it is based on any sameness in the person of the provider." * Whether or not we agree, his book makes interesting reading.

Discipline

Your baby is learning from your actions, your words, your tone of voice. He enjoys attention.

Any unhappy baby will soothe if held and rocked. This is not spoiling him; the young baby who becomes spoiled is the one who is allowed to "cry it out," whose fatigue, hunger, or comfort needs are not met. He is the one who decides he has to fight for his rights. Turning a baby over, perhaps giving him a few sips of water by bottle, or just bringing him out of his room for a bit takes little time. Young babies under 3 or 4 months do not get spoiled by a little attention.

But nevertheless you will be faced by the question, "How much should I let the baby cry before picking him up?" There are no hard and fast rules, but with very young babies it's quite a different matter than with those 1 or 2 years old. While the baby is so tiny, it's better to comfort him fairly promptly. If you are putting him down to sleep and he fuses or cries, you can wait a few minutes, for very often during that time he will drop off.

* Bruno Bettelheim, *The Children of the Dream,* p. 67.

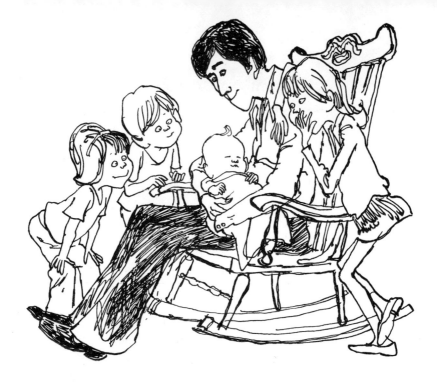

If he is just *waking* from a sleep and cries hard, you may as well pick him up for it's not likely he will settle down.

You will soon learn to distinguish between halfhearted crying, or "fussing," and hard crying. Fussing usually subsides without further attention; hard crying often does not.

When your child has been awake a good while and has had too much handling or too much excitement, he tells you—by becoming cross and irritable. Then is the time to put him in his crib in a quiet room and leave him alone.

As your baby matures and grows in understanding, he will discover the fun of having his own way. He will find out that he has it in his power to make his parents quite miserable. Then will be the time to teach him that parents and other people have rights and feelings, too, and that he cannot have his own way at the expense of the comfort of others.

But he is far too young for this lesson now. He is not yet able to connect his actions with any disagreeable results.

Thumb-sucking and pacifiers

Thumb-sucking used to be frowned upon. Perhaps this was a legacy from the puritanical days when anything that gave plea-

134

sure had to be suspect. For babies certainly derive pleasure from thumb-sucking.

In any event, it was (and, in some places, still is) common practice to put bitter-tasting substances on the baby's favorite sucking finger to discourage him. If this didn't work, stiff cuffs were put on his elbows to make it impossible for him to get his finger to his mouth. The slogan was, "Don't let him get started."

None of the measures used was very successful. The baby sucked the bitter stuff off or promptly started sucking again as soon as the elbow restraints were removed. If his finger was jerked away and his hand slapped, he would cry, but, since he had no way of understanding why he was being slapped, he would comfort himself with his thumb!

Since dentists have assured us that a baby or young child is not permanently changing the shape of his jaw or causing his teeth to come in crooked, there really seems no good reason to fuss about a baby's thumb-sucking. The American Dental Association, in a pamphlet titled *Your Child's Teeth*, reports that "thumbsucking during the first years need not be a cause for undue concern. However, if your child continues to suck his thumb beyond the age of 5, it may affect the position of his incoming permanent teeth, as well as alter the shape of the jawbone." *

Furthermore, your baby probably sucked his thumb before he was born. Dr. Margaret Liley is a specialist in *fetology*, the study of infants before birth. In her book *Modern Motherhood* she wrote, "All unborn babies learn to some degree to suck and swallow while they are still in the womb. . . . Many X-rays show unborn babies of various ages sucking their thumbs." Not much we can do about that, is there?

If you happen to be one of those mothers whose own childhood conditioning makes you really uncomfortable when you see your baby suck his finger or thumb, here is something you might try that won't make your baby feel too frustrated: If you are bottle-feeding your baby, use a stiff nipple with a small hole so

* *Your Child's Teeth*, p. 4.

he will suck for a longer time. He may get enough sucking satisfaction from this not to need to suck his finger.

Nevertheless, later in babyhood or young childhood, when your child is lonely or unhappy, he will look for ways to comfort himself. When he remembers the satisfaction sucking gave him earlier, he will probably try to regain that comfort by sucking on his thumb or fingers or on a soft toy.

Pacifiers fall in the same category. No one has come up with a really good case against them—except the small baby who is apt to lose them easily and therefore to find his finger more satisfying.

Crying

The healthy new baby's crying nearly always indicates hunger, but he soon learns to signal other conditions through crying. Most of the time you will learn to interpret his cries, but not always.

After you make sure that he isn't wet or soiled, and that there are no open safety pins, check him for gas bubbles. If burping him doesn't bring up any air, try placing him on his abdomen. The pressure may help him bring up the bubbles.

If neither gas nor diapers nor pins is the cause, let him cry for 5 or 10 minutes; his lungs won't mind the exercise. But if he persists, try another feeding. He may really be hungry.

Or he may be lonely. A baby who is tired of lying in his crib away from everyone may appreciate being with the rest of the family. Put him in his playpen where he can squirm around, or roll his crib out to where you are and prop him up in his infant seat.

One 2-week-old little girl cried persistently when her parents were chatting at the dinner table, although they could find nothing wrong with her. Then her father decided to move her crib out into the dining area; the infant lay quietly and seemed entirely satisfied.

Babies do seem to enjoy having people nearby and hearing their voices. We know of a 2-month-old child who quietly watched her mother and father as they read stories to her 3-year-old brother.

It is difficult to tell if a young baby is in pain. All babies draw up their legs and get red in the face when they cry. Fortunately, a healthy baby in this age group does not often suffer acute pain. But if your child persists in crying day after day, take him to the doctor or clinic for a thorough checkup.

Occasionally, a baby is quite fretful the first few months for seemingly no cause. This is hard on a mother. If your baby is like this, try to get away once in a while for a shopping trip or an evening out. It will help you a great deal.

Colic. A baby with colic doubles up his legs, cries loudly and wholeheartedly, and gets no relief from being burped or fed. These attacks usually follow feeding by 20 minutes to 1 hour. They may be, or may seem to be, worse at night.

The condition is sometimes called "3-month colic," because that is usually the age at which it starts to disappear. While it lasts it makes both the baby and his parents very unhappy. No one is quite sure what causes colic, or why it disappears (see detailed description in Chapter 10).

FOUR MONTHS TO ONE YEAR

Babies don't need books to find out what they should be doing at any particular age. They just obey their own inner urges.

Jimmy was on his feet and toddling around before his first birthday, ready to creep up the stairs if his mother forgot to fasten the gate.

Jimmy's cousin Ruthie had an entirely different timetable. She apparently didn't care for the idea of creeping or toddling. She managed to get into things very nicely by sliding around on her bottom. But at about 14 months of age, she got up on her feet and walked—and has been walking ever since.

It is risky to try to say exactly what any baby will be able to do at any particular time during his first year. But we can tell you a few things about the usual rate of development between the seventh and twelfth months.

Motor Ability

At 7 months

Can roll from back to abdomen.
Can sit alone briefly.
Reaches for toy, transfers it from hand to hand, looks at it, tastes it, shakes it.

At 12 months

Can scarcely tolerate the idea of lying flat when awake. Rolls over and sits up. Has been able to sit alone for some time. Leans over to pick up object and rights himself.
Shifts from sitting to creeping position, back to sitting.
Has been crawling or creeping for some time—or propels himself around in a sitting position.
Can stand alone, perhaps briefly. "Cruises" sideways by holding onto chairs or playpen.
Likes to pick up small pieces of food to feed himself. Tries to grab spoon when being fed.

Social Development

At 7 months

Likes to be with people.
Watches events going on around him.
Usually shows fear of strangers; may cry at an unfamiliar face.

At 12 months

Tries to imitate sounds and actions of people around him.
Recognizes his own name.
Understands *no* and appears to deliberate whether or not to obey.
Can learn "patty-cake" and moves his hand for "bye-bye." Probably has not mastered the art of waving.
Loves attention. Will repeat any performances that are laughed at.
Is capable of jealousy, affection, fear, anger, sympathy.

If your baby lags noticeably behind this general schedule, menton it to your doctor or take him to the well-baby clinic for a checkup. If he checks out O.K. you have nothing to worry about. If he seems slower than he should be, you will find help in searching out possible causes and remedies.

Your baby is learning so rapidly during this stage of his life that he often goes on to something new while you are still boasting about his last achievement. And he is using up so much energy that he isn't gaining weight as quickly as he did the first 5 or 6 months. By the end of the year he will weigh three times his birth weight.

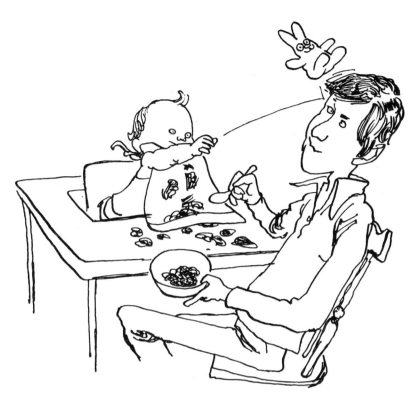

FEEDING

When your child becomes old enough to sit with very little support, it will be easier to feed him if you put him in a chair facing you. As we said in Chapter 1, a low table-chair arrangement seems preferable to a high chair and is certainly much safer. Too many bad falls have resulted from babies leaning over or standing up in high chairs. And yet, we also recognize that a well-made broad-based high chair does have some advantages.

Being in a chair with the family at meals is a very important experience, too important to be mismanaged. It should be a happy time. You must be prepared to be pleasant about it even if your child knocks things off his tray or pours his juice over his head. You can gently but firmly tell him *no*. But no cross words. No slapping. No haranguing. When he tires and begins to fret, take him out of the chair. Never force him to sit and eat food he does not want. Keeping it a happy time will have a lot to do with his table and eating behavior later on. It is one of his first real experiences in family living.

The older he grows, the more your child will enjoy eating

some of his meals with the family. He can usually eat the same foods the family has if you mash up the solids for him.

Somewhere in the second half of the first year you can start giving him foods that are not so finely mashed. At about the same time, your baby will probably enjoy holding and feeding himself a zwieback or one of the commercial baby biscuits. If you are still buying prepared baby foods you can start him on junior foods. You don't have to wait until his teeth appear. Try him with food only slightly mashed, see how well he accepts it, and gradually progress from there. Don't force him. Wait until he is ready to accept "lumpy" foods. You will find that he will go from fluids to semisolids to thicker foods all within the course of a few months. You can afford to go slowly when introducing the more adult-type foods.

The timing for giving solid foods, as well as the amount, can pretty well be adapted to your baby's needs. A sample schedule may give you some guidance.

For the baby who wakes up early:

milk by bottle or cup on waking
midmorning—cereal, or cereal and fruit, milk
lunch—strained meat, vegetable, and milk
midafternoon—orange juice
supper—cereal, fruit, milk
evening—milk by bottle or cup

Remember to let the baby decide how much he wants of any particular food. Remember, too, that it usually works out best to give him his food before you give him his milk. If your baby is refusing food, you can cut down on his milk intake to make him more hungry, but don't cut down too much; he needs from a pint and a half to a quart of milk every day.

As your baby grows older, he will start to show disinterest in one of his feedings and you can gradually work him into a three-meals-a-day routine. The age at which babies are ready for a three-meal schedule varies. Follow your baby's lead.

SELF-FEEDING. Your young explorer will soon start trying to take the spoon away from you to experiment with "do it yourself" feeding. It will take quite a while, and considerable practice, before he is able to get the spoon right side up into his mouth. Scooping up a spoonful of food, turning the arm, and bringing the food to the mouth is a complex skill. Because it takes a lot of practice, give him a spoon of his own to work with while you carry on the serious business of getting him fed. Of course he will be messy. Put a big bib on him. You may want to protect the floor with newspapers.

Around the age of 1 year, many babies can do a fair job of feeding themselves. Of course the going may be too slow to match their appetites, and the spoon is often abandoned in favor of a handier tool, their fingers. They also tire quickly and are soon ready to welcome a helping hand.

Do remember, though, that no skill is learned without practice. Remember, too, that your baby will set his own timing if given the opportunity.

WHEN SHOULD HE GIVE UP HIS BOTTLE? As early as the fourth or fifth month you can start giving your baby sips of water, juice, or milk from a small cup, so that he can learn about cups long before he is ready to give up his bottle. When he reaches the stage of wanting to hold his own cup, try giving him a small cup with a few drops of milk in it. Meanwhile, give him sips from a cup you hold. He will tip his own cup up too far while learning, even turn it upside down. So you'd better make his a plastic or other unbreakable cup. As his muscles become stronger and his judgment improves, he will be able to handle larger amounts of milk in his cup, although he may still be inspired occasionally to turn it upside down to see what happens.

An occasional baby, having discovered that he can drink from a cup, will reject the bottle as early as 8 or 9 months. Others, drinking equally well from a cup, want their bottle until they are 2 years or more. Some are very definite in their opinions: Water and juice are for cups, milk is for bottles! There is nothing to be gained by trying to "break" a baby of the bottle habit. His bottle may be a great comfort to him and satisfy the need some babies have for sucking. Abrupt weaning from the bottle is frequently followed by disruptions in sleep patterns and personality characteristics. Let him give it up when *he* wants to. Sooner or later he will.

He may be especially reluctant to give up his naptime or bedtime bottle. Unless he is so fond of milk that he refuses food, there seems no reason to deny him this comfort. But be sure to use plastic bottles so that you don't spend your time sweeping up glass from the floor when he throws his bottle out of his crib.

TEETHING

During his first year—often around 5 or 6 months—your baby will start getting his baby or *primary* teeth. But some families show a tendency toward very early or very late tooth eruption. So if your mother tells you you didn't have a single tooth until you were a year old, don't be too surprised if your child follows your example.

The first teeth to come through are *usually* the two lower central incisors, though some nonconformists cut their upper incisors first.

Your child may drool—constantly—for weeks before there is any sign of a tooth. On the other hand, some day you may rub your finger along your baby's gums and be startled to receive a sharp bite from a tooth your baby showed no signs of getting.

Will teething make my baby fretful and sick?

Most babies cut their teeth with no noticeable trouble. Teething tends to be blamed for almost anything that happens during the teething age. As a rule, if your baby becomes ill or runs a fever, look for some other cause. Still, it is true that an occasional baby will become fretful because of the ache and tingling in his gums, as the teeth are coming through, and may lose his appetite for a few days.

Babies try to ease the ache in their gums by clamping down on anything they can get into their mouths. A hard rubber or plastic teething ring will be welcomed. If your baby wants to bite and chew on everything available, make sure there is nothing harmful about the object he chooses to "cut his teeth on."

And keep him away from anything on which you don't want to find tooth marks.

Although new baby furniture is painted with lead-free paint, repainted furniture may not be; be careful, then, that your baby does not absorb lead into his system. And keep flimsy rattles and other breakable toys away from him. Parents often give a teether a bone to chew on. A solid bone is fine, but be careful of a small bone that may splinter.

Do not use any medicine or lotion on his gums without consulting your doctor. He will prescribe whatever seems best and will also make sure there is nothing else bothering your child.

Care of baby teeth

If you are giving your baby fluoride drops, follow your doctor's advice concerning when to increase the dosage.

It is an excellent idea to start brushing the baby's teeth with a soft brush and water, if for no other reason than to get him used to the idea. Ruthie's mother was so excited over her baby's first tooth that she immediately bought a small, soft toothbrush. She gently brushed the tooth every day. Soon Ruthie was opening her mouth expectantly when she saw the toothbrush. It is probably not necessary to start brushing *quite* as early as this, but brushing at an early age is good practice for the baby. Nevertheless, don't force it if he objects.

THE PLAYPEN VERSUS FREEDOM

Your baby's horizons have greatly broadened, and his curiosity knows no bounds. He no longer accepts the limited view he gets when lying flat. In fact, lying flat is absolutely abhorrent to him unless he is too tired to care.

It was comical to watch Steven's mother trying to change his diapers, although *she* could not always see the funny side of it. No sooner was his wet diaper removed than he was on his hands and knees creeping off the end of the table. If firmly turned over, he would try to get onto his feet before she could get the safety pin open. Before she could finish pinning the diaper, Steven was making a brave attempt to crawl up the wall.

Some children have more natural curiosity than others, but every baby has some urge to explore his world. If the normal infant lacks such curiosity, it is a safe bet he has been kept in his crib or playpen with nothing to see, taste, or handle. Such babies eventually give the impression of being mentally retarded; indeed, they may become so if the situation does not change. You might liken such a child to a prisoner kept in solitary confinement, with the exception that the baby has not even memories to help keep his mind active.

Playpens are certainly useful and will keep a very young baby contented and safe. But after he has learned to creep and stand he is apt to find a playpen far too confining if kept in it all the time, even if it is plentifully stocked with toys. If your baby goes into a temper when put in his playpen, or gets fretful after an hour or so in it, he is probably trying to tell you he needs more room for his newfound powers of locomotion. So don't let it become a prison merely to serve your convenience. When it is necessary to protect him, use it. You can leave him in it as long as he plays happily there. And you don't need to rush to take him out when he fusses for a short time when first put in. But if he has been there a while and is tired of it, it's best to remove him so that he has a wider world to examine and explore. He really *needs* to find out what kind of world he is in.

Put him on the floor where he can roll, creep, and explore to his heart's content. "All very well," you will say, "but I have no time to watch him every minute. Just as soon as I put him down he gets into all kinds of mischief." And so he does.

The best solution is to babyproof a room or a portion of a room and then let him roam at his own sweet will. Remove any objects that can be broken or damaged. Unplug lamps or appliances and put electrical cords out of reach. You can buy little plastic inserts to plug into floor-level electric outlets; this will protect him from dangerous shocks and burns. Then make sure to provide plenty of things he can handle, bang, or shake.

Pans and covers are great fun to bang together (though you may need to plug your ears). Banging a big spoon against a pan makes a satisfying noise too. Things of this sort are more fun than expensive toys. Blocks are fun to pound together or to put into larger containers. Bells on sticks sound good when shaken. Soft stuffed animals and dolls can be fondled and sucked on.

Before putting your baby down, check his play area for any tiny objects that could go in his mouth. He is just learning to use his thumb and forefinger in a "pincer movement." His special delight will be to practice this new skill. Pins, safety pins, bobby pins, and coins all appeal to his curiosity, but you know where they will end up.

"NO, NO—MUSTN'T TOUCH"

Not too many years ago parents tried earnestly to teach the creeping and toddling infant to "leave Mommy's things alone." It was constantly "No, no," with a light slap on the fingers whenever he pulled books down or threw his mother's best dish on the floor. He would even look guilty—but would be doing the same thing five minutes later.

Following that era of "you must mind" came the inevitable reaction to such strictness. It was then decided *never* to thwart a child, *never* to limit or punish him. Unfortunately this excessive permissiveness planted in the young impressionable mind the idea that there were no rules. Such children became bewildered, hostile, and extremely willful when they grew older and found there were indeed many rules that had to be obeyed. And their parents had made matters infinitely harder for themselves as well as for their children.

The problem is that though every child needs and wants constructive discipline, at this early age of infancy he has not yet built up enough experience to understand restrictions. He does not know that throwing a dish on the floor will break it; how can he? His urge is to throw, to poke, to handle, to taste. Scolding, slapping, and putting him in his crib for punishment only means to him that you don't love him any more. Therefore, the sensible thing to do is to put away the things you don't want him to touch until he is able to understand *mine* and *yours*. It will not be long.

145

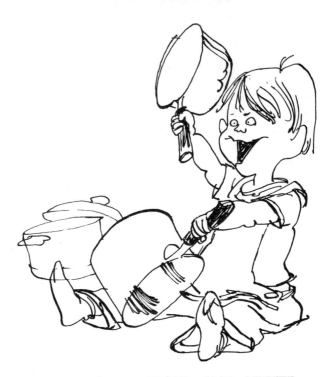

PLAYTHINGS FOR THE CREEPER AND SITTER

After your baby learns to roll over and raise his chest up from the floor, his eyes glisten at the sight of objects just beyond his reach. At first he will roll or wriggle along until he reaches his prize. Then he soon devises quicker and more efficient methods.

Here are some playthings he will now appreciate:

Big wooden spoons, pot covers, metal cups. As we said, what can possibly be more satisfying than banging with a big spoon or pot cover?

Large spools, empty milk cartons, smooth clothespins (the old-fashioned kind), and nesting toys. Your baby is now learning that small articles will fit into larger ones. He will try out this concept for hours on end. You can buy nesting blocks, but your baby will probably enjoy dropping clothespins or large spools into a milk carton and dumping them out again even more. Smooth clothespins are nice for chewing too.

Another good idea* is to hang a shoe bag on the side of the playpen or some other place within the crawler's reach. He will find putting toys in and out of the pockets absorbing fun.

Stuffed dolls and animals. Soft, cuddly dolls and animals are

* From Elizabeth M. Gregg, *What to Do When There's Nothing to Do.*

comforting and may become long-lasting friends. If you make these yourself, use a durable cover and embroider or paint eyes, nose, and mouth onto the material. Use a stuffing that cannot be inhaled or swallowed if the seams should ever happen to burst.

If you buy or are given stuffed toys with button or bead eyes, cut the beads and buttons off before letting your baby have the toy. You would be surprised at how adeptly a creeper or toddler can remove—and swallow—them.

Floating bath toys. These help make bath time fun, though your baby will probably enjoy the wet washcloth as much as anything; it is soft and can be squeezed and sucked on. You may find it easier to give him one to play with while you wash him with another.

Other toys. This by no means exhausts the list of playthings your baby will enjoy—and learn with. Large soft balls and cloth books with large bright-colored pictures are well accepted by the creeping and sitting crowd.

Some pointers to remember

Toys for the "under 1" set should be too large to be put inside the mouth.

Be sure they are well constructed and have no sharp edges or small parts that can be pulled off. Materials should not chip or splinter.

If toys are painted, be sure the color is harmless if sucked. Commercial baby toys can usually be relied on to be safe in this respect. If you make the toys yourself, use safe materials.

GAMES FOR BABIES

Babies love to imitate and are delighted when they can put their hands together and play "patty-cake." They soon learn how to open and close their fists in imitation of "bye-bye."

One game that most babies learn and repeat over and over is that of "peek-a-boo." Babies from a few months on into young childhood are entranced by this game. It usually originates when the mother or caretaker drops a light cloth over the baby's face, then quickly removes it, or lets the baby remove it by his own efforts. The baby wriggles with pleasure and bursts into laughter.

147

Some psychologists believe that all babies should be played with in this manner. It is a universal game of infancy and seems to furnish joy to all babies.

BABY-SITTERS

It is frightening for a baby who has learned to recognize familiar faces to waken and see a strange person looking down at him. And yet you will want to leave your baby at times with someone else. And if you are working, you will have to leave him frequently.

Introduce your baby to a sitter gradually. Let him see you and the sitter together many times before you leave him alone with her, so that he will accept the new person.

There are many things to consider when choosing a baby-sitter. Before you leave your baby with someone outside your family, read the material on sitters in Chapter 6.

SAFETY CHECK FOR THE UNDER-ONE GROUP

Is the playpen solidly constructed? Are you certain your baby cannot pinch his hands at the corners?

Before you put your baby on the floor, do you carefully inspect for any small objects—pins, safety pins, bobby pins, small toys—that he could get into his mouth?

Do you keep any stairs in your house carefully blocked off?

Are there any lamps, dangling cords, or any other objects he can pull over in his play area?

Are electrical outlets within his reach safely covered with plastic plugs?

Do you keep *all* plastic bags or sheets of plastic out of his reach?

Do you keep him out of the kitchen, or safely strapped in his table-chair, while you are cooking or preparing meals?

Do you always remember that he is in the exploring age, and keep household cleaners, medicines, etc. where he *cannot* get them? (See Chapters 4 and 17 on poisoning and other accidents.)

If he is in a high chair, do you put a safety harness on him, and even so never leave him alone?

4

The Toddler
and Preschooler

FROM INFANCY TO YOUNG CHILDHOOD

At 1 year of age your child is occupied with perfecting the skills he learned during the previous months. He gets around on all fours faster than you could have believed possible. Even if he is already walking, he may drop to his hands and knees when he wants to get somewhere in a hurry—such as to that bright object across the room.

When a baby first tries his skill at walking he keeps his legs wide apart as if to provide a solid base for his upright position. He loses his balance frequently, and sits down suddenly. He can, and will, creep up stairways, and his sense of caution is not as well developed as his desire to explore. So if you don't want him falling down the stairs he's crept up, make sure there's a gate at the *foot* of the stairway.

Within a few weeks after your toddler has discovered the joys of walking, his balance will improve. By the time he is 2, he will be running. His gait may be somewhat awkward at first, but now he can *walk* up stairs, taking one step at a time and holding on.

Again, your child's curiosity will grow in proportion to his ability to get around. And he is determined to imitate the people around him. As his balance improves he will be able to reach many of the things you had previously considered safe, so watch out—or you may find him helping himself to your cup of coffee while your back is turned!

To you, busy enough already, it sometimes seems the last straw when your child pulls all the books from the bookcase, empties the wastebaskets on the floor, or does any of the hundred and one things he will do as soon as your back is turned. To be sure, he never is quite certain which of his actions will bring a frown and a sharp "No, no" from you. He understands *no* but he really doesn't stop to consider. His developing nature *demands* that he find out how things work. He can hardly stop to eat or sleep, even when he is so tired he can't keep his eyes open. What! Miss an opportunity to learn more about this dazzling, newfound world? Not if he can help it.

Some night when he is safely asleep and looking angelic again, imagine what it would be like if he sat quietly in his playpen all day, never showing curiosity, never rebelling. Maybe right now you think it would be heaven, but would it really? Would you like to have a child who never showed interest in his surroundings, in what was going on around him? We doubt it.

So put up with him a while longer—until his judgment starts to catch up with his mind.

DISCIPLINE FOR THE ONE-TO-TWO GROUP

We are not advocating that you let your toddler get away with whatever he wishes. It is just as important for his healthy development that he learn to respect the rights of others as it is that he learn "what makes things tick." But he does *have to learn*: he is not born with either kind of knowledge.

When he pulls the cat's tail to find out if it will come off, he is not being malicious. He is just doing to the cat what he has done to his stuffed animals. He needs to be told that he is "hurting the cat." How would he know? And don't expect him to remember for long. If the cat turns and scratches him, he may leave her alone for a while, but he is not yet able to connect "pulling cat's tail" with "cat scratching me."

Some people ascribe malicious motives to the older infant or toddler who bites or hits someone. You've probably heard someone say, "When Johnny bites, bite him back—it's the only way he'll learn." Yes, he will learn from that, but only that you are being unkind to him, not that he should not bite. As a matter of fact, you may actually be teaching this young imitator that biting is socially acceptable!

Then how do you teach him to behave? By saying *no* in a voice that tells him you mean it—and by persisting. He may not seem to pay attention the first time, or quite possibly the twentieth, but he is learning that certain actions are prohibited. He may not know *why* you don't want him to play with the light cord, but he does know you disapprove.

At the same time, remove him from the situation. If he is biting or hitting, take him away by himself for a few minutes. Don't prolong his isolation from his playmates; he very soon forgets why he has been taken away. If he is playing with a forbidden object, put it where he cannot reach it and substitute a toy. (Don't be surprised, though, if he proves all the more determined to go after the forbidden object.) Don't worry if he throws a tantrum, and don't spend a lot of time trying to make it up to him.

Rather than strain your voice and your patience saying No, try to anticipate trouble and remove the cause, whenever possible. Put away precious and breakable objects until he is old enough to understand and control his impulses to some extent.

And while you are out to protect the cat, don't forget the need to protect the new baby sister. Remember, no young toddler should be left alone with an infant; he may "love" her a little too violently. After all, she *is* taking his place as baby in the family.

In spite of all theorizing, busy mothers can be provoked beyond limits. A quick slap, along with the firm *no*, is not going to convince your toddler that you no longer love him. In fact, it may clear the air and relieve tensions. But do try to keep slapping to the minimum. Toddlers should find life an exciting and pleasant experience, setting the background for the belief that life is meant to be enjoyed.

151

INDEPENDENCE OR DEPENDENCE?

As your baby begins to learn that he, himself, can control his actions, can actually make things happen, this becomes his ruling desire. He has an overpowering urge to try out everything, to find out just how far this newfound independence will extend. But at the same time his lack of experience makes him uncertain and sometimes even fearful of things that are new or different. The way he copes with the situation is to compromise. He will go ahead and explore as long as he knows that you, or another familiar adult, are within sight or easy reach.

Just a few short months ago he thought that objects existed only when within his sight. He had no concept of things existing without relation to himself. Hide something you do not want a 7-month-old to have and he will not search for it. He may be persistent in snatching your glasses off, but if you take them off in front of him and let him see you put them out of sight, it will never occur to him to go after them. To him they no longer exist.*

The same holds true for the people in a baby's life. Once out of sight, parents are really gone. He has no idea that they are just away and will come back.

But now your toddler is no longer a baby. Now he will go at once to the place where he saw you hide what he wants. He knows it is there even though he cannot see it. In the same way, he knows you are a person, existing somewhere, even if you are out of his sight, but he likes it much better if he can reassure himself quite frequently. And he still needs to know you are there to protect him if he ventures too far.

Give your toddler as much freedom as he can handle, but don't push him or force him into situations for which he is not ready. Let him set his own pace. He may be afraid of the dog next door, or scared of the noise the vacuum cleaner makes. But he's working on ways to handle his fears. If you leave him alone he will muster up his courage and eventually venture forth to pet the neighbor's dog or to push the button that makes the vacuum cleaner roar.

* Selma Fraiberg's *The Magic Years* explains this in a fascinating manner.

He has also learned to recognize his family and friends. Nevertheless, when visitors come, let your young child take his time about becoming friendly. Don't be embarrassed if he ignores their greetings or even cries and hides his face. After he has become used to their presence and has decided for himself they are to be trusted, *he* will make the friendly overtures, possibly by presenting the visitor with one (or many) of his toys. Not permanently, of course—he will soon take them back—but this is his equivalent of shaking hands.

Don't worry if he is timid about meeting other children at this age. It is a natural stage he is going through. Don't try to push him into relating to others; that will only frighten him and make him more timid.

An only child does not have the chance to participate in the intimate give-and-take of family life, and he may have trouble growing out of this shy stage. Nursery school or a day care center will help him greatly, for there he will have a chance to learn to relate to others of his own age, as well as to adults other than his mother.

Who disciplines your child while you work?

Mothers who work have a particular problem at this age because they must share the child's management and discipline with others in this period of growing independence. A mother's day-long absence from the toddler-age child is not the biologic norm. Necessary, yes—for many possible reasons. Normal for the child, no. Therefore, if you work you must plan to do your best to see to it that as normal and happy an environment as possible is supplied.

You may prefer to have someone come into your home to care for your child: a housekeeper, aunt, or grandmother. One mother with two children had a job in a university research lab miles from her home. She found a widow who lived near the campus, a woman whose children were grown and gone and who was lonely. For a modest charge the widow took on both the 3-year-old and the new baby. The mother would take the two children with her in the morning, drop them off with the widow, and get to work by nine. At noon she would have lunch with the children and give a bottle to the baby. At the end of the day's work, she would pick them up and take them home. The widow had her weekends free. The mother had her working hours free.

There are many other arrangements. The important thing is for you to know what kind of person will be taking your place for the greater part of the day. You cannot expect that her rules and routines will be identical with yours, but if you are to feel comfortable about leaving your child, there are important areas where your rules must be kept.

Make sure your day-care mother really likes children and has some understanding of children of this age. Make sure, too, that when she sets limits as to what your child is permitted to do, she is reasonable in her demands.

Two-year-old Mary was a strong-willed child. She did not like her cereal and refused to eat it. When the woman caring for her insisted, Mary threw her spoon on the floor in a fit of temper. For punishment, she was made to sit at the table until the cereal was gone but was not given another spoon to eat with. This was behavior as childish and stubborn as the child's own had been.

Whoever is caring for your child must take the responsibility for making decisions and handling all the little problems that come up. She must be watchful of your child's safety, yet allow the independence needed at this age.

When you have chosen as carefully as you can, remember that the day-care mother is actually taking your place in the child's life while you are away. There are some things you will have to watch for in your own behavior:

Don't be jealous. It's not easy to see your child respond to another with love and trust. Just be thankful that you have someone whom your child can love and realize that he loves you no less.

Don't undermine the day-care mother's influence. "You don't have to do that when I'm home" is fatal to any kind of training. The bewildered child doesn't know which way is right, so he either has a tantrum or decides not to obey at all.

Don't take sides. If the day mother is too strict or too lenient for your taste, accept it before the child and then discuss your ideas of discipline privately with her.

Don't criticize. Mothers often expect more perfect behavior from the person caring for their children than they would have shown themselves.

Do be frank and firm about any practices of child rearing you believe are best for your child. Again, discuss these things when your child is not listening.

It is not easy to find a person who will come into your home and give your child the care you want him to have. Nor does it always work out to take the child into someone else's home for care. You may find a day care center will more nearly suit your child's needs. Advantages of day care centers and nursery schools are discussed toward the end of this chapter.

PLAYTHINGS FOR TODDLERS

Trains. Two or three shoeboxes strung in a line make a satisfactory train to pull along. If they are painted bright colors, they are even more fun. Leave the tops off so the toddler can give his toys a ride.

Picture books. Cut out big pictures of animals and paste them on sheets of stiff cardboard. Punch holes along the side and tie together with a shoelace or some yarn.

Dump box. Keep a supply of small objects, such as spools, small boxes, or plastic bottles. Give your toddler a cardboard box or container and see how much fun he has filling it up and dumping it.

Stuffed dolls and animals. Draw a simple pattern for a doll or animal. Cut two identical pieces out of stout cloth, such as denim. Sew the side and top edges together, leaving the bottom opening for stuffing. Pieces of old nylon stockings or strips of soft rags make good stuffing material. Sew up the opening.

With a bit of yarn or embroidery floss, sew on eyes, nose, mouth, perhaps ears or whiskers. Don't use buttons or dangling strands of wool for this age group.

Boxes or wastebaskets. Many children up to the age of 2½ or 3 years are fascinated by removing things from one container and putting them in another. Provide two empty cartons and a third that is partly full of old blocks, small rocks, and other things that are easily and safely handled.

Show the child how he can take a piece out of one box, move it across the room, and put it in another. Little flaps or doors on the boxes make it even more fun. Children will spend considerable time just moving things back and forth. They will be learning a first lesson in putting things away—and in sorting shapes, sizes, and colors, but don't stress that yet. Let it be fun.

A *kitchen drawer or cupboard of his own.* Most mothers necessarily spend a fair amount of time in the kitchen. A toddler can make getting a meal a major operation for you. He doesn't want to be in his playpen; he wants to be in and out of drawers and handling lots of *things* as you are.

A separate floor-level cupboard or drawer filled with old utensils, a couple of empty boxes, some clothespins, and other odds and ends will keep him busy.

Reserve his playing in this area for those times when you are busy in the kitchen. Then both of you can be busy separately, and yet he will feel near to you and the activity. Do watch where you step—he's not yet ready to put everything away.

RELATIONSHIP WITH OTHER CHILDREN

The child just growing out of infancy is still completely self-centered. He has not established himself firmly enough to consider others. And yet he enjoys the companionship of other children of his own age.

Watch a few creepers or toddlers together in the same play area. Each one is happily playing alone with his toy, not joining with another in any project. They notice one another; you can be sure of that. The toy Jimmy has is sure to look better to your child than the one he is holding. Indeed, he is quite likely to throw his own on the floor and grab for Jimmy's.

And it is more than the toy that interests him. He obviously enjoys the presence of his friends. He may go over and fervently embrace another toddler. But in another minute he is just as likely to be biting someone or bopping him over the head.

When your child gets involved in a biting, pushing, or hair-pulling incident, the best thing to do is to stop him quietly and provide him with a new interest. As he grows a little older, he will learn that others feel pain just as he does. But he does not know it now. Again, it doesn't hurt his stuffed doll when he bangs it around; how can he know it hurts a real child? Besides, his own pleasure is important to him, not someone else's.

Of course you cannot let him continue to bite, scratch, or hit. And along with stopping him and giving him something else to do, you can certainly tell him, "That hurt Jimmy," as he solemnly watches the tears roll down his friend's face. But don't make a big thing of comforting Jimmy in front of him. Your child will think that you have withdrawn your love from him and given it to Jimmy. This is not the point you want to make.

Be patient for a few months more—say "No, no, don't do that," and keep reminding yourself that he is not being purposely naughty. In a few months you can take him away from the group for a short time in order to help him learn how he must behave if he is to get along with other people. But right now his memory is short and cause and effect are not clear to him. Still, he *is* learning.

LEARNING TO TALK

No infant or child will learn to talk adequately if he is never spoken to. As we saw, babies learn the first elements of speech by having their babbling sounds repeated to them. They watch the face of the adult intently during this give-and-take. They also listen to their own sounds and repeat these to themselves.

As the baby grows older, the speech of adults is one of the principal ways through which he learns about himself and his world. He understands a great deal before he masters the difficult technique of speaking himself.

At about the end of his first year, the average child has learned to make many of the sounds he will need for forming words. While he is making sounds for the sheer pleasure of it, he discovers that certain combinations bring unexpected results. He is both surprised and pleased at the excitement his parents show when he tries out *mamamama* and *dadada*. Soon he finds that the magic sound of *mama* brings attention from the most important person in his life.*

When he finally grasps the idea that certain combinations of sounds belong to certain objects, he is on his way to true speech. Before they reach this goal, however, most children go through an imitative period of talking. Your child comes up to you and repeats a long line of jargon, complete with nods, smiles, and gestures. It *sounds* like true speech, except that you can find few if any intelligible words in it. This seems to be entirely an imitation of adults, much in the same way your child sits and carefully "reads" the newspaper, like Daddy. If he really has something to communicate to you, he will do it by the use of a word or by leading you toward the object he wants. The jargon, however, is preparation for talking, and as such it is valuable to the child.

Nonfluency (stuttering) in early childhood

Between the ages of 2 and 5 years, many children experience some language difficulty. The child is making a great effort to use his rapidly increasing supply of words to express his ideas and experiences. His supply is not equal to his needs, and so he often finds himself without the words to express his thoughts (even as you and I).

In this situation he does what we all do when we cannot think of the word we want. He hesitates, repeats, backs up, or fills in with "I—I—I—I," while he gropes for a word to use. He may even give up altogether at that particular time.

This kind of "stuttering" or lack of fluent speech is quite normal for children within this age group and may last for several months. It seems to happen more often in boys than girls. Maybe this is why women have the reputation of "never being at a loss for words."

Treatment: Let him alone!

It cannot be stressed too strongly that the best way to handle

* See Selma Fraiberg's *The Magic Years*, pp. 112–115.

your young child's stuttering is to ignore it. You must understand that this is a normal phase in his development, not draw attention to it. Never make him repeat; do not tell him to "slow up," "stop and start over," "now think what you want to say." These admonitions create a problem for him rather than correct one. *Never* scold or punish him for "not talking right." Scolding or punishing him is one of the best ways to make him into a real stutterer. On the other hand, you should give your child full attention during his speech attempts. Don't speak for him, turn away, or interrupt. Listen and respond in a normal manner. It helps if you do all you can to prevent others from poking fun at him or criticizing. Explain to critical friends and relatives that this is a normal phase for young children and does not mean that your child will become a stutterer unless people convince him this is where he is heading.

Nearly every child who passes through such a period of nonfluency will develop good speech *if* his difficulty is ignored in the manner just described. It is the child who is ridiculed, shamed, and belittled or made unduly conscious of his nonfluency who is in real danger of becoming a true stutterer.

TEMPER TANTRUMS

Your child is still preoccupied with his own desires and is determined to gratify them at all costs. His persistence, when he really tries, can outlast yours. So it really is better to keep opportunities for a clash of wills at a minimum until he can understand a little better. That is why we have stressed the importance of keeping temptation out of the sight and reach of inquisitive toddlers.

But there are a hundred and one situations your child can cook up (or so it seems) that will require intervention—often the forcible parting of your child from something he wants.

Your child has found his big sister's crayons and has decided to decorate the wallpaper. No, a sheet of paper won't do; he wants the wallpaper.

He has been playing so hard that he is cross and tired. No, he is not going to take his nap!

Your child has just discovered the prize flower garden of your next-door neighbor.

He decides his friend's toy is much nicer than his own and appropriates it.

You remove your toddler from his determined purpose. You are the authority; there is not much he can do about that. What *can* he do? About the only thing left is to go into a fine rage. He throws himself on the floor and kicks, screams, and pounds. And he doesn't care whether he happens to be at home, on the street, or in the supermarket.

Obviously, you would prefer to avoid such a tantrum—and you often can, with a little foresight. But no one has perfect forecasting abilities, and so when you must impose your will on your child, try to make sure it is for reasons of health, safety, or respect for the rights of others. Then be firm and consistent.

If you can manage to go about your business and ignore the exhibition your child is giving with such enthusiasm, do so. He will probably not put on a show for long if no one is interested. Pick him up from the street or supermarket floor and carry him away from the scene, if possible. In any event, try to "keep your cool." Two hot heads invite disaster.

Don't try to reason with your child while he is in a rage. His emotions are so strong he can't hear you. But stay near him. Don't shut or lock him in his room. After the storm has passed, resume business as usual.

Be consistent. If the prohibition was worth enforcing, stick to your guns. Don't give in because you are weary or he has a bad cold. If, on reflection, it really wasn't important, you may have to change your rules next time.

An occasional tantrum will happen in the best of families. If they are frequent, however, you'd better look to the causes. Are you providing your child with enough opportunity to play and explore so he doesn't have to look for dangerous or forbidden ways to satisfy his urges? Does he have a playroom of his own or a place where he can explore at will, without danger? He needs to climb, to romp around, to explore cupboards and drawers. If he has no outdoor play area, what can you do to provide activity indoors? Maybe there is a low solid footstool he can jump from, or a large toy he can climb into or over. He needs to use those big muscles.

Are you too strict? Are there too many "no's" and "mustn't do that's" in his life? Or are you inclined to be a bit inconsistent. Does what brought forth a "mustn't touch" or "stop that" at one time, bring out a "cute" at another? This says to your child, "You got away with it once; try it again."

Parents are inclined to be much more lenient with a child who has a chronic or long-term illness. Certainly, you need to consider the discomfort and frustration his illness brings. But you are doing your child a great disservice when you let down rules because he is sick.

This shows up sadly when a chronically ill child goes to a hospital for treatment. A little girl was very sick and the nurses, who knew her well, were full of sympathy for her. They tried to make her as happy as possible, but she was so accustomed to having every passing whim satisfied that it was impossible to please her. What she *really* wanted was to be made to feel well, and when no one could do that she became more and more angry.

Another child, who had hemophilia, tried to climb up onto the hospital window sills, wandered into treatment rooms, and tried out all sorts of things that were forbidden. He had a ready answer for any prohibition, an answer that worked completely with his parents. He simply threw himself on the floor, went into a screaming rage, and started banging his head. He knew his parents were afraid that he would bruise himself. The hospital attendants finally put him into his well-padded crib, drew the curtains, and let him work it out. But it took a long time. As soon as he quieted a bit and someone stuck her head in, he started all over again. Eventually he gained control over himself and everything was fine—until the next time.

Let us hasten to add that we do not ordinarily recommend putting a child in his bed for punishment. Beds are for sleeping or resting or for recovery from illness. In the described case, however, it was the only safe solution to a sick child's problem.

TOILET TRAINING

After your creeper has become an upright person (however uncertainly), he uses much of his second year to perfect his standing and walking skills. As he progresses he finds he can do many more things now that he is upright and his hands are free. His energy—as well as his curiosity—can be directed toward new kinds of learning.

There are areas in which he is *usually* ready to start to learn but which carry over into his third year and even later. One of these is toilet training.

All too often, undue importance is attached to the process of toilet training. There is hardly another subject in the field of child raising where so many firmly fixed ideas, right or wrong, are brought to bear. At its worst, it can be a cause of major family hang-ups, especially if strong-willed grandparents try to tell you how much better things were in *their* day. Listen to them, but hear them not! Even if you make no effort at all, sooner or later your child will be toilet trained. Therefore it is not a thing that is ever worth fighting about.

If you get into a battle with your child over toilet training, you will not win. You will, for a considerable time, be defeated. This is not at all the same thing as saying you cannot *help* your child to become toilet trained. It is only to say that if you get into a contest about it, you will lose the early rounds. Your child will soon sense that here is one area where you *cannot* have the last word. You cannot *make* him, by any means whatsoever, produce when and where you want him to. But if you go about it right he will do it for you with no battle at all in his own good time. To repeat, children *always* become toilet trained. We urge you to put your major efforts elsewhere.

Here are some of the things you are almost sure to hear on the subject:

"My Susie had a bowel movement every day at the same time when she was just a few months old. I held her on a potty each time and soon had her trained to use it."

"I tried that, but after a few weeks Ruthie had her movement at different times right in her diaper. She hadn't learned a thing."

"I have heard about babies being trained to use a potty for

both wetting and bowel movements by the time they were a few months old. You do it by keeping track of the times your baby wets or dirties himself and holding him on a potty at those times. That's what I'm going to do when my baby comes. I'm not going to spend all my time washing diapers."

"I just read where such early training may do his personality a great deal of harm later in life."

"Wait until he is older, but don't force him. It will make him stubborn."

"Be firm; he has to learn you mean business. Make him sit there until he goes. He is only being stubborn."

The most sensible approach is geared to the child's own rate of development, his ability to control his body, and his readiness to learn. It is true that you may catch a bowel movement by sitting your young infant on a potty, but that is *all* you have done. The first time his pattern changes—as it will—everything will be undone. Your baby moves his bowels and wets his diapers when his body tells him to. Waiting until he is able to understand a little will certainly be less frustrating for your child and much easier for you.

Daytime bowel control

By the time he has reached the age of 2—or shortly thereafter—your toddler will probably have achieved at least a measure of daytime bowel and bladder control. Let's look back and see how he has done this.

He has been developing rapidly, both in control of his body and in understanding. Sometime during his second year of life he realizes that he can relieve the discomfort of a rectum full of bowel movement, or feces, by pushing the material out. Of course his muscles have always done this automatically. But he has just discovered that he himself was responsible for the relief he felt after the bowel movement.

Now he gives you clues showing that he knows his bowels are going to move. He gets a queer, absorbed look on his face, or he goes off into a corner by himself, or he starts straining.

163

You can take advantage of his awareness by sitting him on his potty chair. At first, it is true, he uses the chair only because he happens to be sitting on it. But he is much older than the 5- or 6-month-old baby. He *knows* that he is making his bowels move.

When he performs correctly, praise him. If this new action of being put on the potty chair diverts his attention and his bowels don't move, take him off in a few minutes. No doubt he *will* soon fill his diapers. Don't scold or show disapproval at this point. It takes a while for him to figure things out.

Another change in his awareness is working in your favor now. He has learned to value your praise, to understand that he has done something to please you. And in spite of how it may seem at times, he really is very happy when you are pleased with him. After all, from the beginning of his life you have been associated in his mind with pleasure and satisfaction, for you have taken care of him. So he values your acceptance and praise highly.

After a few successes, he will realize that having his movement in the potty or toilet is the thing you are pleased about. All right, he can do that. Perhaps he will believe that the product he has made all by himself—the bowel movement he is now giving you —is what pleases you. You have shown pleasure before when he gave you things.

From here on it will not be long before he is able to indicate to you when his bowels are *about* to move. He will soon start running toward his potty. Most of the time he will be able to hold out until he reaches the proper place. He will have lapses; who doesn't during any learning process? Scolding him will not help, especially if something he has eaten has given him an urgency he can't control. But if he seems to you to be taking a perverse delight in rebelling against this means of conforming, take him to the potty chair and say gently, "Remember, this is where we make a bowel movement."

Messing with his feces. The product of moving his bowels is not displeasing to a young child. He has not learned to associate shame with it. In fact, the color, texture, and even the odor may be pleasing to him.

He may try using his feces as finger paint. If he does, you

should neither show disgust nor let it continue. Just clean up the mess and pin his diapers more firmly to prevent further leakage. Give him something else to play with while you are cleaning up. He will soon learn for himself that feces are not used for play.

Potty chair or toilet seat? A potty chair is certainly convenient for starting training. If it is used only for toilet purposes, the little child soon learns its meaning, and the transition to a toilet seat later will not be difficult.

If you want to do away with the need for emptying and cleaning a potty, you can put your child on a small seat set over a regular toilet seat. But many small children are afraid of a flush toilet, even though they will gleefully flush *your* possessions away. They seem to fear that *they* may be flushed down the same way.

Much has been written about the "rejection" a small child feels when he sees the gift he gave you flushed away. If you are concerned about this, wait to empty the potty or flush the toilet until he has gone off to play.

Daytime bladder control

There is a common—and true—saying that the mother who times the frequency of her baby's wetting and slips him on the potty is training herself, not the baby. A baby will use a potty if his mother catches him in time, but he will remain serenely unaware of any "training" and will keep on wetting his diapers whenever his bladder is full.

The first sign of readiness for bladder control comes when your toddler is able to connect that puddle on the floor with something he did himself. If he has seen older children use the toilet he will begin to see a connection there. Perhaps Mother would be pleased if he used the toilet too!

Soon he will start running to you to indicate his need to urinate—*after* it has happened. Even when he is able to get to you before he wets, it will take a while longer before he can hold off until he gets to the toilet chair.

There is not much point in starting training for urine control until the muscles that keep the child's bladder closed have become strong enough to let him stay dry for 2 hours. This usually happens around the age of 18 months but may be later. Girls seem to get this control a little earlier than boys.

If you have waited until your child has shown his awareness of his need to urinate, and is staying dry for 2 hours at a time, you can start training with hope of success in a fairly short time. You don't have to wait every time until he tells you he needs to go. Often he will be so absorbed in his play he will ignore the warnings. Make a practice of putting him on the potty chair or toilet every 2 hours in the daytime. If he does not use it in about 5 minutes, take him off. Otherwise, his being forced to sit for a long time becomes punishment. This will not be helpful in making him anxious to please you.

Try to keep a proper sense of proportion about it all. Don't get upset or worried if your child is slower than your neighbor's children in learning bladder control. It may be embarrassing— and probably will be—when you take him visiting to hear your relatives say, "Haven't you got that child trained yet?" But you can take comfort in knowing that he is following his own timetable of development. You might also reflect on the fact that very few indeed are the healthy, well-adjusted people who do not conform eventually.

Most young children find it difficult to urinate when they are away from home. In fact, some tighten up and may even have to be taken home. If your child is at least partly trained, take his potty chair along when you go on long visits. But even then don't expect him to be able to urinate if you are not with him. Eventually he will probably urinate involuntarily.

Little boys of 2 or 3 who have watched their fathers or older boys stand up to urinate will try to be big boys too. If there are no males in your household, perhaps you can find a male relative or friend to set the example. If not, your child will learn in nursery school or in other public places.

Training pants. Training pants are useful in reminding the child to stay dry. An incident that occurred in the children's hospital brought this out quite clearly.

Because Susie was able to stay dry during the day, the night nurse thought she should stay dry at night as well. When she did not, she was put in diapers at night. One day her mother brought her some frilly new panties. Someone forgot to take them off at bedtime, and Susie stayed dry all night. She was not going to wet the pretty new panties! Nor did she thereafter whenever she wore panties instead of a diaper.

Night control

Complete night control usually comes later than daytime control. It is seldom achieved before the age of 3 and may come much later.

Limiting fluids at bedtime may help, but don't make such a point of it that your child feels uncomfortable or guilty about wetting his bed. Waking him up to urinate is again training his parents. He is usually too sleepy to know what is happening.

When too much emphasis is placed on staying dry at night, a conscientious, eager-to-please child may actually stay awake worrying about it. Eventually, when you reach the point of telling him to "go to sleep and forget about wetting the bed," he will do just that.

When an older child is still having trouble, a parent needs to look for causes, but for the young child who is just gaining control all you really need is patience.

CURIOSITY ABOUT HIS OWN BODY

When your child was a very young baby and saw his two hands waving around before his eyes, he had no way of knowing they were his own hands and that he himself was making them move. When he saw his feet, he grabbed at them, probably brought them to his mouth, and sucked on his toes.

In a short period of time he became aware that these playthings were parts of himself. And, born curious, he began to explore more of his body. When his fingers touched his genital region, he was simply continuing his exploration, discovering that this too was part of his body. If you slapped his hand, frowned, said "No, no," or pulled his hand away, you were only impressing on him that there was something special about this region—and he would try again to find out what was so special.

As a toddler, your child carries on his exploration. As he sits on his potty chair or lies in his crib, his hands stray to his genitals occasionally. This area is sensitive to touch just as the region around his mouth has been since birth. Handling it produces a pleasurable sensation and he prolongs it for brief periods before dropping off to sleep. Since he has no inhibitions—and no guilt—he may quite openly handle his genitals in the living room if the mood overtakes him.

Although you will probably hear such handling called *masturbation*, in this young a child it hardly deserves such a label. After all, the word carries unpleasant connotations for most people, but in the young child this interest is entirely normal.

Excessive preoccupation with his genitals and the sensations produced is not usual, however. It is a sign that something is wrong in his life. Is he feeling unloved, unwanted, so that he has to turn to himself for love? Are you expecting too much of him too soon, shaming him for "being a baby?" Or is it, quite simply, that he has nothing else to do?

Sex play. It is not at all uncommon for a small boy to help his girl playmate undress, or for a girl to examine her boy playmate. It is all part of the curiosity about the way bodies are made.

If you call this "nasty" or "bad," if you punish your child or become angry, you may turn what was originally a normal curiosity into something quite different. As it is, children seem to sense their parents' disapproval of such games and generally choose some place out of sight for their experiments.

But though we don't want you to implant guilt in a young mind, neither do we ask you to approve of socially unacceptable behavior. We suggest that when you come upon it, you quietly say, "We don't do that," help the children get dressed, and send them off to a new interest. This phase will pass and your child will lose his intense interest in his body and become absorbed in the world around him.

Sex fears. It is open to question whether all little boys think their little sisters were not "finished" because they do not have a penis, or whether all little girls feel cheated. But what seems definite is that all small children wonder about the difference and may ask about it. Don't worry about the question. Use plenty

168

of love, common sense, and understanding, and you can't go too far wrong.

The small child who inquires about the difference between himself and his baby sister needs an explanation geared to his understanding. It is obvious that the best teaching can be done by parents who are relaxed and natural, and who can fit their teaching into the context of daily living. This is not always as easy as it might seem. A mother may be able to accept whole-heartedly the idea that she should answer her child's questions frankly and simply, but she may still be thrown for a loss when her child chooses the Sunday she has guests for dinner to ask, "Mommy, where do babies come from?"

If you are somewhat unsure about how to answer children's questions, there are excellent books for helping children from preschool age to adulthood. A short list is given at the back of the book.

OTHER WORRIES OF THE YOUNG CHILD

A child with a rich imagination is most fortunate, for it will prove an asset to him all his life. But that same imagination can create fearful situations for him. After all, the young child does not understand the difference between fantasy and reality, because he does not have the experience to help him reason things out. And he takes stories of catastrophe at face value. As his knowledge increases, he will know that man-eating tigers and bears do not live in his neighborhood, or that a volcano is not going to erupt under his house. But right now he cannot be sure.

A small child was at school the day the rumor spread that a mad dog had appeared in the next village and was headed in her direction. When she got home, she met her mother in the yard and breathlessly told the news. Her mother brushed it off as the wild tale that it was and went into the house to finish her work. But the child stood rooted to the ground in fear, fully convinced that her mother didn't care if that dog ran up and bit her! It took a long time before the child could have a dog run up to her without cringing; she would go out of her way to avoid one.

Another child was taken shopping by his mother. While the mother was busy at the counter, he wandered off. Found, in tears, a few minutes later, he maintained that he was not lost; his mother was lost. He was convinced that his mother had walked off and left him, as that was the way he perceived it.

Nighttime fears

Fear of the dark is a common temporary anxiety of young children. When we are surrounded by everyday things we can see, our imagination is held in check. For the child, darkness is an inability to see and, given a good imagination, many scary things are possible.

Stories your child hears, television scenes, bits of adult talk all return to haunt him in the dark. Don't belittle them or tell him not to be silly. As far as he knows, he has every right to be afraid of shadows in the dark. Think about your own fears. Are you so brave when you hear a noise or see shadows on the wall?

There is no easy way to tell you how to deal with your child's nighttime fears. In fact, he may even be reluctant to discuss them with you. But try to explain to him the reality of things as much as possible. Comfort him if he wakens frightened from a dream. Don't try to make him "brave" by closing his bedroom door and turning off the light. Let him have a light in his room, or his door into the hall open.

A 3-year-old girl saw a television documentary on an invasion of locusts. A few nights later she began to have screaming spells

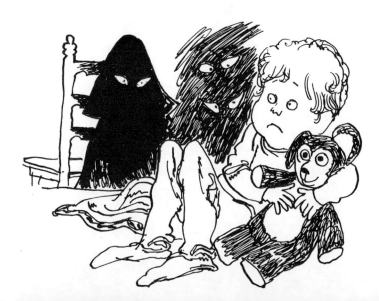

because, in the dark, she could not see that a swarm of locusts was not in her room. A small night light soon relieved her anxiety.

Your child needs all the love and assurance he can get. Don't push the assurance on him when he doesn't need it, but have it available when he does. When he wakens crying because of a fearful dream or fancy, go to him and sit at his bedside. Reassure him that everything is all right. You may need to stay with him until he goes back to sleep. This is a little hard on a working mother—and father, too—but the child will eventually outgrow this stage.

Don't, though, let him get into the habit of climbing into your bed when he wakens during the night. This disturbs both your rest and his and soon leads to his wanting to sleep there every night.

Fear of animals

Remember that if you were only 3 feet high and a beast the same size suddenly jumped at you, you would be afraid too. So don't force your child into any situation. Let him see you pet the cat or friendly dog but don't expect him to do the same. In fact, restrain the animal until your child wants to make the first move.

Remember that fear is never a reasoned thing. What you *do* is much more important than what you *say* to a frightened child. If he is afraid of a worm, it will not help to make him hold one to prove that the worm is harmless. At another time, it may help to let him see *you* hold a worm, but without any comment or any effort to make him do likewise.

A playful puppy or kitten in the house may help him, or even pictures of animals playing with children. Some 2-year-olds have quite a menagerie of stuffed animals and carefully compare each one with pictures in their storybooks.

Some children appear to have no fear of animals, even strange ones. Don't encourage your child to go up and pet any strange animal. Let him admire the dog or cat from a distance, but explain that he should pet only animals he knows.

Fear of death

Small children do not understand the meaning of death and seldom show fear when confronted with it. They may grieve over the death of a pet or feel lonely at separation from a friend, but their grief and fear is over the *separation* rather than the death. A small child cannot understand not being alive. If a parent or relative dies, or if he is faced with his own death, it is again the separation that he fears, and he holds resentment against the person for leaving him.

A group of nursing students were trying to increase their understanding of the meaning of death to a child. They were asked to think back to their own childhood experiences. One told of falling into a drainage ditch and being carried down by the water to the conduit pipe. She thought she would drown, but her only concern was that they would miss her at home. Another told of standing beside her father at the age of 3 and watching the burial of her baby sister. The picture was vivid in her memory, but she had no remembrance of fear, only wonder. Still another nurse told how, as a child of 6, she was upset because she couldn't cry when everyone around her was crying at the death of a relative. She knew it was the proper thing to do, but she didn't understand why.

Nor does the thought of his own death concern a young child, if he thinks of it at all. And boys play at being dead quite cheerfully.

However, when an older child with a serious illness is faced with the fact of his own death, there are other considerations. They are discussed in Chapter 7.

Television—a monster to be controlled

Spokesmen for the television industry have made many statements defending the programming of violence. They have said that there is no evidence that children are harmed or led to aggressive acts by watching murder and mayhem on the screen.

Psychologists who have studied the impact of television on young children have reached some rather different conclusions. It has been found that in some areas children spend as much as 60 percent of their waking hours watching television. By the time a child leaves high school, the hours spent watching TV may exceed those spent in the classroom.

Under such conditions parents and teachers are no longer the prime source of the child's information, and he may become more and more bound by what he sees on the screen. The TV tube becomes a principal architect of the child's world and of his understanding of his own relation to that world. The danger of violence leading to aggressive behavior is real.

There is also danger in sitting as a passive observer while countless acts of socially unacceptable behavior are shown. The child becomes so used to the portrayal of violence that when it happens in his own world his natural tendency will be to accept it, to simply sit by and watch.

Commercials also produce distortions of the child's view of the world. Cleverly designed conditioning techniques prey on the youngster's ability to distinguish between what is real and what is fantasy. In this way elements of misjudgment are implanted that may be difficult to erase.

One of our young patients panicked after he had become sick at his stomach in the office—panicked not because he had been physically ill but because he was afraid that what he had vomited would make holes in our rug—stomach acid, you know!

Small children accept—and even relish—hearing scary fairy tales as long as at the end the good "all live happily ever after" and the bad are either banished or, preferably, converted into good people or good animals. Some especially sensitive children, however, cannot tolerate even the happy ending kind of story and should not be exposed to any frightening tales. And for all children there is a vast difference between listening to a story and seeing it played out on television. A small child cannot tell himself that what he sees on television is not happening. He sees and hears a gun go off; he sees the victim fall "dead." How can he *not* believe his own eyes and ears?

The child who saw her favorite television performer in person and asked him solemnly, "How did you get out of the television set?" was displaying the workings of a child's mind. The marvel was not in the man's being in the box—she could see he was there—but how he had managed to get out.

Television presentations are far too real to a child to justify your letting him watch those things you would not want him to admire or imitate. This goes for children's cartoons as well. Watch a sampling of a series of cartoons or children's stories to see for yourself what they are. Violence, whether in cartoons or stories, is harmful to children.

Fortunately, there are a few excellent television offerings, programs which hold a young child's attention, entertain him, and teach him as well.

There is no excuse for using television as a baby-sitter, tempting as it may be at times. And it hardly makes sense to let your child turn on the TV set just because he cries if you don't. After all, you wouldn't let him run into traffic just because he's in a hurry to cross the street. Why should he be the "boss" of the family where television is concerned?

Sitting still in front of a television set for hours does not give your child the opportunity to develop his body as he needs to do. Set a limit of an hour or perhaps two while he is small, and choose the program for him to watch. As he grows older the time can be increased within reasonable limits.

EATING HABITS

Only a short time ago, your child had a ravenous appetite. His whole body fairly quivered with his eagerness to eat. Now, quite suddenly, he seems to have lost all interest in food.

"Is he ill? He doesn't eat enough to keep a bird alive."

It really doesn't help very much to tell a worried parent that all children go through this stage. But perhaps we can at least see to it that it doesn't come as a surprise.

Throughout his babyhood, especially during his first 6 months, your child's principal business in life was to grow, both physically and mentally. To do this his system demanded food—and more food. His principal pleasure in life was filling his stomach.

Now his growth has slowed down and his interests have broadened. So you must stop comparing his appetite to that of his early months. Instead, think of him as he is, a child of 2 or 3 or 4. You will find his appetite fits his size, his age, and his own individual growth pattern very well.

174

You can be sure of one thing: The best way to spoil a young child's interest in food is to nag and command—in short, to make eating a big issue. If you heap a child's plate full and then state inflexibly, "You must eat everything on your plate; think of all the hungry children," you'll end any pleasure he might have had. How all the hungry children will help his appetite is a mystery to him; he would willingly give his food to them if you would let him.

Dr. Miriam Lowenberg puts the matter well:

There's no need to get into wrangles with a small child about his variations in appetite. (This is fortunate, because even if there were a need, there'd be no use. Arguments will only increase his obstinacy.) . . . When a child sees a plate heaped with as much food as his mother hopes he'll eat, it turns his stomach a bit. . . . But if a child sees *less* than he will probably eat, it makes him feel like saying, "Is that all I get?" This is the spirit we want. We want him to have to ask for seconds.*

A balanced diet?

Some parents demand that their children take one bite of every food offered them. Why? Such a tactic will only increase a child's obstinacy. All very well, you say, but what about the "balanced diet" he should have? First of all, let's consider your growing child and his quite normal variations in appetite.

A healthy child, if offered wholesome food, will take care of his nutritional requirements. But if he is urged to eat more than he wants, he will realize that refusing food brings him extra attention—and this will become something of a game for him.

You can further spoil his appetite by setting a bad example or by making mealtime an unpleasant occasion. If his father says, "Carrots again; you know I hate them," how can you expect your child to accept them with enthusiasm? And how would your appetite be if someone spent the entire mealtime criticizing your table manners? Your children learn good manners through practice and imitation, *not* by nagging.

* Benjamin M. Spock and Miriam E. Lowenberg, *Feeding Your Baby and Child*, pp. 232, 235.

"If you don't eat your vegetables, you can't have dessert." Use this tactic and your child learns to set a very high value on desserts and to consider vegetables nuisances to be disposed of quickly. He may decide, "When I get older, I'll never eat carrots again. I'll just live on cake and candy."

The most important thing you can do is to learn to take a relaxed attitude about your child's appetite. If he is healthy, full of energy, and not losing weight, why are you worried?

Do you really think he is starving to death? Take a sheet of paper and write down every single thing he has eaten for the last 24 hours. Since he has eaten so little, and you have worried so much, you should have no trouble remembering.

Yesterday's lunch: just ½ of a chicken sandwich. Oh, yes, his milk, an 8-ounce glassful. Afternoon snack: 3 little pretzels and a small glass of orange juice, about 2 ounces. Supper: let's see, he drank ½ cup of soup, ate about 3 teaspoons of mashed potato. For dessert, 3 dates. Bedtime: his 8-ounce bottle of milk. Today's breakfast: ½ egg and his 8 ounces of milk. And his vitamins (count these, too).

Now try this experiment. What is Johnny's size in comparison to yours? Let's say he weighs 20 pounds and you weigh about 120 pounds, or 6 times his weight. Suppose you ate the same things he ate, only 6 times as much:

Child (20 lbs.)	Mother (120 lbs.)
½ chicken sandwich	3 chicken sandwiches
8 oz. milk	48 oz. milk
3 small pretzels	18 small pretzels
2 oz. orange juice	12 oz. orange juice
½ cup soup	3 cups soup
3 teaspoons potato	18 teaspoons potato
3 dates	18 dates
8 oz. milk	48 oz. milk
½ egg	3 eggs
8 oz. milk	48 oz. milk

By the end of those three meals and two snacks, you would feel stuffed. After all, you would have had 4½ quarts of milk alone!

We're not pretending that this was a carefully planned set

of meals. All we are saying is that you must view your child in proportion to his own size and requirements.

If you need an outline for a balanced diet for your toddler or preschooler, the following is suggested:

Breakfast
cereal or toast
fruit or fruit juice
egg (poached or boiled) if he tolerates them
milk (part may be used on cereal)

Midmorning or afternoon snack
milk or fruit juice
cracker

Lunch
meat, fish, or poultry (may be in a sandwich); peanut butter
   may be substituted occasionally
vegetable or fruit (the child of 3 or 4 may enjoy his vegetables
   raw, but be careful about giving raw vegetables to 2- and
   possibly 3-year-olds, as they may not chew them properly
   and may choke)
potato, or occasionally spaghetti
milk, part of which may be in the form of custard, Junket,
   yogurt, or occasionally ice cream

Supper
cereal or bread
egg occasionally
fruit
milk

It should be pointed out that a child who goes on a food jag, making a meal of one particular food, will eventually right himself, especially if he eats at the family table where he sees others enjoying other foods. So if he refuses his vegetables, don't worry. See that he gets his vitamins daily. Eventually he will start trying out vegetables of his own accord if they are available to him and he is not pressured.

One precaution is needed here. Sometimes a toddler drinks so much milk that he is not hungry for solid foods. If this continues day after day he is likely to become pale and anemic. You can help prevent this by giving him his solids first, by making sure to offer him a variety, and by limiting his milk. It is not wise however, to cut out milk entirely without his doctor's approval. If his refusal of food persists, take him to his doctor for a checkup.

Mealtime rules—do we need them?

Certainly you must set standards in this as in any other area of child raising. After all, your child does not have the experience or the maturity to set his own rules. But he will test your limits to find out if you mean them—and will benefit from them *only* if they have a purpose. So don't make a rule on the spur of the moment just to satisfy a whim. All you will be doing then is teaching him that rules apply *sometimes*.

The rules you set should help your child live in harmony with others and should respect his rights as well. Here are the most important ones for mealtimes:

1. Keep mealtime pleasant. Set a good example without nagging or preaching. (But do insist he wash his hands before meals.)

2. Let your small child eat at least some of his meals with the family. He will learn much from the others—both good and bad.

3. Serve him small portions or let him serve himself. However, don't insist he eat everything he took; he didn't know how much he would be able to hold. You can help him decide how much to take.

4. Do not insist he try something he does not want. He will probably do it on his own some other time.

5. When he is finished, take his plate away without praise or scolding.

6. Do not make dessert a prize for good behavior or a punishment for misbehavior. It's just part of the meal, usually a nourishing part as well.

7. Be firm about snacks between meals. If he has crackers, cookies, candy, soda pop whenever the mood comes on him, he will spoil his appetite for a regular meal. Use your good judgment here and stick to it.

8. Again, plan your meals to present an adequate diet, but don't worry when your child goes on a food jag. If he has a healthy appetite for his age, his own body will see to it that he picks the food elements he needs over the long run as long as you make them available.

9. Make sure your child has regular physical checkups.

10. Avoid talking about his "poor appetite" in his hearing. This only makes the subject interesting to him and encourages picky eating.

11. Accept eating accidents as cheerfully as you can. They *will* happen in the best society. But do not accept disagreeable behavior, disobedience, temper tantrums, deliberate misbehaving. Most of the time, we hope, he will imitate the good manners of the others. You cannot, of course, expect him to ignore the bad manners.

Some young children do not do very well when eating the evening meal with the family. They may be tired or overexcited and find it difficult to sit still and eat quietly. If so, it is better for them to have their meals quietly by themselves earlier, perhaps joining the family for dessert.

But if you are working and want the companionship of your family at dinner, just remember that a child of this age has a small appetite and make his portions tiny. If he wants to leave the table when he has finished, let him. If he wanders back while you are still at the table, do not make a big thing of it. A young child is not likely to clown around and act up if no attention is paid to his antics. If he becomes tired and cross, remove him from the table and try giving him his evening meal early for a few days.

DENTAL CARE

It usually is not difficult to get a small child to brush his teeth after meals. He tends to see this as a grown-up thing to do. But as he grows older he thinks he has more important things to do, and tooth-brushing seems just a nuisance. Still, *you* know the importance of dental care and have to see to it that it becomes a part of his life like bathing and sleeping. Incidentally, he probably will rebel against all of these at some time. A little dirt behind his ears is not likely to ruin his future health, but neglect of his teeth can bring about serious problems.

At what age should I take him to the dentist?

Start him going to the dentist when he is between 2 and 3. Decayed baby teeth are unsightly, sometimes ache, and may become infected. They frequently have to be pulled long before the permanent teeth are ready to come through the gums. Early loss of baby teeth may cause the permanent teeth to come in out of position. The earlier you take your child, the more the dentist can do to prevent trouble. Make the first trip simply a get-acquainted one. Let him look around the office. Everything there is so strange to his experience that he needs time to adjust.

Dentists who work with children know how to make friends with them. But some children mistrust the unfamiliar so much that it takes a while to convince them to open their mouths and cooperate. Nothing will be gained by threatening, excessive coaxing, or shaming.

Dentists like to start painting the child's teeth with fluoride as early as he will accept having work done in his mouth. But this can't be done without his cooperation, for if he cries or struggles he will salivate so much that the fluoride cannot be put on.

Even if your child has been taking fluoride drops since early babyhood, he will still benefit from local fluoride applications to his teeth. The drops strengthen the teeth while they are being formed but do nothing for them after they have come through the gum. Fluoride put on the teeth helps preserve them and prevent cavities.

180

ACCIDENTS AND POISONING

One unfortunate result of your child's urge to find out everything for himself is the frequency with which he has accidents and injuries. The child between 1 and 5 is most likely to be the victim of home accidents, accidental poisonings, and burns. It is the combination of his urge to explore and his lack of experience that leads him into so many potentially dangerous situations. Warning him has little value; his memory is short and his limited experience does little to help. You must do his thinking for him until he is mature enough to foresee possible hazards for himself. In other words, the best preventive measure against harm to your very young child is to childproof your house or apartment *before* he reaches the experimenting age. Let's start with the kitchen.

Avoiding accidents in the kitchen

Be sure all pans on the stove have their handles turned in. Few things are more tempting to pull than a handle sticking out over the edge of the stove. If you always *turn saucepan handles in,* you will find yourself doing it as a matter of routine.

Make your kitchen out of bounds whenever you leave it while you are cooking or baking. Take your young child with you if you are called away, even "for just a minute" to answer the door or telephone.

Parents do not always realize that nearly all cleaning agents are harmful if taken internally. Your toddler is delighted with his newly acquired ability to eat and drink from a cup or dish. He acts as though every bottle of liquid were labeled "drink me" and every solid substance "eat me." Detergents, cleaning agents, and floor and furniture polish may contain ammonia, kerosene, chlorine, or other chemicals. Toilet bowl cleaners and drain openers have lye as an ingredient. Oven cleaners contain caustics that burn the throat and stomach. In fact, your cleaning closet may be an arsenal of chemical poisons for your young child.

To avoid taking even a shadow of a chance, *store cleaning materials out of reach.* Always leave the materials in their original

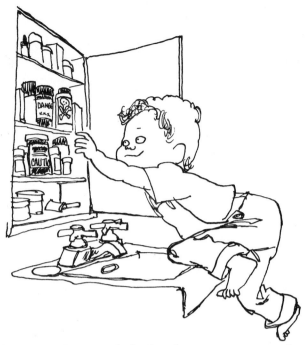

containers. Never put them in Coke bottles, cups, or open jars, for these become an open invitation to drink.

In spite of the warnings on many cans and bottles, mothers and baby-sitters frequently do not take them seriously. "He couldn't possibly reach them, or open that cupboard door." Oh, but he can! You would be surprised at what he can do when he really puts his mind to it. *Don't take chances!*

Avoiding accidents in the bathroom

If your toddler was ever sick enough to need medicine, you know how hard it was to persuade him to take it. But you had not *forbidden* him to eat or drink it! Anything forbidden has an irresistible glamour not necessarily restricted to toddlers and young children. The same medicine you despaired of ever getting down him will probably seem most attractive if he finds and opens the bottle himself.

Some drug manufacturers are using bottles with safety tops that are difficult to open unless you know how to manipulate them, but even these are not as childproof as they would seem. For one thing, the safety precautions will not work if you do not put the cap back on securely. For another, a determined young child can cope with some of the devices. It might be a good idea to give a responsible older child an empty bottle, minus label,

182

to find out how long it will take to solve the puzzle. In this way you can determine just how difficult—or easy—it would be to open the bottle without first reading the directions. No medicine bottle is completely childproof, especially from an older child. So even when using a bottle with a safety cap, *keep all medicines out of reach of children.*

Medicine cabinets present another hazard: Here are some pointers to keep in mind.

1. Discard all leftover medicine unless you are sure you will be needing it again. The fewer medicine bottles around, the less chance for accidental poisoning.
2. *Never* put medicine in the garbage. Pour it down the sink or flush it down the toilet.
3. Keep your medicine cabinet locked when you have small children about.* And make sure all your medicines are kept in the cabinet. If you are taking pills two or three times a day, it will be a temptation to keep them within easy reach. It's a nuisance to unlock a cabinet every time—but it's more than a nuisance to rush your child to Emergency to have his stomach washed out.
4. Cosmetics, hair-dressing lotions, wave sets, and fingernail polish and remover are not the most healthful drinks either. Keep them away from children.

Avoiding accidents in the bedrooms

Be sure that medicines do not appear in the bedrooms under special circumstances. Grandmother has come for a few days' visit. She doesn't sleep well, nor is she used to having small children around. She may unthinkingly leave her sleeping pills or her heart medicine on her bedside stand.

Uncle has diabetes, but he may not make himself sufficiently at home during his visit to put his urine-testing tablets in the locked bathroom medicine cabinet. His tablets can cause severe burns if swallowed.

* There are cabinets on the market that require two adult hands, and know-how, to open.

Chronic lead poisoning

During the late 1930s, it was found that hundreds of children in this country were suffering from chronic lead poisoning. Investigation showed that nearly all of them had licked, chewed, or eaten lead-based paint from walls, furniture, or toys. The results were extremely serious. Many of the children died, and those who lived suffered severe disabilities—most frequently, brain damage—so laws were passed prohibiting the use of lead-based paint on indoor walls and furniture, and people turned their attention to other matters. And yet we have recently been dismayed to discover that lead poisoning in our city children is still frequent and, according to the Children's Bureau, reaching epidemic proportions in some places.

The bloodstream carries lead throughout the body. At first, the symptoms are merely loss of appetite, anemia, malnourishment, and listlessness—and so the cause is seldom suspected early enough for treatment. By the time the brain becomes affected and the child has convulsions, mental retardation, cerebral palsy, or other nervous conditions, it is often too late to do anything.

Chronic lead poisoning occurs primarily in children between the ages of 1 and 6 who live in old, deteriorating homes, often in substandard housing in the core areas of our big cities. These small children will often chew or eat anything, including the plaster and paint flaking from walls, woodwork, and window sills. In 1960 there were over 30 million housing units in the United States that had been built before the use of lead-bearing paint was outlawed.* Furthermore, even cities which have building codes designed to protect tenants from exposure to such paint frequently do not enforce them—sometimes because of indifference, sometimes because of lack of adequate substitute housing.

The only way this man-made disease will be wiped out is through the concerned action of all citizens. PTAs, volunteer groups, and news media all need to join in to see that building codes are effective and enforced and that the public is educated. A booklet called *Facts about Lead and Pediatrics*, published in 1969 by the Lead Industry Association, is available to anyone

* *Children*, Jan.–Feb., 1970, p. 3, a Children's Bureau publication.

interested in helping to stamp out this menace to children. In one city, screening tests, such as those offered for the detection of diabetes, are given by the health bureau.

An X-ray device has recently been invented which, if placed against a wall, can detect the presence of lead immediately. This will cut out the need for the current time-consuming, complicated laboratory tests on plaster and paint. When these machines become generally available, all of us should make it possible for our local health bureaus to purchase a sufficient number to test every urban dwelling place.

Other hazards

ELECTRICAL OUTLETS. The child who has become good at using his thumb and forefinger for poking is greatly tempted by electrical outlets. After all, he has seen his parents push plugs into them. What fun! Young children are often obsessed with a desire to try out something, and if you forbid them to do it you may only increase their desire.

One mother, noticing that an electrical cord was frayed, disconnected it but left it where it was. When Jimmie decided to connect it again, his mother thought he was old enough to learn to mind, and so she said "No, no," quite severely. A half hour later when she found him trying again, she slapped his hands and put the cord out of sight. Jimmie found it and went back to work on it. This time his mother threw it in the garbage, but Jimmie fished it out and tried yet again!

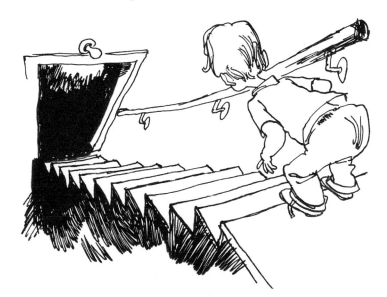

What should she have done? Childproofed. Electrical outlets within your child's reach—and remember, he can climb—should be covered with the plastic plugs made for that purpose, plugs that have to be twisted carefully to be removed.

Be sure to disconnect lamps or other electrical appliances in your child's play area and put them out of his reach. Otherwise you will find him pulling them down on his head or teething on them. Too many babies are hospitalized with mouth burns from chewing on connected cords.

PLASTIC BAGS. By now, everyone has been well warned of the dangers of plastic bags. If you need additional warning, try putting your head inside one. The minute you try to pull the clinging stuff away from your mouth and nose, you will understand the danger very well. Better have someone standing by in case *you* should panic. Suffocation is *not* always a long, slow thing.

ORNAMENTAL PONDS AND SWIMMING POOLS. Every year creepers and toddlers fall into pools and drown. Very young children generally have no fear of the water because they have had no unpleasant experience to frighten them.

Swimming pool covers, high fences, and locked gates are all good preventive measures. But once in a while someone forgets to lock the gate, a child climbs the fence, or a napping infant wakens and creeps to the water side—and drowns in a foot of water.

One of the best safeguards for the toddler and small child is to teach him to swim, preferably before he develops any fear of the water. In her excellent book, *Teaching an Infant to Swim,* Virginia Hunt Newman explains her method of teaching water safety to infants. She emphasizes that one *never* leaves a small child unwatched at pool side or beach, even if he has learned water safety.

Children under 1 year old have been taught to float and swim. It is much easier to learn at an early age. In the apartment complex where one of the authors lives, there is an outdoor heated pool. Every day a young mother brings her 6-month-old son to it. Holding him securely under her arm, she walks in the water. The baby kicks out and moves his arms vigorously in a dog-paddle stroke, laughing and enjoying himself enormously. In some places, the YWCA or other organizations have swimming classes for the "diaper set."

FIRE. Many children have lost their lives or been permanently disabled by burns. If there is a cigarette smoker in your family, keep the matches out of reach. Fire has a fascination that is as old as mankind—and remember, children love to imitate.

You should be aware of the hazard of children's clothing that has not been made fire-resistant. The federal Flammable Fabrics Act of 1953 (broadened in 1967) set standards of fire resistance, but it is still grossly inadequate, for it requires the testing only of a square of material and not of the whole garment, and it covers only children's sleepwear size 6X and under. A new federal act scheduled to go into effect in July, 1973, is much more strict, although it too applies only to young children's sleepwear. But at least it requires the testing of the whole garment rather than just the fabric. (The garment is hung in vertical strips and exposed to flame for three seconds; if it is charred over more than 7 inches, it is rejected.) Unfortunately, there are reports that this new regulation is being reconsidered by the Commerce Department as too strict and too difficult to maintain.

Parents have a duty to insist that adequate laws be not only passed but *enforced.*

Though playing with fire is the most common cause of burns, the small child may also be scalded by pulling down the coffee-pot, or a cup of hot coffee, so don't leave him alone in their vicinity.

If all of these precautions seem too much for you, remember they are temporary. It will not be long before your child reaches the age where he can understand your warnings and take over some of the responsibility for his own actions. But remember, too, that it is far easier to childproof your home *before* your baby turns into an inquisitive toddler than to panic over potential dangers as he explores.

THE PRESCHOOLER

There is no special day to pinpoint as the day your toddler became a preschooler. But the change comes somewhere between his second and third birthday, when he begins to lose his baby ways and commences to imitate the adults and older children around him (though many of his learning attempts, such as toilet training, carry through into his third or perhaps fourth year).

PHYSICAL CHANGES IN THE THREE-YEAR-OLD

Your 3-year-old is losing his chubby look and becoming taller and thinner. He can climb stairs by alternating his feet unless the individual steps are too high. (By 4 years, he can usually go downstairs the same way.)

He can feed himself and can probably pour from a light pitcher without spilling, but he will need help to cut his meat. He can run smoothly, jump, and ride a tricycle. He is able to string large beads and put together a jigsaw puzzle of large pieces. He enjoys building a tower of blocks and will soon be building bridges, trains, and houses.

He is beginning to learn to share and to wait his turn with other children. He enjoys companionship and is happy to have a playmate, but he still spends much of his time playing alone, alongside his friends, rather than in cooperation with them.

Nevertheless, he is developing a sense of belonging to the group. In his own home he finds pleasure in doing small errands: grown-up things, like putting silverware on the table or drying a dish. His play becomes largely an imitation of the work of adults. He is the milkman, or the daddy going to work, while his sister may bathe and dress her doll babies, help her mother dust the furniture, and use her own small broom or carpet sweeper vigorously. There seems to be no real distinction at this age between a man's and a woman's work, except as a child learns from his parents. There is nothing sissy about the boy who carefully tucks a doll in its carriage or the one who is willing to play at being the baby himself while his sister tucks him in.

188

PLAYTHINGS

Play is the business of children. It is through play that a child learns to live. His senses are developed through play, his character traits formed. In fact, his play years constitute a training ground for living in the adult world.

It is up to you to supply the child with objects to stimulate his curiosity. Playthings that allow a child to use his imagination freely are the most helpful. A cardboard box can become a train, a house, or a satisfactory building block.

You need not worry about teaching the young child, as though he were in school. There will be time enough for that later. But you can supply him with materials that will stimulate his mental and emotional development. You can assist him in learning to understand his world. And you can give his imagination food to grow on.

Be selective. Toys that do nothing may be fun to look at but soon lose their interest. The toys that a child can manipulate in some manner are the ones that will capture and keep his interest. You can spend a great deal of money on children's playthings. But you can also make toys for him—or provide him with the simple ingredients for making his own.

Homemade toys

Doll houses are not hard to make. Any good-sized carton will do. Turn it on its side, leaving the front open. Cut windows and doors in the sides. Paint the walls and floors or paste on gaily colored paper. Toy furniture can be fashioned from cardboard boxes. Matchboxes make good beds. Small boxes easily become stoves, TV sets, and refrigerators. The likeness doesn't have to be too real. The family to live in the house can be found in the ten-cent store.

Dressing up is probably the greatest fun of all for preschoolers. Keep a box of old dresses (the fancier the better), hats, purses, scarves, and bits of jewelry. Keep some dress-up clothes for the boys too.

Finger painting is an excellent occupation for the small child but, let's face it, it's messy as well. Try putting a large square of

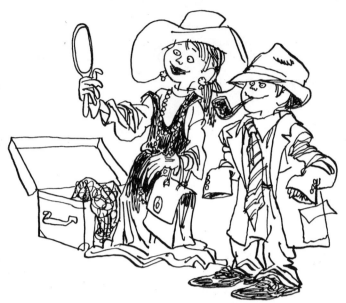

oilcloth under the table and another one *on* the table. A piece
of shelf paper makes a good canvas for the finger painter. Wipe
the surface with a wet cloth or sponge before he begins.

Have three or four small jars of different-colored finger paint
ready. Pour a little from each jar on the paper. Show your child
how he can spread the paint around with his fingers. He may be
a bit shy at first, but once he has experienced the joy of making
swirls, streaks, or just handfuls of paint on the paper, you will
soon find you have a number of paintings to be hung for exhibit.
Let them dry a few minutes before hanging.

To make your own finger paint, mix ½ cup of cornstarch with
¾ cup of cold water. Soak one envelope of plain gelatin (or one
tablespoonful) in ¼ cup of cold water. Add 2 cups of hot water
to the cornstarch paste and cook over medium heat, stirring
constantly. Remove from heat and blend in gelatine. Add ½ cup
of mild soap flakes and stir till blended. Divide into small
amounts and color with food colors. If you wish to keep for a
time, put into small jars that can be tightly sealed.

Play dough, too, is great fun. After the dough is well kneaded,
the child can roll a piece out or shape it with his hands. A toy
rolling pin and a couple of cookie cutters will help. (Oilcloths
on and underneath the table will make you happier with the
results here too.) To make play dough, mix 1 cup of salt, 2 cups
of flour, and add water to form dough. If sticky, add more flour.
A small amount of vegetable oil will make the dough more

190

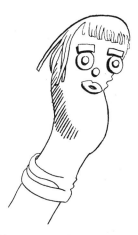

flexible. It should be about the thickness of cooky dough. Add food coloring if desired.

Hand puppets can be made in the shape of people or of animals. Stitch a bag-shaped piece of cloth to fit over a child's hand, or use an old sock. Sew or paste a face on the part that goes over the child's palm. If you cut a small mouth in the material, the child can stick the end of his finger through to make the puppet talk.

Matching pictures, or picture lotto, is an easily constructed game. Find four pictures in magazines of people, animals, food, or flowers. Paste each picture on a card about 3 by 3 inches. On a large piece of cardboard, about 12 inches square, paste four identical pictures from magazine ads. Give your child the picture cards and let him match them to the pictures on the cardboard. If you make three or four such sets, your child can play a game with his friends, to see who gets his pictures placed first.

Or you can make two sets of identical individual cards and have your child match them. But don't put too many cards in a set or you will confuse him.

Puzzles can be made by pasting simple postcards or pictures on cardboard backing and cutting them into three or four parts to be reassembled by your child. Parts should be large and cut in simple shapes.

Imaginative play

Your child has only recently discovered that things really exist as objects and are not just the results of his own magical thinking. He does not know what makes most events happen, and he still has a lingering notion that he—or someone else—causes them by believing or wishing them into being.

Magical happenings are perfectly real to him. He finds it easy to believe that the tooth fairy leaves a coin under his pillow in exchange for a tooth, that Santa Claus and the Easter bunny exist. As far as he is concerned, stranger things happen every day. His father comes home from work with a story about his day that is no more real to your child than the story *he* is telling about *his* day: "I went out to play and there was a *lion* right in our back yard." Well, the dog was big enough—it could have been a lion!

Imaginary playmates are quite common. A child can find acceptance and comfort with one because he can make his "friend" act just the way he wants him to. Imaginary pets become quite real, too, even though you may find it somewhat startling to be told, "Don't shut the door on Ginger's tail," or, "Will you open the door and let Ginger in, please?"

Some children find an imaginary pet helpful in overcoming their own fearful imaginations. Little Jannie * had a Laughing Tiger, a gentle, quiet, and obedient beast who always did as he was commanded. In this way, she learned to overcome her fear of ferocious wild animals that just *might* be hiding under her bed in the dark.

Imaginary friends or pets are quite normal up to the age of 5 or a little beyond. It is surprising to see the great detail with which such friends are brought into the child's life. One day a 3-year-old boy went to the doctor's office to have a large splinter removed from his foot. When he was put on the examining table, he insisted that space be made on the table for "Charlie." His mother explained that he and Charlie were quite inseparable and that now and then a little food had to be laid out for Charlie. While novacaine was injected, he kept up a steady line of talk with his friend: "Don't worry, Charlie, it's not going to hurt me." The splinter was removed without tears and the patient left the room full of smiles. A moment later he burst back through the door and held out his hand. "Here's a nickel," he said to the doctor. "Charlie wants you to have it."

* Selma Fraiberg, *The Magic Years*, pp. 16–23.

The story of Robbie

Robbie, an only child, at the age of 3 shows the general characteristics we expect to find in a child of this age. Yet he clearly demonstrates the fact that every child has a personality all his own.

Robbie received a set of blocks for Christmas and enjoys playing with them. He builds a tower and has fun knocking it down. But when he sees the tower all gone, he cries. His mother says, "He wants the momentary thrill of knocking it down, but he can't face destroying what he has just created."

Robbie's favorite toy is a horse on wheels that he has had for a long time. He rides his horse all over the house, talks to it, gives it water to drink, and offers it a bite of his cookie. It is really his friend.

Robbie has many toys, but he still enjoys playing with pots and pans and piling up cans of vegetables. He loves to "help" his father on weekends, using his own hammer and screwdriver and painting with his own brush, minus paint.

It is not only girls who feel proud to have responsibility as members of the family. Robbie has helped to set the table for some time and now considers this his job. When he has more important things to do, his mother does not force him, but this does not happen often because he has a job to do.

Every Wednesday he trots around with a big paper bag and empties the wastebaskets. He is helping to get the trash ready for his friend, the trash collector, whom he watches for and waves to every week.

A child who is warmly accepted as a real member of the family can hardly help developing a sense of pride and self-respect. Robbie is off to an excellent start in life.

NURSERY SCHOOL OR DAY CARE CENTER— AIDS IN DEVELOPMENT

As a child passes from babyhood to childhood, the wise parent loosens the tie of dependence in proportion to the child's ability to stand on his own two feet.

If your child is naturally shy and cautious, don't be impatient and don't tease him; it will only make him crawl further into his shell. Give him opportunities to meet new people and new situations. A nursery school or day care center can help. Start with a few hours a week and stay in the room with him, if you can, until he develops self-confidence. Throwing a child into the water was never the way to teach him how to swim. But don't be fearful on his behalf. You want him to be self-sufficient, to find out many things for himself. Just remove the dangers in his surroundings as far as possible and then encourage him to strike out on his own.

Perhaps your child is outgoing, bold and reckless. He probably needs to be restrained. Make sure you teach him how to get along with others, to respect their rights and their property. Here too a good nursery school can be helpful.

There are pros and cons about nursery schools, and you should be aware of them. Nursery schools and play groups are especially important for those children who do not have other children of their own age as playmates. Children need the stimulation of other children and need to learn how to get along with others.

But any such group in which too much formal teaching is attempted may do the child a disservice. When he gets to regular kindergarten or school, his teachers may be hard-pressed to find things to hold his attention. Boredom may develop at this level and set up a pattern of indifference that is hard to overcome through the early grades. Therefore nursery schools should confine their teaching to healthy constructive play and developing the give-and-take of social interchange.

Furthermore, you must be prepared for the fact that various infections will be passed from one child to another. They are usually not serious and, in the long run, the child builds some immunity from this experience. But do not be surprised if you encounter one cold after another, earaches, swollen glands, tonsillitis, and other minor afflictions. Group activity at this age places a lot of susceptibles together. Despite all this, nursery schools, on balance, are good for children.*

The sharp difference in meaning between a nursery school and

* The leaflet entitled *Questions and Answers About Nursery Schools*, listed in the references under the heading Special Circumstances, should be helpful here.

a day nursery or day care center has largely vanished. A nursery school gives day care; a day nursery cannot avoid doing some everyday teaching. But there are, of course, differences between individual child-care facilities. Some accept infants and toddlers; some start at the preschool age. Some nursery schools or day nurseries are open all day to accommodate working mothers; others limit the hours for any one child to two or three a day. Many are cooperative nurseries, accepting the mothers as helpers.

Until recently the feeling was strong that babies and young children under the age of 3 needed to be at home with their mothers. This overlooked the fact that not every young child gets in his own home the opportunity that he needs to learn and to grow mentally. Today many children are brought up in small apartments with little or no opportunity to roam, to explore, or to learn to live with other children.

We found out, through such programs as Head Start, the advantages a few hours daily in the company of other children under trained leaders has for children from disadvantaged homes. After that it did not take long for people to realize that such programs could fill the gap modern living creates in the lives of other young children as well. For all small children need other children—to play with and to learn from.

According to Laura Dittmann, "Day care can be a positive factor in the young child's life. . . . There seems to be no reason why a baby cannot profit from the interest of more than one person, if there has been a sensitive effort to make the transition without shock to him." * Children from comfortable homes, as well as children from impoverished homes, may well find their environment enriched.

The mother who does not have an outside job may choose one of the cooperative nurseries, in which she can help for a few hours a week. The mother who returns to her job or profession can be assured that by putting her child in a nursery school she is giving him the opportunity to learn about his world—and to enjoy the experience more than he would if cared for by neighbors or in a private day care home.

* Laura L. Dittmann, *Children in Day Care* (Children's Bureau Publication No. 444), p 52.

The Child Welfare League of America believes that day care should be available to all children, offered as freely as public school and limited only by the wishes of the parents. Parents should have an opportunity to participate in the programs.

Generally, day care centers adjust their hours to the needs of working mothers. They do provide day-long care, although usually only for children whose mothers work the routine Monday-through-Friday 9–5 week. Nursery schools, on the other hand, are usually set up in half-day sessions for children over 2½ or 3 years. Here the distinction between the two facilities should end, and usually does. The concept of custodial care versus learning environment is outmoded.

An occasional toddler, used to the loving attention of his mother at home, may not adjust well to the group experience of a day care center. There is no point in forcing such a child to stay in such a facility if after a few days' trial he is still unhappy. He undoubtedly will be better able to accept the hours away from his mother if he is cared for by a motherly, understanding person in his own home or in hers.

What to look for in a day care facility

A good day care service provides a program designed to help the child develop mentally and physically. It also maintains a good relationship with the parents of the children.

Visit the center while children are there. If it is a good one, your visit will be welcome. Listen to the children as they chatter, sing, and play. Are they free to romp, to select their toys, to experiment?

The teachers in a good center are friendly, affectionate, and enjoy being with young children. They provide opportunities to question, to investigate, to make choices, to be creative. They do not set up regimented, inflexible programs for the children. They do, however, provide activities and encourage the children to participate.

The teacher of a 3-year-old group announced, "We are going to make play dough. Everyone who wants to make play dough come to this table." And make play dough they did. One tot was the flour girl, pouring her measure of flour into the mixing bowl. Others were salt boy, oil and coloring girl, and water boy. The teacher kneaded the dough; then each child rolled out a portion and made imaginative objects from it. Nor were the children above tasting the dough at intervals.

Not all the 3-year-olds joined the group. One boy chose the opportunity to be the daddy, pushing a doll around in its carriage. Another was a doctor, encouraging the daddy to bring the doll to the hospital for an operation. Others decided to spend their time painting.

Teachers in a good nursery understand how to be firm or gentle, consistent or flexible, as the occasion demands. Equipment is ample and suited to the needs of small children. Although children are encouraged to be creative, they are not allowed to run wild. Programs are supervised, and the daily routine kept regular enough to make the children feel secure.

Health and safety regulations are maintained, and the staff knows how to deal with emergencies.

What to avoid in a day care facility

Watch out for a center or school that permits no visitors. Programs so supervised and regimented as to leave no room for individual creativity will not help your child grow and are as bad for him as centers where children are left entirely to their own devices, where no attempt is made to provide programs or to initiate activities, and where the only attention an individual child receives is disciplinary.

DAY CARE IN YOUR OWN HOME

Many working mothers prefer to have their infants or young children cared for in their own homes. There are advantages to this arrangement. The child does not have to adjust to new surroundings, and there is someone in the house to keep it clean and tidy. Mothers of school-age children may look for someone to keep house, give the children noon lunch, and be there when they come home from school.

However, such arrangements are difficult or impossible for many mothers, unless they have a relative willing to come in.

Most women who are competent to care for young children charge more for such service than an average working mother can pay. Where older children are concerned, few women going out to do day work are willing to take on the added responsibility of looking after them. The average working mother is more likely to go outside her home for acceptable child care.

DAY CARE IN A PRIVATE HOME

Many women who offer to care for children in their homes have children of their own. They are thus able to care for their own children while earning money caring for others. If you choose this plan, consider carefully the surroundings in which your child will spend most of his waking hours. Here are some things to look for:

1. Find out how many other children are being cared for including the woman's own. Is she attempting to look after too many children? If your child is a baby or toddler, will she have time (and inclination) to hold and cuddle him, talk to him, let him play out of his crib?

2. Observe the prospective day-care mother as she deals with the children in her home. Is she at ease, calm, kind but firm? Does she maintain discipline in an understanding way?

3. Be suspicious of a house that is always neat and tidy, with an unused atmosphere. Where do the children play? Are they accepted as part of the family?

4. See what toys, books, and playthings are available for the children. Do they have plenty of space to play freely?

5. Check for safety features: for small children, fenced-in yards, protected stairways, covered electrical outlets, suitable cribs. In short, look for the same precautions you would use yourself.

6. Ask for a general outline of the meals she serves the children. Are the foods those you want your child to have? Find out what happens in case of illness.

7. What provision is made for the care of the children if she has to go out or becomes ill? Does she have your pediatrician's phone number as well as the phone number where you work? Be sure she understands she is to call your doctor in any emergency as well as to notify you.

Make every effort to assess the home carefully before you place your child in it. Some women consider a baby adequately cared for if he is routinely fed and changed. Some treat the boarding children as outsiders, giving preference to their own children.

You cannot, of course, be certain that you will never have to move your child into another home. But do keep in mind that a child is better off if he can settle down and feel secure. Even though the home may be somewhat less than ideal, if your child is happy, is receiving good care, and is eager to go each day, you can relax. Don't be picky about unimportant details.

Unfortunately, satisfactory homes are very difficult to find. You may find that your child will be much better served in a day care center or nursery.

SHORT-TERM CARE: HOMEMAKER SERVICE

In many communities, homemaker service is available to families needing special help in their own homes and has helped many families in crisis situations. Homemaker service may be provided by a public agency, such as a family service agency, or by a volunteer group, such as the Children's Aid Society.

Under such a program, responsible and sympathetic women are trained to go into homes to provide temporary help. When the mother of the family must be away or is incapacitated, the homemaker acts as substitute mother until she returns. Or if a young mother is overwhelmed and bewildered by her new responsibilities, the homemaker offers encouragement and practical advice.

A blind mother may receive homemaking help in caring for her baby daughter. As she grows confident, the homemaker will drop in less frequently. The homemaker may spend only an hour or so or may be on call for 24 hours.

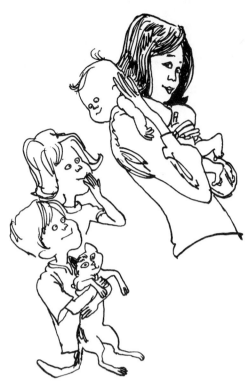

Homemakers receive basic training for their jobs and work under the supervision of a professional person, who may be a nurse, social worker, or home economist.

Fees for such service may be on a sliding scale, according to the recipient's ability to pay, or there may be a flat rate for all.

JEALOUSY OF THE NEW BABY

You should, of course, tell your child that he is going to have a new brother or sister. But don't belabor the point ahead of time. Let him feel your tummy where the new baby lives. Tell him you are going to the hospital to get help in bringing the baby out where everybody can see her. *Don't* tell him he is getting a baby sister or brother to play with. He will think you are letting him down when he finds out he cannot play with her.

If your child is to graduate to a larger crib or another room, make the change a few weeks before the new baby comes home. That way he can feel proud of his new status without feeling dispossessed. And plan to have someone take your young child for an outing when the new baby is coming home, to give you and the baby time to get settled down and relaxed. Then, when he gets home, you can give him the love and attention he needs

200

from a mother he has not seen for several days. He can be taken in to see the baby, to feel her soft hands and pat her face. But try to be casual about the baby when your young child is around.

Don't fan the fires of jealousy by repeatedly paying attention to the new baby while making the number-one child stand aside. Don't diaper the baby while telling the displaced child to run along and play. Either let him take part in what you are doing or do it in private while he is doing something else.

Many young children become jealous when they see a new baby breast-feeding. You cannot always feed your baby privately, so if your older child is in the room, simply explain that the baby is getting milk the way he drank his before he had a nice cup of his own to drink from.

It is only natural for a child to feel at times that his new brother or sister is getting more attention than he or is better liked. And there will be times when he is right!

After all, *he* has always been your baby. What happened to make you want a new one? Sure, he wanted to grow up to be a big boy, but his attitude now seems to be: If being a big boy means that this little thing, who can't do anything but sleep and cry, is going to get all my mother's attention, I'll go back to being a baby too.

So if the young child regresses into baby ways for a while, take it in your stride. He may go back to wetting his pants, though he has learned to stay dry, or to wanting the bottle he has given up. Let him: A few wet pants or a few pulls on a nipple will probably convince him that the new ways were much better. But don't shame him or tell him he is acting like a baby; that is his intention.

You will not help him any by saying; "This is our baby now and you're her big brother," for other adults and older children will emphasize the change: "Aha, so you're not your mommie's baby any more," or "Your mother has someone else to hold in her lap now; you're too big to be a baby." These comments are not calculated to make a child feel secure and comfortable.

The best way you can help your child during this difficult time is by being considerate of his feelings. Remember how it felt when *your* best friend suddenly found a new best friend? Your child is experiencing some of that now. You know you love them both, but you will have to work patiently to get this across to your child.

To 2-year-old Billy, the advent of a new baby was bewildering. His mother was just too busy to hold him any more. When he tried to climb up into her lap, he was pushed away and told to sit on the floor. Of course he whined and begged; he still wanted to be the baby himself. His mother was so overwhelmed with all the responsibilities of keeping a clean house and caring for the new baby that she ignored Billy. She needed someone to point out that Billy's feelings were more important than a clean kitchen floor.

Your older child is quite likely to say something like, "O.K., let's take her back to the hospital now." Or even if he is trying to make a big fuss over the baby as the rest do, his feelings of anger may be too much for him: the big hug he gives her turns out to be hard enough to make her cry.

And when his feelings get beyond control, he may slap or pinch her. It is just not a good plan to leave a tiny baby alone with a small child. You cannot let him hurt the baby, of course, and you should be there to stop him if he tries. But don't put temptation in his way.

Thoughtful visitors and relatives will include him in their greetings and remember to bring him a small gift when they come bearing gifts for the new child. But just in case they don't, keep a couple of gifts on hand for him at such times.

Never, while you all live together, *never* hold one child up to the other as a model. Don't openly compare them in any way. When they are old enough, let them compete against outsiders but minimize competition against each other.

When you're feeling distraught over the seemingly endless signs of jealousy on the part of your first child, remind yourself that he would be abnormal if he felt no jealousy. But unless you manage to pour fuel on the fire it will, ever so slowly, burn lower and lower as the children grow older. It won't go out, but it will get down to such a very low flame that family loyalty will all but extinguish it.

202

DISCIPLINE VERSUS PUNISHMENT

Your child's understanding of words is developing, as well as his ability to use them. He is getting away from the closed circle of his home. And he is discovering for himself that others have rights as well as he. He can listen to reason and is beginning to understand right and wrong. He is certainly quick to see when someone else does wrong:

"Billy hit Susan and made her cry."

"Joey stole a cookie—I saw him."

But he is not nearly as concerned about his own actions. He is only beginning to develop a conscience about himself. His own wishes are still most important to him, even when he knows a thing is forbidden. So he will continue to please himself first unless you make an effort to teach him a better way.

Discipline should be the means by which a child is helped to learn socially acceptable behavior: self-control and self-direction.

All too often we hear, "This child must be disciplined," meaning solely, "This child must be punished." Discipline should mean much more than that.

At its best discipline is preventive, for good discipline reduces the need for later punishment. But if it is to be preventive, it must be started quite early.

Parents often feel that the whole question of discipline is complicated and difficult, but that is only because in recent decades there have been such widely divergent views on the subject.

Near the end of the 1940s a school of psychology developed that suggested nothing should be done to inhibit the development of the young child's psyche. There was great concern about the Rights of Infants and a corresponding downgrading of the Rights of Parents. To say *no* to a child was supposed to frustrate and damage. The idea of discipline in child management reached a low point.

Perhaps it was a reaction to a preceding time of overstrictness, a time when it was felt that children should be seen and not heard. Whatever the cause, the new concept of permissiveness in child management gained a considerable following.

Children raised in totally permissive homes are allowed to break rules at will. In fact, there are seldom even rules to be broken. These children may appear quite happy in their early years, but their happiness doesn't last. For when they have not been taught the need for rules at home, they become confused or rebellious when they confront rules in school, the community, or society as a whole.

The permissiveness so popular in the 1940s has yielded a significant percentage of uncertain and rebellious young adults. We have seen this many times as we have watched families evolve. Indeed, many young adults have acknowledged the lack of security they experienced as children when there were no definitive limits to their behavior.

Psychologists, educators, and pediatricians now recognize these mistakes of the past and generally agree that every child needs rules—rules that must be obeyed until changed by mutual agreement of parents and child. Along with rules, there must be respect—respect for the parents by the child and for the child as a person by the adults in his life.

The parents must take the first step by setting fair limits on all phases of the child's behavior and sticking to these limits. Parents must teach children to live by family rules so that they can later live by the laws of society.

You must start by not being afraid to say *no*—and by not being afraid to admit a mistake if you make one. You are human; you may make a decision too hastily. Your child will respect the rules and do his best to obey them if he knows he can appeal a decision he thinks unfair.

Certainly the laws and attitudes of society are not always good or right. But we cannot break them or have temper tantrums because they do not suit us personally. If we sincerely believe a law is wrong or unjust, we can follow the rules for getting it changed.

Many times parents will complain to a doctor that their child has been in one serious situation after another. They say, "I did everything for him. How could this happen?" Yet the record shows early signs of trouble, usually stemming from lack of firmness: parents who lost control because they did not apply the brakes; parents who gave in whenever their child cried out at them in momentary anger.

You will not gain your child's lasting love and respect by giving in to all his demands. It may cost him his freedom or his life if he must learn too late that society cannot give in to all his whims. That's why early firmness on your part is truly preventive discipline.

But you can say *no* to your child without saying it in anger:

"I'm sorry, but you cannot do that."

"It is bedtime now. No more play tonight."

Firmness passes strength from parent to child. Firmness with fairness. Few children become happy, well-adjusted adults without it.

Parents can be too strict

Even the best of parents sometimes demands better behavior or obedience from a child than he can manage. And so the child in self-defense may decide that it was his other self, someone he calls "Jimmy," who broke the lamp or who "made him" pick Mrs. Brown's flowers. This can be a sign that the child is on the verge of developing a conscience, but if your child is doing this, examine your own demands. Are you giving him too many don'ts and must nots? Do you say, "Johnny is a naughty boy," too often and, "Johnny is a good boy; he put his toys away," not often enough? Children grow and thrive on approval.

5
The School-Ager

EARLY SCHOOL AGE

Your 6-year-old is about ready to declare his independence—as *he* sees it—of home and parents.

Of course he is still very much dependent on his parents for all the necessities of life, as well as for support and guidance. But these he takes for granted. Ideally, he has always had them. He is ready for the larger world of the schoolroom.

The child who is outgoing and adventuresome will step out boldly; the shy, timid one may need a friendly nudge from you to get going.

PHYSICAL HEALTH AND DEVELOPMENT

The early school years are normally free from serious illnesses, though one of the common childhood diseases may pass through a classroom or entire school, keeping your child home for a few days.

Colds and sore throats do pass freely from child to child. Fortunately, school-age children are somewhat less prone to complications from these than are babies and toddlers. You may do well, though, to keep your child indoors for a few days it he has sniffles, fever, or sore throat—if only not to expose others. You will of course want to keep him away from close contact with the baby as much as possible whenever he has any sort of infection.

If your child appears really ill with fever, cough, earache, or loss of appetite, phone your doctor and follow his advice.

NUTRITION

Your child's appetite will have picked up from his toddler days. But now he may fall into the habit of dashing into the kitchen and grabbing a handful of crackers or cookies and then not being hungry at mealtime. No one wants to deprive him of that peanut butter sandwich after school or an ice cream cone on a hot day. But he does need *you* to set the rules on indiscriminate eating between meals.

A healthy, active child is usually hungry enough at mealtime. He may have certain food preferences; he has every right to them. There are enough choices within any of the necessary food groups to make a firm "you eat that or else" quite unnecessary. But when a child makes a habit of munching on cookies, crackers, candy, or other snacks, only to be "just not hungry" when mealtime comes, that is a different story.

Make rules about between-meal snacks, but don't be a policeman. When the snacker declares at mealtime, "Mom, really I'm not hungry and Dick is waiting for me to play ball," just quietly remind him that the next meal will be served in five hours. Let him make his own decision not to eat, but when he bursts in an hour later, "starving," remind him of the rule and make the kitchen out of bounds. He may tell you, "You are the meanest mother in the world; you don't care if I starve to death." But no healthy child will suffer too much from waiting for the next meal, and he may learn some good eating habits.

The basic needs

Your school-age child needs an adequate, well-balanced diet for health and normal growth. Children learn about the "basic four" diet in school. They tend to accept the teacher as the ultimate authority, so don't be startled when yours announces, "My teacher says I should have a dark green or yellow vegetable every day—how come we don't have one tonight?" You probably have served such a vegetable faithfully for weeks, only to hear, "Oh, Mom, do I *have* to eat it?" and have finally decided to call a truce for a day. Children are not inclined to be reasonable at all times.

Let's take a look at the necessary food elements and then see how they can be supplied.

Protein is what the child's body uses for building material, for muscles, for organs such as the heart and brain, and for all body tissues. Much of the malnutrition found in children around the world is due to insufficient protein.

Carbohydrates (starches, sugar) furnish energy, which the child uses in abundance. It is much like the fuel in an engine; he needs it to keep going.

Vitamins keep the body in running order; they act as safeguards against deficiency diseases such as rickets, scurvy, and beri-beri. Once common conditions, these now are rare in the United States, precisely because we guard our children against them.

Calcium is a necessary component of bone structure. The young child's bones are growing rapidly. As he takes in calcium through his food, it is processed into hard strong bone, capable of making a firm framework for his body.

Iron is needed to make the hemoglobin in the blood, the substance that carries oxygen to all the body cells and prevents anemia.

Iodine is necessary for the thyroid gland to function properly. In certain parts of the world the soil is lacking in iodine, causing a deficiency of iodine in the foodstuffs grown in that region. Use of iodized salt is the simplest way of ensuring adequate iodine intake.

Other minerals are needed in minute quantities. Any well-balanced diet will provide enough of these minerals for healthy children.

208

A balanced diet

Let's start with a word of caution. As important as a good, nutritious diet is for your child, it is more important for you to be flexible about his eating. One meal or one day that doesn't meet all the suggested requirements is not going to harm him. Let your child have some independence; let him indulge his food jag for a few days.

Dr. Haim Ginott says "Eating problems in children are often created by mothers who take too great a personal interest in their children's taste buds." He states that a mother does best for the child when she lets him eat as much or as little as his appetite demands, unless the doctor has advised differently. "Clearly," he says, "eating falls within the child's realm of responsibility." *

With this in mind, let's see what *does* constitute a balanced diet that we can offer a child.

MILK PRODUCTS: 3 or more glasses daily. Milk furnishes the calcium needed for bone growth. It also furnishes valuable protein, vitamin A (whole milk), riboflavin, and other nutrients. Many milk products are reinforced with vitamin D.

Milk does not have to be taken in liquid form as a beverage. It counts poured over cereal, or when taken as cheese, ice cream, puddings, sauces, or yogurt.

> 1-inch cube American cheese = ½ cup milk
> ½ cup cottage cheese = ⅓ cup milk
> ½ cup ice cream = ¼ cup milk
> ½ cup yogurt = ½ cup milk

MEATS: 2 to 3 ounces twice daily. This will supply about half the needed protein.

You can vary the meats with fish, eggs, cheese, cottage cheese, peanut butter, dried peas, beans, and lentils. The following are equivalent in protein to 1 ounce of meat: 1 egg, 1 ounce cheese, 2 ounces cottage cheese (about 2 rounded tablespoons), 2 tablespoons peanut butter, or ⅓ cup dried beans, peas, or lentils. (The National Dairy Council states that the vegetable proteins should be supplemented with some animal protein.)

* Haim Ginott, *Between Parent and Child*, p. 76.

VEGETABLES AND FRUITS: four or more servings daily. These foods supply vitamin C, vitamin A, iron, and other minerals.

Foods supplying vitamin C should be served daily. Good sources are oranges or orange juice, grapefruit or grapefruit juice, tomatoes or tomato juice, cantaloupes, strawberries, and greens such as broccoli, kale, and turnip and mustard greens.

Sources of vitamin A include greens, carrots, sweet potatoes, tomatoes, apricots, and cantaloupes.

Other vegetables are important for their variety, as well as for their mineral and vitamin contents. Potatoes are a valuable source of energy.

BREADS AND CEREALS: four or more servings daily. These should be made with enriched or whole grain cereals. They supply protein, iron, vitamin B, and food energy. Include bread, cereals, rice, cornmeal, grits, spaghetti, macaroni, and noodles.

BUTTER OR MARGARINE AND SIMPLE DESSERTS. These belong in the food plan as well.

Again, remember that neither you nor your child will gain anything if he is forced to eat a food he does not like. There are plenty of substitutes available.

Eating breakfast

Some 6 percent of American children go to school without breakfast.* Yet the children who have eaten breakfast seem to do better during the forenoon than those who have not.

It is unfortunately true that in many homes in our country children go to school without breakfast because their parents do not have the food to give them. We have recognized the need to provide school lunches, and day care centers often give breakfast to their children. Provision should be made for the school-age child too.

But all too often, even in homes where the food supply is no particular problem, children go off without breakfast. They may dawdle over getting up and dressing, then have to rush off to catch the school bus. (Quite often this is the example set them

* A *Source Book on Food Practices with Emphasis on Children and Adolescents* (National Dairy Council, 1968), p. 14. A pamphlet.

by the adults in the family.) Why not make it a firm rule that your child has to get up in time to eat breakfast, even if he has to go to bed earlier to make up for the lost sleep? He will stop dawdling—especially if you help set the breakfast example.

DENTAL CARE

Even before he loses his two front teeth, or perhaps at about the same time, your child's permanent 6-year molars erupt through his gums. They appear right behind his primary molars. Count back six from the center of his mouth: The sixth tooth is his permanent molar.

These 6-year molars are often mistaken for primary teeth, since they appear so early and do not replace any others, but they are important members of the permanent set. They preserve the shape of the dental arch while the rest of the permanent teeth are erupting. If they are neglected and have to be pulled, your child will never grow another set to replace them—and yet they are, of course, very important for chewing food.

The primary teeth are replaced by the permanent teeth throughout childhood. The front central incisors are the first to fall out—and to call forth the tooth fairy. The wisdom teeth are the last to appear, if they appear at all. Frequently, they do not even form in the gums.

You can expect your child to have his entire set of permanent teeth—except for the wisdom teeth—by his thirteenth year.

Dental care includes routine visits to the dentist, brushing the teeth after meals, and a good nutritious diet.

Research has shown that sugar, in the form of candy and other sweet foods, is the major cause of tooth decay. It is wise to control the amount of sweets a child eats and to restrict those he does eat to mealtime or other times when he can brush immediately afterward.

However, don't set such rigid sweets rules that you deprive your child of some of the pleasure of childhood. And don't make him overly concerned about his health. Here, as in all matters pertaining to the raising of children, liberal doses of good, ordinary common sense are needed.

STARTING SCHOOL

Children in the United States are expected to enroll in the first grade at the age of 6. School districts differ in one respect: some will take a child if he has his sixth birthday during the coming term. Others will require him to wait until the first term after his sixth birthday. This usually depends on how crowded the schools are, rather than on the individual readiness of the child.

If you have a choice, don't push your child before he is ready.

Bobby would not have his sixth birthday until November, but as the first grade enrollment was low his mother was invited to enter him at the beginning of the term in September.

Some children are ready early for the first grade and are proud to be enrolled. Bobby was not. An active boy, he took a dim view of going to school—ever. When asked how he expected to grow up to be successful without knowing how to read or write, his reply was, "Oh, I'll learn soon enough when I need to." Then he dashed out to ride his tricycle around the house.

His mother wisely declined the invitation to send him early. He was well into his sixth year when his chance came again. By this time he had forgotten all about not wanting to go to school and was as eager to learn as nearly all young children are.

Most children who are developmentally ready for school enjoy the experience—assuming, of course, that they have well-prepared and understanding teachers. They enjoy the importance of being "a school child." Of course, occasionally they have lapses. First-graders can turn back into babies at times when they are tired or when things have not gone well.

Older school children may develop stomachaches and other illnesses that disappear mysteriously as soon as the school bus leaves. Don't think that the aches are not real; they usually are. They come when your child remembers the homework he didn't do, or thinks about the way his teacher hurt his feelings yesterday or humiliated him in front of the class. Teachers are human too, you know.

If your child gets this kind of going-to-school sickness, treat it with a casual, "I'm sorry your stomach aches. Better hurry." If these incidents happen frequently, you had better heed the sig-

212

nals and seek out the cause—with the child and his teacher.

Perhaps one or two subjects are too difficult for him because of some lack of previous preparation. This will be especially likely if your child has been moved from one school district to another.

Susie confided to her mother, "They're doing 'times' in arithmetic, but we were only finishing 'add and take away.' " A word to Susie's teacher was all that was needed. She at once arranged for some individual help until Susie got caught up in arithmetic.

Sometimes an unnoticed physical condition keeps a child from doing the kind of work of which he is mentally capable. Billy, who had been out of school with a long illness, was required to have a physical examination before entering school again. Billy had read all the books he could get his hands on during his illness. Therefore his mother was considerably startled, and most uncomfortable under the nurse's questioning gaze, when Billy was not able to read any of the material held up before him. A further eye check revealed that he had become very nearsighted. Had this condition gone undetected and untreated, he certainly would have been labeled a slow learner. Through his frustration, he would soon have hated school.

The same thing happens to children who are hard of hearing. Unless the child is noticeably deaf, the condition is rarely detected until the child starts school. He appears not to be paying attention and to be willfully disregarding instructions. He soon is in real trouble. For his part, he cannot understand why his teacher mumbles and does not speak up. He too soon hates school.

There are other reasons for trouble in school. Your child may be small or larger than the others, or not feel accepted for some other reason. If one particular child is reluctant to go to school, you and his teacher will need to get together to find out the reason. You may even need additional help. Remember, healthy, well-adjusted children are curious about the world they live in.

Reading difficulties (dyslexia)
Some 5 to 15 percent of children have difficulty in learning to read and write by the usual methods of teaching.

A great deal of the learning process is based on reading. No matter how high his intelligence, the child who cannot learn to read reasonably well in the first grade of school soon finds himself dropping behind his classmates. Try as he will, he simply cannot understand written communication as well as his classmates and cannot communicate as well in writing. He soon becomes restless, disinterested, disappointed, frustrated, and a problem to the teacher.

Most specialists in this area believe that the difficulty is largely perceptual, a problem called *dyslexia*. The child actually sees things differently. Perhaps it is that his brain cannot interpret correctly what his eyes see. The eye itself is not at fault, for most such children have perfect sight; the trouble lies in the interpretation of the visual images. Dyslexic children seem to lack the ability to coordinate what they see, hear, and wish to write.

Dyslexia varies greatly in severity, and the rate of progress of individual children will also vary greatly. Many improve with age. It is at least partly a problem of delayed maturing of certain coordinating functions of the brain: symbol identification, symbol coordination, and use of written symbols. (An older word for dyslexia was *strephosymbolia*, literally, "twisted symbols.") The great tragedy is that by the time these children mature to the point of overcoming their problem, many have become so frustrated that they've simply given up. They are apt to be among the dropouts.

How do you recognize the dyslexic child? When they are beginning to learn the written language, almost all children reverse occasional letters and words. Confusion of *was* and *saw*, *p* and *d*, and *m* and *w* is quite normal at the first-grade level. And the first-grader produces bizarre sounded-out spellings of simple words such as *hrr* for *her*. Handwriting, too, begins crudely.

But the dyslexic child fails to improve in these matters while his classmates make steady progress. "Ralph seems to do well with everything but reading and copying." Such a remark should serve as a warning bell. As pressures build for Ralph to do better, he may do worse.

The parent who finds a child persisting in the reversal of letters and words and doing poorly in writing, spelling, and simple reading should seek help early. First grade is none too soon, for the frustrations build up rapidly. The inability to compete with his classmates may overwhelm the child and set the stage for severe emotional maladjustments to the whole learning process. Simply to state that the child is a "late bloomer" may be to lose the race before it is well started.

Many of these children later compensate for their difficulty and, after a struggle, find an area of success for themselves—often in work that does not require extensive reading and writing. But they should have every bit of help that is possible. Without such help, school for them is one long misery.

If dyslexia is recognized early, a great deal can be done about it, and much of the struggle and unhappiness in school can be minimized. What is needed is great understanding, patience, and special teaching methods. If you detect, or even suspect, the symptoms of dyslexia, have your child evaluated by a reading specialist or by a clinical psychologist. If dyslexia is present, he will need perceptual training—much of it given orally instead of by written word. In many schools there are teachers who have the training and equipment to help children learn, at least in the early stages, largely by hearing. They use various perceptual reinforcement techniques. Sometimes they let the students do their homework and their exams orally until they mature to the point where they can overcome or adjust to their difficulty. Admittedly, such help is not everywhere available. If you are frustrated at the local level, write to your State Board of Education. Some states have programs available that are not a matter of general public knowledge. And, while seeking help, parents should never forget that many highly successful people were dyslexic as children.

HOW CHILDREN LEARN

We are learning a great deal about how—and why—children learn. The Swiss psychologist Jean Piaget contributed to our knowledge by observing his own children. His 3-month-old daughter lay kicking in her bassinet, and the cloth dolls over her bassinet danced. As soon as she realized that it was her own movements that made them dance, she smiled and tried again.

This was her first sign of acting with "intention," of deliberately repeating an action that brought exciting results. Piaget concluded that the more new things a child sees and hears, the more he wants to see and hear. Any mother has observed the same thing. But we have not always put this knowledge to use. And that's a shame, for when we do, exciting things happen.

When a young baby can see the consequences of his own actions, he will repeat the action until it becomes familiar and then go on to use it in new situations. For example, a baby waving his arms about accidentally slaps a bell dangling before him and makes it ring. He stops his movement and listens. Soon the same thing happens again. He shortly learns that he can make the bell ring by deliberately slapping it. As soon as he has proved this to himself, he tries out this action on other objects.

When their interest has been captured, children love to learn. Learning to them becomes as engrossing as any sport. Most of us, looking back, can remember this eagerness.

It is this eagerness of childhood that is the hope for human beings. The creativity of a child is amazing. It can be nourished by loving care, an environment in which a child can grow, a policy of noninterference. Unfortunately, it is easily repressed or stamped out by such things as restrictive poverty, malnutrition —or the actions of adults whose own childhood hopes and aspirations turned sour.

Reading

There have always been nonreaders, slow readers, and children who read only what they are obliged to read. But in today's world, reading is a necessity.

We want our children to be competent in the world of language. We want them to be able to express their thoughts effectively and to understand the thoughts of others. However, for a child to continue to read, he must find satisfaction in it.

There are many reasons why children read: Curiosity, adventure, a quest for information, or just for fun are some of them. Josette Frank says that a child who reads for pleasure, who becomes immersed in a book, is "living with the people in it. He sits with them, so to speak. To his great joy he finds he may re-visit them at will." *

One might add a further joy. If he chooses, he can carry on where the book leaves off, through his own creative imagination.

On the other hand, some children find greater pleasure in do-ing, in active physical participation, than in reading. There will always be those who do not find reading their chief pleasure, but whose interests or hobbies may lead them to want to learn more through books.

Some children learn to dislike reading because of "required reading." These same children have surprised teachers and par-ents when allowed to pick books for themselves in the school library. Or a child may be turned away from reading at an early age by too many restrictions: "Don't tear your book, don't mark it up. See, you got your book dirty. I'll have to put it away."

HELPING CHILDREN ENJOY READING AT AN EARLY AGE. How can you help your child learn the enjoyment that comes with reading? Not by starting actual reading instructions too early; it is doubtful that teaching a 3-year-old to read has any partic-ular merit. But much can be done by your own attitude toward learning. Stimulate his curiosity, put new experiences in his way. "Read" the toddler's picture book with him, then take him on the bus he just saw pictured. Let him learn to identify the dog and cat in the book, and introduce him to the real animal.

Encourage the child by your example. Even if reading is not your own chief pleasure, you may surprise yourself at the growth of your interest when you turn to the encyclopedia or reference book for answers to your questions.

Don't be discouraged if your child is a slow reader to start. Each child has his own rate of growth. If you are worried about him, talk with his teacher or his doctor.

Read to your child. It is hard to find a small child who does not love to be read to. And reading to him is one of the best ways to awaken his curiosity. Tell him stories. Listen to *his* stories and encourage him to read aloud to you. Include him in the family conversation.

* Josette Frank, *Your Child's Reading Today,* p. 14.

217

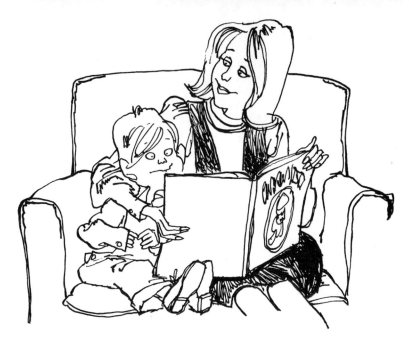

Don't make the mistake of reading aloud a story that is too young for your child, or he will become bored. And don't read him a story that he could read himself. Try reading him a book that is slightly beyond his own ability; it may open up new ideas for him and make him eager to read such books for himself. You do not need to stop and explain every big word. If he gets the gist of the story, he will be satisfied. Of course, you must not err in the opposite direction and bore a child with something he cannot comprehend at all.

One 4-year-old greatly enjoys the family reading hour each evening. He particularly enjoys having his parents read books that are on a third- or fourth-grade level. During the reading hour, his 5-month-old sister lies quietly with her eyes fixed intently on the reader. Of course she does not understand what is being read, but she enjoys the cadence of the spoken word. She is growing up in an atmosphere of reading. It is a part of her environment, as natural as anything else she sees or hears.

THE CREATIVITY OF CHILDREN

Go to one of the art shows given by the public schools. You will come away with greatly increased respect for the creativity of children, even very young children. The imaginative photography, painting, ceramic, and craft work will surprise you. Perhaps it will remind you of when you too thought big. Perhaps you did not have the opportunity or encouragement these children have to express their ideas and fantasies.

We seldom see very deeply into the minds and dreams of our children, but once in a while we are fortunate enough to get tantalizing glimpses of what is going on beneath the surface. Most children are too shy and reserved to let those close to them see their secret thoughts. In more impersonal surroundings, though, they quite freely describe the world as they see it.

There are few things more helpful for understanding and empathy with childhood than these occasional glimpses. Here are some samples:

> Sometimes when you meet your relatives
> you think you are a lollypop.
>
> *by Paul Uhlis, age 13* *

> Last year I was watching the cars by my house.
> They were slippin' around just like tails
> swishin' on cats.
>
> *by Brian Hoban, age 7* †

These are delectable samples of the vision and expression of children given an unfettered opportunity to express their thoughts. The children are not precocious; they are not showing off on a television show or being prompted by zealous adults. They are just being themselves.

One does not have to go to books, however, to get a sampling of a child's thoughts. Here are some written by a child in a letter to her grandmother.

Awake in Action

> I feel like a wild horse
> that's hobbled.

* Richard Lewis, *Journeys—Prose by Children of the English-Speaking World*, p. 126.
† *Ibid.*, p. 48.

I feel like a bomb
that's been thrown.
I feel like the wind,
as fast as lightning and faster.

I feel like jumping, running, a somersault.
I feel like a horse,
I feel like the wind,
I feel like a bomb,
I feel Awake in Action!

I feel alive,
I feel like me:
Western Peggy
with her horse
of the wind.

by Karen Haynes, age 8

YOUR CHILD FINDS HIS PLACE IN HIS SOCIETY

In the middle school years, when your child is about 8 to 10 years old, he becomes absorbed in others of his own age. His greatest desire in life is to become one of the group. Boys, as a rule, relegate such tasks as bathing, dressing up, or changing their clothes to the very lowest level of importance. Girls are more likely to have an eye for pretty clothes and a fresh appearance. It is of course the culture in which a child lives that determines the child's values.

Ceremony at the Washstand
Junior wets his fingertips,
Looks in the mirror, frowning,
He quickly dabs his eyes and lips,
And runs no risk of drowning.*

BUT WE STILL NEED RULES

Your child nearly always has to be told to wash up for lunch or

* Sheldon White, *McCall's*, August, 1969, p. 95.

dinner. It would be against his code to wash without being told. And you may have to send him back to wash the *backs* of his hands as well as the palms.

Bathtime will be met with groans and protests. If you can unbend a little and not insist on too many baths, the groans may continue as a matter of pride but resistance will be less. You will still have to infringe on his independence and check neck and ears.

Your child will no doubt carry his disregard for neatness into his own room. He may toss his clothing around anywhere, but he will still insist on the privacy of his own possessions. He doesn't want anyone messing around with his things. Signs go up on doors: "Keep Out—This Means You!" "Beware of the Dog," and "Danger, High Voltage." It's all part of growing up.

Setting up rules

No parent can allow general bedlam, but there is a way of avoiding it: Parent and child sit down together and draw up rules. Each side learns to give a little when necessary. And a child is far less apt to break rules he has helped to make.

An interviewer held a number of discussions with groups of children on the subject of ideal parents. Nearly all the children agreed on the need for rules at home. One girl expressed it this way: "I think that I have a much better idea of what's good for me in some ways than my parents do, but the thing is that there are some ways in which they're probably right and I think they're wrong, but I'm not sure what they are. Am I clear?"

"Do you mean you'd be nervous if there were no rules?" she was asked. "Yes," she said, "I'd be really scared."

A younger child defined perfect parents as those who would "give me whatever I want." When asked if he thought he'd "want whatever he wanted," he answered, "No." *

Practically all the children taking part in the discussions of their ideal parent agreed that it was proper for parents to punish when discipline broke down. There was, however, no agreement on what punishment should be.

---

* Sam Bloom, "The Perfect Parent," *McCall's*, August, 1969, p. 51.

Because children do have a strong sense of fair play and justice, it pays to listen to their thinking.

Discipline while you work

If you are a working mother, you may have to arrange for the care of your child after school and perhaps for an hour or so in the morning before he leaves home. Part of that arrangement involves deciding how your child is to be disciplined when you are not at home.

Some mothers have their children go to a neighbor's or friend's home after school. If you choose this system, work out all rules carefully with your neighbor ahead of time. Then tell your child that he is to obey the neighbor's rules while under her care. And your neighbor has an obligation to be home every day your child is there and to take responsibility for him.

Some working mothers are fortunate enough to find a college girl who will live in and care for the children before and after school. This often works out well. Again, though, you need to define what you expect of her and where her responsibility lies. Do you want her to discipline the children and punish misbehavior, or do you want her to leave that for you? Of what sort of discipline do you approve?

If neither of these choices is convenient, and if there are no nearby relatives who can care for your children, look around to see if there is a day care center in your locality for before and after school, and often on Saturdays as well. This may be the best solution of all.

Children are not mature adults and will at times get into mischief while you are away. Seven-year-old Freddy was doing well with his sitter, a young woman who came into his home every day. She sent him off to school in the morning and was there until his mother came home about 5 p.m.

Freddy knew the rules: He was to tell her where he was playing and with whom, and he was not to go off the block he lived in. One day Freddy came in to ask if he could play with two boys just up the street. Yes, he said, his mother knew the boys; they often played together. But when Freddy's mother arrived home,

Freddy was nowhere to be seen and a search of the block brought no results.

It was much later when Freddy came home to his worried mother. On questioning he admitted that the boys lived three streets away, and he had never played with them before. Freddy's mother was very angry with him and let him know it. Later, when both calmed down, she was able to discuss his lying and disobedience. But Freddy needed more than that; he needed to know that disobedience brings punishment. Freddy was confined to his yard and house for a week.

ALLOWANCES

The subject of allowances is frequently a cause of friction between parent and children, especially when your child's friends receive more money than he does.

Most parents are willing to give their children an allowance in amounts relative to the financial resources of the family as well as the child's age and level of maturity. If money is scarce, you have to say quite frankly, "This is the most we can afford." When a child is really accepted as a functioning member of the family organization and knows how things stand, he can understand and cooperate. Just do not expect mature judgment from him. You are still the guide and the head of the family. If you must say, "I'm sorry, you cannot have as much money as your friend Ruthie," then just say it.

If your child is old enough, it will be good experience for him to have enough allowance to cover such things as bus fare, school lunches, and other everyday expenses. He will need your help; you cannot let him go without lunches because he spent his money early on something that took his fancy. You probably will have to tell him, "First put aside enough for lunches," or bus fare or whatever. After that, you will do well to keep hands off. As he will tell you, it's his money.

Judy must have that ring she saw in the window. Bobby won't ever again be happy without that tiny marked-down transistor radio. You may remind Judy she already has six rings. You may feel it your duty to tell Bobby the transistor is pretty flimsy. But there you should stop. At the end of the week, Judy is wishing the new ring lying in her drawer were back in the store so she could have enough money to go to the movies with her friends. Bobby bemoans the radio that lasted two days and remembers how he had planned to save for a new gadget for his bicycle. Both are richer for the experience, and little by little they learn the value of spending wisely.

What an allowance is not

An allowance is not pay for chores done. Your child as a member of the family group has certain responsibilities to that group. He should not be paid for doing his work as though he were a hired helper. If he shirks his work there has to be an accounting, but this has nothing to do with his allowance.

An allowance is not a reward for good behavior, nor is it a weapon for punishing bad behavior. You give your child an allowance because he is part of the family and needs to have the means for handling his own affairs as far as his ability allows. Punishments and rewards have a part to play in raising children. They have no bearing on the child's allowance. Don't take away his allowance because he has misbehaved. How can he learn to be a good planner if he can never be sure what his resources will be?

However, when your child has thoughtlessly or mischievously damaged someone else's property, he must bear the responsibility for making good the damage done. If he prefers to find jobs to earn the money, let him make the decision, but it must be an honest job, not one made up for the occasion. The principle here is not dictating the use to which he puts his allowance but taking responsibility for his act.

Your job, of course, is to help your child become a responsible and reliable person, and it may come to a firm statement: "You will have to pay for this out of your allowance." This is a different matter from giving or withholding an allowance according to whether he has been good or bad.

Finally, an allowance is not something you give with one hand but control with the other. After necessities are allowed for, no strings!

224

GROUPS AND CLUBS

The middle years of childhood are noted for the formation of secret clubs. These are all-girl or all-boy groups. However much Johnny may actually admire Susie, the code of a school-age child demands scorn for the opposite sex.

There is a period when secret words and codes, known only to the initiated, are important. The purpose of the club is a secret too, perhaps even from the club members themselves. It is the formation of a group, free from adult management and interference, that matters. The purpose can be decided later.

TELEVISION

Television has become a major factor in the lives of children. Its potential for education is tremendous, but so also is its potential for vacant and uninspiring entertainment.

One study of television-watching habits in the United States reported that 75 percent of the families studied used television as an "electronic baby sitter." *

A child will believe his teacher rather than his parents any day if there is a disagreement between them, for the teacher is the authority. Television assumes this same authority. "It's got to be true. I saw it on TV."

Just as you would not let your child loose in dangerous surroundings, so you should not let yourself be guided by him as to how much or what he watches. If you believe certain programs are harmful, wasteful of time, or set bad examples for your child, don't be afraid to forbid them. Undoubtedly he will grumble. "The other kids watch it. I feel like a jerk when I don't know what they are talking about." But you, not his friends, are his guide through childhood.

It is, however, not very realistic to use a time limit for watching TV as the only rule. Otherwise, your child will be forced to stop in the middle of a program that was worth watching or will watch something you disapprove of while using up his daily limit.

* From "Through the Video Screen Darkly," *Christian Science Monitor,* February 28, 1969.

RESPONSIBILITIES IN THE HOME

No child should be allowed to think he is a guest in his home. He has responsibilities as well as privileges. It should give him a sense of pride to feel that he is needed, even though he may not show it. Praise for work well done is in order, even if he did only what he was expected to do.

There is one slight precaution. If your child has a regular chore, he should be thanked for doing it but not overly praised. Excessive praise for carrying out routine matters of ordinary responsibility may set up an expectation for praise that is nearly insatiable. Later on he may feel thwarted in school or at work when he isn't given any praise for ordinary assignments. But of course work exceptionally well done or outside his routine deserves a special thank you.

And be careful with the faultfinding. "Son, the garage looked clean and tidy today. Next week I'll try to find time to help you clear out a couple of shelves to make more room."

After all, you wouldn't know what to do with a perfect child. You just want one you can live with happily.

HOMEWORK

By and large children seem to accept homework as necessary, but you will have to help set the rules for time and place. You may need to say, "No TV unless you do your homework first." Or a compromise may be in order: "Homework right after [his favorite program]." Once you and your child have agreed on the ground rules, make them stick. After that, however, homework is strictly his responsibility. Don't fall in the habit of doing his homework for him. Be willing to help with a specific problem, if asked, but let it end there. If you think too much homework is being assigned, take the matter up with the school teacher or principal.

FREE TIME

Leave plenty of time for your child to use as he pleases. One of our worst hang-ups today is that we try to keep our children busy every minute. We give them little if any time to grow, to dream, to be themselves. They need room to breathe. A child who lies and dreams for an hour is doing what his nature tells him to do. Or when he and his best friend sit and waste time doing nothing at all, leave them alone. Don't always feel you must invent activities for your child. Let him use his own inclination—and imagination.

SEX EDUCATION

Intense interest and curiosity about the genitals is normal for the small child but quite abnormal when it carries over into the ninth or tenth year. Normally this preoccupation fades during older childhood, to reappear as the child approaches adolescence.

Your child may giggle over mention of body functions, thinking jokes concerning elimination are very funny. But his major interest is far removed from these. The unfortunate child who has not been able to outgrow his infant curiosity is indicating that something is wrong with his environment or his development. He needs someone to find out what is wrong and to set him on the right track toward sound mental health.

In general, girls accept teaching best from their mothers, and boys from their fathers. If yours is a single-parent family, use the various printed aids for support. Of if you feel you cannot help your son in any meaningful manner, enlist the aid of your minister or rabbi or some male friend whom the boy admires and respects.

Whether sex education should be taught in the grade schools will probably be argued for a long time to come. Much depends on the person teaching it.

School-age children should be told of the physical changes to expect in puberty well in advance. Remember that some girls start their menstrual periods as early as age 10 or 11. You wouldn't want your daughter to have the shock of experiencing her first period before she knows what is happening. Yet this happens to girls surprisingly often even today. Boys, too, need to be prepared for the changes in their bodies. If you leave this information to their schoolmates to supply, don't count on accuracy.

One thing you can be very sure about: Your child is being

bombarded on all sides with a type of sex education, whether you wish it or not. You can also be assured that he is highly curious, even if he never opens his mouth about the matter. The best policy is to see that he gets frank, accurate information, whether it comes from the home, school, or church. Surely the best-qualified source is the one that should take major responsibility.

It can't be stressed too often that you should give a frank and honest answer to any question—not an evasion.

PROBLEMS OF CHILDHOOD

Adults are inclined to look back on childhood as a period of carefree happiness: no problems of importance, no money worries, no hard work.

But the truth is that everything looms out of proportion to an inexperienced child. Pleasures are keener, to be sure, but problems too become acute. Children are apt to worry about their fears and troubles all by themselves—and to try to find solutions without asking advice. Unfortunately, in their inexperience, the solutions they try are not always acceptable to society.

In another sense, however, they do ask for help, although not in words. Their very behavior is a way of saying, "I'm confused. I don't know how to handle this. Please help me." Because they do not put their plea into words, we have to learn to understand their behavior. What is making Bobby tell lies, steal, or refuse to go to school? Why does he beat up little kids and run away from boys his own size?

Let's discuss some of the symptoms of the underlying problems children may be having.

TELLING LIES

It has been said, "Parents are enraged when children lie, especially when the lie is obvious. . . . It is infuriating to hear a child

228

insist that he did not touch the paint or eat the chocolate when the evidence is all over his shirt and face." *

Think about that a minute. Are you angry because he lied or because he is implying that you are stupid? You may even shout, "Do you think I'm stupid? You've got chocolate all over your face!"

In any event, you worry a great deal, and with reason, when your child tells lies. You want him to have the courage to face up to the truth. You want him to grow up to have self-respect and to respect others. No one who uses up his energy making excuses and distorting the truth because he cannot admit his mistakes is going to develop into a well-adjusted, confident person.

Why do children lie?

There are, of course, many reasons. In the case of the very young child, as we have seen, lies may not be intentional; he sees so many things happening which he doesn't understand that the line between fact and imagination is not always clear. He may really believe his own story. But the child who grows into the middle years of childhood still asserting that his tall tales are simple truth is indicating there is something wrong in his life.

FEAR. One reason for lying is just plain fear of the consequences. (Adults are far from innocent of this: "No, officer, I did not know I was going so fast.") Fear of the consequences of his act can be great enough to overcome completely your child's developing conscience. You should not condone the lying, of course, nor should you ignore his wrongdoing. But are you sure that you are not asking him to act beyond his capacity? Are you making too much out of what, after all, may have been an accident? Listen to him and find out the facts in the case, before you pass judgment. When a child knows his parents will be fair, will listen, will not punish out of all proportion to the offense, he has little need to lie.

---

* Haim Ginott, *Between Parent and Child*, p. 58.

THE PUNISHMENT OF TELLING THE TRUTH. Dr. Ginott*
reminds us that, in some families, when a child admits to his
mother that he hates his brother, he is spanked for telling
this truth. If expediency then dictates that he declare he loves
his brother, he is rewarded with a hug and a kiss. Unfortunately,
he still hates his brother. The spanking did not teach him love.
It only showed him that it is better to please his mother than to
tell the truth. He may even decide that lying is rewarded and
telling the truth is punished. Why not try to understand why he
hates his brother—and help him overcome his feeling?

LACK OF SELF-RESPECT. A child who has a poor opinion of
himself will search around for some way to make himself important in the eyes of others.

Bobby was small for his age and not at all certain that he could
meet his schoolfellows as an equal. He desperately wanted to be
accepted. But the neighborhood boys made fun of him, picked
on him, or ran off and left him alone. His father was too busy
to pay much attention and just told Bobby, "Stand up to them.
Don't come to me crying like a girl!"

To make the boys like him, Bobby decided to treat them all
to ice cream and tell them he had a big allowance because his
father was such a rich man. So Bobby took the change his mother
had left on the table. But the boys still didn't accept him, his
father still thought him a sissy, and now his mother had found
him a thief. More than ever, Bobby needed help in building up
his self-esteem.

One of the soundest pieces of advice for helping a child respect himself was given by a pediatrician some time ago. "Let
your child know that to you he is the best, the finest child in the
world. You couldn't possibly even think about exchanging him
for *anyone* else."

You are not saying he has no faults, no limitations. You *are*
saying that you are glad that he is your child and that you think
he is wonderful. Don't you really? Don't you pick at him because
you think he's a wonderful child and you want him to live up to
your picture of him? Try praise instead of faultfinding and see

* *Ibid.*

what happens. There is certainly some area in which he does well. Tell him so. Give him something real to pride himself in. He will find that, when he has a healthy self-esteem, others will respect him also.

TRAPPED INTO TELLING A LIE. Johnny has been playing ball with the boys in Mr. Jones' back yard. His mother sees him there and sees the ball he throws go right through the Jones' kitchen window. Suddenly there isn't a boy in sight in the neighborhood.

When Johnny goes home very quietly, some time later, he is greeted with: "Were you playing in Mr. Jones' back yard after I warned you not to?"

Johnny sees the fire in his mother's eye, and his courage fails him. "No, Mom, I wasn't. I was over at Sammy's all afternoon."

"Don't you stand there and lie to me, young man! I saw you there, and I saw you throw the ball that broke the window, too. Now you've lied to me on top of everything else. Just wait till your father gets home!"

Poor Johnny. But who made him lie? If his mother already knew what happened, why did she invite the lie? Sometimes we actually challenge our children to their worst behavior. It would have been better if she had said firmly, "Johnny, I saw you boys playing in Mr. Jones' back yard again this afternoon. I saw the ball you threw go through the window too. It's too bad you disobeyed and it's too bad the window is broken. You will have to pay for it out of your allowance."

Johnny would not have needed to lie, but he would have learned that disobedience doesn't pay.

Setting a good example

Children have a strong natural sense of justice, of fair play, of honesty. They see through hypocrisy and injustice very quickly. A child who sees fair play and justice practiced in his home will not forget it. If his parents are not afraid to admit they are wrong, or to take a stand for what they believe is right, his own belief will be strengthened.

Children never go halfway. They accept what they find wholeheartedly. When children from such homes go out into the world they will not accept lying and cheating as the way to get on in the world. It is the children who have seen deception, "white lies," and unfair practices in their own parents who will say, "It may not be entirely honest but it's the way to get ahead in life. Everyone does it."

STEALING

Here also we have to distinguish between the very young child who has as yet no sense of property rights and the older child who knows what he is doing.

You do not ignore the very young child who takes his playmate's toy. You say, "No, that's Billy's," and you give it back to Billy. Then you help him find a toy of his own. "This is Johnny's, and that is Billy's," you say. Slowly both children build up a sense of "mine" and "yours." But when Johnny is found carrying Billy's stuffed animal out to the car, you do not call it stealing. You just tell him he has to give it back.

You continue to teach the child as he grows older. He sees a candy bar or small toy on the store shelf and he sticks it in his pocket. After all, he reasons, it doesn't belong to anyone. So now you have to tell him that we don't take *anything* that is not ours. "The candy bar is not yours. Put it back." If he brings crayons home from school in his pocket, don't laugh to yourself because he fooled his teacher. Just tell him, "Those crayons belong to the school. Take them back tomorrow."

We do not believe that it is always necessary to make a child confess publicly that he took something. Public humiliation seems a punishment out of proportion to the misdeed. If your child can put the candy bar back on the shelf, if he returns the crayons to their box, he is learning that he cannot take things.

Older children frequently steal for the same reasons they lie: to make themselves powerful and important in the eyes of their companions. Or perhaps a child envies another's possession and decides to help himself. Once in a while, however, a child gives in to an overwhelming impulse without really thinking much about it.

Joey was brought up in a children's home, a good enough institution, but still an institution. Occasionally, but not often, when he thought about it he felt quite sorry for himself.

One day while he was walking through a department store, he saw a small mechanical toy that took his fancy. Somehow it slipped into his pocket. Almost immediately, he felt a hand on his shoulder and heard the store detective say, "Come with me." In the office he was asked, "Why did you take the toy?" Joey was badly frightened, but children are resourceful. He told a sad tale of living in an orphanage, with no toys or love. He did so well he nearly convinced himself.

The store detective said, "All right, I believe you. But this toy is not yours; you will have to give it back. After this when you really want something so badly, come to me. We will work out a way for you to get it. You can depend on me. But don't ever again take anything not yours."

Throughout his life, Joey was convinced that the understanding treatment he received that day kept him from ever again stealing anything. The story—it is a true one—could have had a different ending. He could have been preached to, threatened, made to feel that he was going to turn out "no good." And he might have done just that.

OTHER SIGNS OF POSSIBLE TROUBLE

It is risky to say that certain kinds of behavior are indications that a child is having difficulties and needs help. Every deviation from what is normal behavior for his age does not mean problems; he may just be going through a phase.

There are, though, many kinds of undesirable behavior that, if persisted in, are likely to be warning signals. We have already mentioned continued reluctance to go to school, lying, and stealing. Temper tantrums which come frequently after the child has reached the more reasonable age of childhood are another sign. Even if the child is using them only to get his own way, they are not healthy and the child is not happy.

Persistent nervous mannerisms—grimacing, blinking, constant throat clearing—may be the result of too much pressure on your child. Sometimes when children are pushed ahead too fast in school, or are too strictly disciplined at home, these mannerisms result. But they may also have a physical cause. Talk to your doctor about them.

Aggressive behavior, bullying, excessive timidity, sleepwalking, and insomnia are other kinds of behavior that may be your child's way of saying, "Please let up on me a little." It is often difficult to interpret such behavior correctly, so this is the place where professional help is most valuable—before something really serious results.

CHILD GUIDANCE

What happens if we do the very best we know how and our children still get into serious difficulties? "What did I do wrong?" we ask, or we lament, "I knew everything wasn't as it should be, but there was nothing else I could do." And that may truly be the case.

The child may have had a long illness that kept him away from the normal companionship of his age group. Children hospitalized with long-term illnesses often need help with their future adjustment. They have not participated in the regular give-and-take of childhood, and the result all too often is deep emotional scarring.

But it helps neither you nor your child to say, "If only I had done differently," or, "If I had understood what was happening." The most important question is, "What can I do *now?*"

One answer lies with the child guidance clinics that have come into existence in recent years in most cities in the United States, as well as in many other countries. The clinics have helped to prevent many distorted or seriously damaged personalities and have also helped numbers of children with serious problems to make a better adjustment to life. Many schools have a child psychiatrist on their staff for the same purpose—that of helping children who need help.

In a child guidance clinic, a child psychiatrist or psychologist will work with your child individually, getting to know and understand him. With a young child he will often use play therapy; that is, he will let the child play freely and work out his feelings in his play. Eventually, under guidance, the child learns to adapt and bring his feelings under control.

The psychologist will usually give your child certain mental tests to try to discover where his difficulties lie. After getting at the source of trouble, he and the child work on ways to eliminate it.

Although the child is seen alone by the psychiatrist or psychologist, and often also by a social worker, the parents also have interviews with those working with their child.

A child guidance clinic may be connected with the school system or with a social service agency or with a hospital outpatient department. Your school principal, doctor, or nurse should be able to help you contact a clinic in your community. Or check with your local health bureau or social service center.

THE ADOLESCENT YEARS

A child moving from the middle years of childhood into adolescence goes through a transition period when he is no longer a child yet is not an adult. Frequently, he would like to be both. The rapid physical and emotional changes create considerable uncertainty in his mind.

During this age of emerging from childhood into adulthood, your teen-ager needs privacy to sort out his thoughts. Daydreaming helps him try on for size the many concepts of his adult life. So when your previously cheerful and gregarious child becomes solitary, asking nothing so much as to be let alone, let him be.

Your young person needs to be respected, to have a chance to become self-reliant and independent. It is not easy to see a child who depended on you so much for direction and guidance suddenly take the controls in his own hands. It is particularly hard when you realize how uncertain he actually is. You long to do it for him, while all he wants is for you to get off his back.

Think of when he was a baby starting to walk. He tottered; he fell or sat down suddenly; he even got bumps. Yet the only time you interfered was when he ran into danger. Now you have to let your budding adult learn to walk by keeping hands off when he totters and bumps himself, but be available when he needs comfort and protection.

The main thing to remember is that we must change with our children as the world changes, but stand as a tower of strength where real values are concerned.

PHYSICAL CHANGES

The first two years of adolescence are called the *prepubertal period*, a period which ends, as the term suggests, with puberty.

Puberty is the stage in which a person becomes capable of reproduction. In a girl, it is marked by the appearance of her first menstrual period. In the boy, it is signaled by the appearance of seminal emissions.

Boys usually arrive at puberty a year or two later than girls do. A boy enters this phase somewhere between the ages of 10 and 16. For girls the beginning of puberty usually arrives between the ages of 9 and 15.

When a boy starts his sudden growth spurt, his frame becomes heavier and more masculine in build. Usually he has an appetite to go with it and indulges it—unlike the girl adolescent who may value slimness of figure over satisfaction of hunger. Growth of pubic hair, overactive sweat glands, and appearance of underarm hair signal the approach of puberty, as do those troublesome adolescent pimples, *acne*. The girl's figure begins to fill out. Her breasts start to enlarge and her hips to broaden.

Regardless of what a girl has learned from her schoolmates or from advertisements, she needs correct, matter-of-fact information from her mother. She needs to know how to take care of herself and what sort of menstrual supplies are available in the stores. In fact, she will be very grateful if her mother has long since given her a starter set of napkins and belt, put away ready for use when needed.

It is important also that the boy understand about emissions. He may have so-called dry ejaculations before puberty. After he becomes sexually mature, the ejaculations contain semen. Frequently these occur at night and are known as wet dreams. The boy needs to be told—preferably by his father—that a wet dream is just nature's way of getting rid of surplus semen; it is nothing to worry over or to be embarrassed about. He should understand that he is now growing into manhood.

DELAYED ADOLESCENCE. A boy is apt to suffer more than a girl if puberty is delayed. Some boys become so disturbed they consider themselves abnormal. If late maturing is a family trait, tell your son; it will reassure him to know that all the others made it eventually.

You may have little success persuading him that he is merely on a slower timetable. While most boys do catch up in time, you cannot say, "I *know* you will," with any authority. Your son realizes this.

What you can do is take him in for a complete physical examination, special tests if necessary. Man-to-man frankness can give him the medical assurance he needs.

His pediatrician is the most logical person to help him. He may, however, be sensitive about continuing to go to a "baby doctor"; if so, his doctor will recommend someone who takes an interest in adolescents. Let your boy talk alone with the doctor, and make sure he knows that whatever passes between doctor and patient is confidential. Your son will talk much more frankly when he knows you will not be asking, "What did he say?" and, "What did you tell him?"

If your daughter is late in showing signs of maturity and is embarrassed because she still has a flat chest while all her friends are wearing bras, get her a first-stage bra. If the bra lies pretty flat and she begs for padding, let her have it until she is able to supply her own. What harm can come from that?

MASTURBATION. Just as your son must learn that seminal emissions are normal and that erections occur frequently during adolescence, he needs to understand that young people, both boys and girls, have always relieved sexual tension by masturbation.

Many parents are as upset as many young people about this subject. They shouldn't be. For as Dr. Haim Ginott has written, after reviewing all the serious conditions once thought to result from the practice of masturbation, "Today we know that masturbation does not even cause pimples." *

In adolescence, sexual passion is at a peak, and sources of

* Haim Ginott, *Between Parent and Teenager*, pp. 168–169.

arousal are many. Masturbation is a common outlet. In the adolescent it serves the purpose of exploring and experimenting with new sexual feelings, and it may aid in giving the adolescent control over them.

The pamphlet *Masturbation* published by the Sex Information and Educational Council of the United States (SIECUS) states, "Medical opinion is generally agreed today that masturbation, no matter how frequently it is practiced, produces none of the harmful effects about which physicians warned in the past." * Psychological damage, if it occurs, is the result of the child's having been taught that what he is doing is wrong and bad.

Excessive masturbation may be a symptom of problems that the person cannot handle. The pamphlet tells of a 10-year-old boy who masturbated whenever he had any free time. Careful psychological examination showed that his failure to achieve in sports and games had brought him ridicule and teasing from other children when he tried to join them.

On rare occasions, persistent masturbation may be caused by skin irritation, and a physical examination certainly should be made. More often, though, the problem is one of adjustment.

TROUBLES DISCUSSING SEX. A mother may find it hard to speak about sex with her son, especially if she doesn't have a husband to help her. Or a father may have great difficulty discussing sex with his daughter. That's when a counselor or family friend can help. There are also excellent books available for your teen-ager to read or for you to read yourself. Unfortunately, there are also some very poorly written books on the same bookshelves, so read the books over for yourself before you recommend them to your child. The reference list at the end of the book includes several books geared to the teen-ager and adult.

INFORMATION ABOUT THE OPPOSITE SEX. We take it for granted that boys and girls know about each other, but do they really understand? Does your daughter realize what she does to a boy when she encourages him to a point and then turns away? She is not likely to think this out all by herself; she is not a boy. In

* SIECUS Study Guide No. 3, 1970.

238

the same manner, your son needs to have sympathy for a girl's feelings.*

NUTRITIONAL NEEDS

It goes without saying that these boys and girls need lots of food, and food of the right kind. The rapidly growing adolescent boy needs more protein, calcium, and other nutrients than at any other time in his life. The teen-age girl's needs are only exceeded during times of pregnancy and lactation. †

Young people who have gone through school have certainly learned the benefits to health and well-being of a well-balanced, nutritious diet. It is, however, a mistake to believe that people change their habits solely because they learn of better ways.

Questionnaires answered by groups of students show that "Although they generally knew which foods were nutritionally valuable, they frequently did not consider them personally desirable." Although students in one study gave health reasons for the use of milk, meat, vegetables, cereals, and fruits, they chose their own food on the basis of preference and taste. ‡

Of course, this is not surprising. Do we, as adults, always eat what is good for us rather than the foods we crave? Somehow, the very words "it's good for you" turn us off.

How can you help your teen-ager toward health?

One way *not* to do it is to say, "Eat what I tell you to. I know better than you what you need." Insisting on your superior wisdom will get you nowhere at all. Try, instead, to treat your teenager as an intelligent individual capable of making his own decisions and dealing with life's problems.

Many teen-agers today, through their interest in ecology, have become interested in growing and eating uncontaminated, unadulterated foods. Natural foods, organically grown, have become a popular cause among the young.

* You will find the book *He and She* by Kenneth Barnes helpful.
† The section on nutrition in Chapter 5 will help refresh your memory on the basic nutritional needs.
‡ *A Source Book on Food Practices with Emphasis on Children and Adolescents* (National Dairy Council, 1968), p. 13.

In case the terminology is confusing, *organic* foods are foods grown without pesticides or artificial fertilizers (only natural fertilizers are used); *natural* foods—such as whole wheat flour, brown rice, molasses—are as unrefined as possible and free from any extraneous matter. All natural foods, however, are not organically grown. Encourage your son or daughter to help plan family meals, even to help with the marketing and cooking. Be available for consultation, but otherwise keep hands off. Young people enjoy accepting responsibility.

Don't worry about the refrigerator raids and snacks that seem to take up so much of your active son's time. He needs a great deal of food. Just see that he has access to the kinds he needs. Prepare necessary food items in as attractive and enticing a manner as possible. Try for variety. How about an imaginatively arranged bowl of fruit prominently placed on the kitchen table? Too often vegetables are overcooked and served so poorly as to dampen the spirits of the most ardent food enthusiast. This is no way to make health through good nutrition popular.

This brings us to a word of caution. Nutrition in itself, however desirable, is but one factor of importance. In itself it cannot assure total physical and mental health or social success. Diets, cosmetic products, foods, or what have you cannot alone ever make a boy or girl over in the image of his ideal.

The Problem of Breakfast.   Much has been written about the importance of eating a good breakfast. It is important to supply energy for the morning, especially for young people. The National Dairy Council points out, "The most basic fact about American breakfasts today seems to be that a substantial weekday morning meal, with all the family members eating together, is not important to most families in comparison with other desires and demands that occur at the same time." * It would pay many of us to look into ways of changing this pattern.

Health foods.   The wave of enthusiasm for so-called "health foods" has attracted some fast-money operators. There are legitimate health food stores where you get your money's worth. But

* A Source Book on Food Practices, p. 14.

240

you must be careful. Ordinary foods are frequently repackaged as special health foods and sold at marked-up prices.

There is still nothing better than a simple well-balanced diet, and there is no more virtue in exotic tropical fruits than there is in plain oranges, apples, dates, or other ordinary foods. Green vegetables, whole wheat muffins or bread, and a little plain cheese will do you as much good as the most expensive imported health foods or gourmet specialties. Buyer, beware!

UNDERSTANDING YOUR TEEN-AGER

The frightful problems confronting young people today cannot be dealt with in a book such as this. The subject is far too involved. But we can and must consider a primary problem, how to understand the teen-ager.

Probably every teen-ager thinks at times that his parents don't understand him—and he is right. The problem starts when your teen-ager decides that he cannot talk to you as he did when he was a child; you will not understand, so why try? It is not surprising that he feels this way, for he does not understand himself. Above everything, he wants to be accepted as an adult—and yet he cannot help looking back over his shoulder and wishing for the security of his childhood.

No doubt you understand him a lot better than he thinks. But it will not help to tell him so, or to assure him that he will see things differently later.

LEARN TO LISTEN. You have to start by freeing your mind from any or all notions that your ways are always best. Adults have to learn to listen before they can have any meaningful communication with the younger generation.

And that is precisely what young people have been saying to us for a long time: "No one listens to me." We really have not listened, you know. We thought we knew all the answers.

Not that parents should sit meekly by and accept the young as their teachers and guides. Not at all. If living does not add to useful understanding and opening of the mind, what is it good for? You can enter into lively discussions with the young, can present vital issues as you see them, and still *listen*. But if you

241

try to set them straight without ever hearing what they have to say, you will only strengthen their conviction that you are not interested in them.

So begin by learning and trying to accept the feelings of your young son or daughter. You don't have to agree with them. You can say, "I respect the way you feel, and I am not going to tell you that you are all wrong. But this is the way *I* feel, and these are my reasons." First, though, make sure you have some pretty good reasons for your beliefs or you will find yourself backed into a corner.

If the point is one in which a serious issue is involved, it may end with your "I'm sorry, but these are the rules of this household. As members of this family, we all must obey its laws, unless we have mutual agreement to change them. As the head of the family, I cannot agree to a change in this matter." Your teen-ager will respect you for taking a firm stand, as long as you don't get bogged down in making rules about nonessentials.

THE BIG ISSUES—ALCOHOL, DRUGS, SMOKING. This is the place where you as parents have to take a stand. Do you want to teach your child how to drink socially, when, and how much? Or are you strongly opposed to the use of any alcoholic beverages?

Do you feel he should be forbidden to smoke at all? Or just not cigarettes?

Do you understand the dangers in the use of both hard and soft drugs? Can you present him with the facts and make your own position crystal clear? Don't be swayed by "But they all do it"; answer, "This is one family that does not."

It is true that your son or daughter may try the forbidden thing anyway. But your child will not turn away easily from your teachings if you have made them meaningful.

Those children whose parents have helped them learn trust in infancy, self-control in preschool years, and independence as children will have what it takes to establish their identity as adolescents.

PARENTS' RIGHTS

Oh, yes, you have rights, too, even as the parent of a teen-ager. You have a right to peace of mind, which includes the right to know where your child is and who he is with. You have a right to set a reasonable time for your child to be home, and a right to be notified if for some reason he is going to be delayed beyond the set hour.

You have a right to the major voice in setting rules, the right to be obeyed, and the right to enact penalties for breaking the rules. In fact, you have the responsibilility as well as the right. You have the right, and the duty, to say, "This is our home and these are the rules we live by. While you live at home you are expected to follow them."

But be sure the rules are meaningful, or you may find yourself out on a limb. Does it really matter if he wants to grow long hair and a beard? There are much more important things in life; keep your rules for them. Your teen-ager is a member of the family with voting rights too. He is trying to become an adult, and he must have freedom to do so. But he does not have the right to infringe on the rights of other family members.

THE AGE OF IDEALISM

If adolescence is a time of rebellion, it is also a time of idealism: the time of life, perhaps more than any other, of enthusiasm, eagerness to be of service to others, and dedication to a cause. Maladjusted young people who rebel against accepted moral standards for no other reason except that they are standards are still a minority in spite of the attention they receive. Young people want and need to be active. When their energy is channeled into useful areas of social service, they become absorbed and satisfied.

Frequently, the young person's confusion about basic values results from his seeing an adult world shot through with materialism, greed, and hypocrisy. Totally lacking in experience himself, he goes overboard and throws the baby out with the bath. The adolescent fortunate enough to have parents who set an example of honesty, decency, compassion, and regard for the rights of all people has a foundation to build on that is not easily destroyed. He may be badly rocked by pressures from the outside world, but he certainly has a far better chance of coming through without being wrecked.

6
Special Circumstances

THE ONE-PARENT FAMILY

The one-parent family is far from rare in our society. Sometimes it is a temporary condition caused by the illness of the other parent or by absence on a job or in the armed services. But in many homes it is a permanent way of life—the result of divorce, death, or of a single woman bringing up her child alone. Some adoption agencies have modified their placement practices and allowed qualified single people to adopt children.

While one parent is away from his family, it is important that he feels included in everyday happenings. It is also important for the children to feel that the absent mother or father is still very close to them. The children will enjoy writing or dictating letters and drawing pictures for Daddy or Mommy. Family sound tapes are especially nice, so that the parent can hear his children talk and sing. In any case, pictures of the family and everyday accounts of family life will make both parent and family feel closer together.

Unquestionably, it is difficult for a mother or father to bring up a child alone. A growing child may feel a responsibility toward his mother if she is alone—may be thoughtful and considerate of her and take pride in his ability to be a real support to her—and yet, at the same time, feel a resentment he does not admit even to himself. Why does he have to be the one to work so hard for what he gets, to give up pleasures others take for granted?

Too much responsibility should not be put on his immature shoulders. He needs companionship of his own age, and time to profit from it. He may need an older person of the sex of the missing parent to lean on. But with a little thoughtful planning, he has as good a chance of growing up into a well-adjusted adult as does any other child. As a matter of fact, his chances may be better than those of a child who has both parents but whose own rights are ignored or denied, for the child whose parents are unable to create a secure, harmonious family life for him may be very neglected.

The important thing is not to become overanxious to make it up to the child for the lack of a parent. To overprotect a child for whatever reason will prove more harmful to him than the condition itself. It will be far better to work out a harmonious relationship between yourself and your children. After all, you share the hardship, and you all must contribute toward making this a strong, secure, loving home.

CHILDREN OF DIVORCE

It is not the legal divorce that causes unhappiness, confusion, and perhaps delinquent behavior in the child of divorced parents as much as the unhappy situation that existed in the home before the divorce.

When divorce occurs, it is most important that the parents avoid sharing their bitterness with their child. If you are the parent with whom the child will live, explain that when people marry, they hope they will be happy together, but that it doesn't always work. When it doesn't, parents often find it better to live apart. Carefully explain that the absent parent still loves him, and assure him he will still see and visit frequently with that parent (if this is true).

There are, unfortunately, situations in which visiting the "other" parent is consistently a highly traumatic experience for the child. If this is the case, it will take all the strength parents can summon to do what is best for the youngster. In our experience it is the most difficult aspect of the whole problem and, if not handled with mature wisdom and skill, often does permanent harm to the child's emotional makeup. In solving it the best professional guidance is often needed.

MAKING A LIVING—
AND BEING A HOMEMAKER AS WELL

It takes ingenuity to combine the roles of provider and homemaker. One of the main problems is to secure the proper kind of care for your children while you are away from them. But assuring safe, affectionate, competent care for your children is not a problem unique to the single parent. The mother who works, for whatever reason, faces a similar situation.

What you must do is examine the different kinds of child care available in your community. You should learn as much as you can about the benefits and possible disadvantages of each in order to make an intelligent choice.

As we said, we are beginning to understand the benefits any child can derive from companionship with others, perhaps in a different setting. We are not seeking substitute mothering. Rather we are concerned with the supplement to the love and care the child receives from his parent—and the way both child and parent can benefit from the enrichment the child receives in this manner.

BABY-SITTERS

According to the dictionary, to *baby-sit* means "to take care of a child or children while the parents are temporarily away." The term has been used rather loosely for people who give full-time care to children while their mother works or is away for a long period. In this section, however, a baby-sitter is a person, often a teen-ager, who contracts to care for a child or children for a few hours.

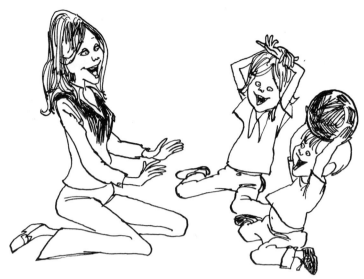

PREPARING YOUR SITTER

After you have satisfied yourself that the sitter is competent to care for your children, make your arrangements in person in your own home. Tell him or her the name and age of the child and have them meet. Discuss the duties: Is the child to be fed, bathed, put to bed? Will some housework be expected of the sitter as well? Generally speaking, a baby-sitter should have one responsibility only, that of caring for your child or children. After all, your child's safety and happiness is your main concern.

If you require a teen-age girl's services during the evening hours, be prepared to see that she is taken home. Although many teen-agers drive their own (or parents') cars, it would not be wise to expect a young girl to drive home alone at night. Her safety is your responsibility. You may, on occasion, have to pick her up as well as take her home.

Introducing the Baby-Sitter to Your Child. It is important for baby-sitter and child to get to know each other before they are left alone. This is especially important for a very young child. He cannot understand his mother's going away and leaving him with a stranger. Besides, it is a terrifying experience to awaken in the dark and see a strange face staring down at you.

You may need to arrange two or three visits while you are home before your small child feels friendly and comfortable with the sitter. Of course, this is not always possible, but at least have them be together a half hour or so before you leave, for a few times.

After your child has accepted the new sitter and all is going well, don't be disturbed if he still cries and tries to keep you from leaving. It is the nature of a young child to try to control his environment. It's the way he learns. But he also needs to learn that other people have rights too. Just give him a kiss and say casually, "I'm going now. I will be home later." Then go. No threats, bribes, or wavering. Otherwise, you might convince him that he really does have something to cry about.

WRITTEN INSTRUCTIONS FOR YOUR SITTER. Leave necessary information and clear instructions for your sitter. Tack up a list over the telephone, or attach it to the phone itself. The following items should be included:

> Your name and home address. In an emergency, a new sitter may "blank out."
> The phone number of the police department.
> The phone number of the fire department.
> The name, address, and phone number where you can be reached.
> The name and phone number of a near neighbor to be contacted in an emergency. (Check ahead to make sure your neighbor will be home.)
> It is also helpful, if possible, to leave the phone number and name of a relative or close friend.
> The time you expect to return. This is important. If you cannot make it, be sure to let the sitter know.
> The name and phone number of the children's doctor. Instruct the sitter to call him if in the slightest doubt.

SHOW THE SITTER WHERE THINGS ARE. Leave a flashlight handy for a possible power failure or for finding the way to a light switch. Test the batteries.

Point out the emergency exits or fire escapes in the building.

Explain where to find Band-Aids and simple home remedies for hurts and bruises.

Say what your child is to be fed and where his nightclothes are. Provide a timetable as well.

If you have a baby, make sure the sitter knows how to diaper, where to find the diapers, and where to dispose of them. Explain

248

how you hold the baby for his bottle, and point out that you never prop the bottle.

Don't expect your young sitter to give any medicines to your child. This can be dangerous. Make other arrangements.

Young people get hungry during a long evening. Tell your sitter what you have left for snacks—and what you do *not* want eaten.

What rules do you want the sitter to follow?

May the telephone or TV be used? Do you object to a friend's staying too? Discourage a girl from having a boy friend visit or from asking a group of her friends in. Caution her against letting anyone she does not know into the apartment or house, no matter who they may claim to be. It's too bad if your uncle gets angry because he was refused admission, but you can be sincerely thankful that she did her job so well.

Also tell the sitter what to say when answering the phone. If you are expecting an important phone call or caller, mention exactly who or what it will be.

Describe the routines and habits you allow your child, and what you forbid. May he have a night light in his room? Or his door left open? How about a bedtime story? Toys in bed, or a bedtime snack? Does your child have any special names for things an outsider would not understand without being told?

If your small child gets lonely and wants to call you up, may he do this?

And how is the child to be disciplined? Explain what works for you.

Sitter service agencies

Sitter service agencies have been set up in most urban areas. These advertise a variety of services: baby-sitting for an evening or weekend, or 24-hour services for longer periods.

ADOPTION PRACTICES

In the past, there were at least six couples eager to adopt for each child available for adoption. Today the situation has changed. There are more children available for adoption, and agencies have come to realize that many of their rigid standards were unrealistic and artificial. So today more children are more easily adopted—though, of course, there are still firm rules.

The Child Welfare League of America sets the standards for many child care agencies. Agencies who are members of the League, as well as nonmember agencies, accept its standards and apply its newer practices (as revised in 1968) as conditions permit. The emphasis is on meeting the needs of the child—on finding the child a warm, loving home.

If you wish to adopt a child you need to know about some of the changes in procedures today. If the agency you consult appears to cling to unrealistic standards, consult another.

Adoption without the help of an agency carries hazards. Skilled adoption caseworkers are in a better position to assess the situation, to protect you against future legal problems, and to give counsel and help.

MAJOR CHANGES IN PRACTICE

Although a stable, two-parent family is ideal for a child, it is now recognized that love, care, and security can be provided in a one-parent home. Unmarried, widowed, or divorced mothers are successfully rearing children. Adoption is no longer denied on this basis alone, nor are unmarried men automatically excluded as prospective adoptive fathers. But an unmarried prospective parent must satisfy the placement agency as to his rightness for a child, just as married couples must do.

Age, income, education, and neighborhood of the adoptive parents are no longer *the* determining factors; they are considered along with all the other advantages the parents would provide for the child. Nor does the fact that the adoptive mother works outside the home automatically disqualify her. It is, however, considered desirable for the child's emotional well-being that she be able to stay home for a period immediately following his placement with her. How long depends on the child's ability to make the adjustment.

Matching color, personality, and cultural background are no

longer required in every case, unless the difference seriously hinders the adopting parents from accepting the child.

The waiting periods between application and fulfillment have been shortened.

Foster parents are no longer automatically barred from adopting the child they have had under their care.

It is now recognized that many adoptive parents are ready to take the same risk as natural parents and do not need guarantees of perfect babies—though the agency will, of course, tell the parents of any known or suspected defects.

INTERRACIAL ADOPTIONS

For those who have love and understanding to share with any child who needs it, there is the possibility of adopting a child of another race or of a mixed race.

It has been heartbreaking in the past to see children of a minority racial background waiting years for a home, often never finding one. Children of mixed racial backgrounds were especially vulnerable; it seemed no one wanted them.

Since some Caucasian families have pioneered in adopting children from other ethnic groups, most of the old predictions have proved false. The argument that such a child growing up in a white family would be happier with his own kind has serious flaws in it. There may be no one of his own kind looking to adopt him. And if he is of mixed background, what is his "own kind"? Certainly his chances for happiness and security are greatest when he becomes a member of a well-adjusted "color-blind" family group.

Families still often have to face the disapproval of their neighbors, even of their relatives. It takes well-adjusted parents, secure in themselves and able to stand any ostracism that may result. There are also many minority people who are fearful that a black, Indian, or oriental child will forget his racial heritage and his pride in such heritage in a Caucasian society. There is, of course, good reason for such fears. Perhaps it boils down to this: Is a child of a minority group going to have a better chance to grow up into a responsible person in an orphanage or children's home or in a family where he will be a cherished member?

Marian Mitchell, a supervisor of adoptions in a child care agency, writes:

> Admittedly, children of mixed racial background will be subject to additional community pressures upon entering school, and later in adolescence. These children, however, would also have to face pressures because of their race, even if they had been placed in Negro homes, or those with a racial mixture. We should no longer be defensive about transracial placements." *

CHILDREN OF UNMARRIED MOTHERS

We now recognize that many unmarried mothers wish to keep their babies, though anyone faced with this decision must assess carefully her ability to care for the child, her acceptance by her family and the community, and her own emotional stability.

Few young pregnant girls are capable of making such an objective evaluation. They are too confused and uncertain about the future. But any girl in this dilemma can find sympathetic, understanding counsel and practical help from the social agencies in her community. Such agencies are frequently also adoption agencies. They put no pressure on the prospective mother to give up her child but do help her to see, realistically, all aspects of her problem. The decision must be hers, or possibly that of her family if she is a minor.

Giving a child for adoption

A mother who plans to relinquish her newborn baby for adoption should not make the final decision, or sign any legal papers, until after her child has been born and she has recovered from the effects of delivery.

If she wishes to see her baby before giving him up, she should be free to do so. Said one 18-year-old, "I wouldn't have felt complete without seeing him!" Seeing the baby helps resolve the problem and helps the girl to know and feel sure of what she is doing.†

* Marian Mitchell, *Child Welfare Journal*, December, 1969, p. 616.
† *The Unmarried Mother* (Public Affairs Pamphlet No. 282), p. 22.

Some girls find relinquishment easier when they themselves take the baby from the hospital nursery to the adoption agency. This is a way of bringing a difficult period of a girl's life to a conclusion. It also gives her pride in her ability to put the baby's welfare first and frees her to start a new life with confidence and added maturity.*

The mother must make the break a clean one, however. She must realize and accept the fact that she will not see her baby again or know who his new parents are. He is no longer hers. She must have faith that the adoption agency will find the baby a home in which he will be secure, accepted, and loved.

A CHILD IN THE HOSPITAL

Not so many years ago, a mother would say to her child, "We'll go out and buy some ice cream," and not mention that their second stop would be the children's ward in the hospital. She thought she was protecting her child, but actually she was protecting her own feelings at the expense of the child's trust and sense of security. The result was a great shock to the child, as parents now realize.

Of course you worry if your child must be hospitalized. Most of us are pretty apprehensive when we ourselves must become patients. How do you prepare your child for such an experience without letting your own anxiety show? Doctors and hospital personnel will do all they can to help, but the major responsibility rests on your shoulders.

PREPARE YOURSELF

You cannot help your child unless you know the score yourself. Your doctor will give you the details of what will happen in the surgical or medical procedures. Ask him questions about anything you do not understand.

* *Ibid.*

Visit the department where you child will be a patient. Some hospitals have a special setup for inviting parents to visit. And some hospitals invite your child along also, so that he can watch the children in the playroom, see what a hospital room looks like, meet nurses and doctors.

If there is no special program at your hospital, ask for an appointment to visit and meet the nurses. You will not be able to take your child along, but you will have the information you need to pass on to him. Don't be backward about asking questions. This is your child's emotional well-being you are concerned about.

WHEN, WHERE, AND HOW TO TELL HIM

Little can be done to get a very young child—18 months or 2 years old—prepared in advance. Because his concept of time is hazy, it is better to wait until only a day or two before he enters. But you can show him pictures of hospital wards, playrooms, nurses, and doctors, and tell him, "Tomorrow you and I are going to the hospital. You can take your teddy bear too." Tell him why he is going, even if he doesn't quite understand. You can't go into detail, but you can say, "Dr. Smith wants to fix your throat [or whatever] to help it get better." When the time comes, he can help pack his bag "just like Daddy does" when he takes a trip.

Visiting hours in most children's departments have been liberalized so that you can be with a small child most of his waking hours. And more and more hospitals allow you to sleep in your child's room, to provide security to the child too young to understand.

The child of 4 or 5 and older, and even most 3-year-olds, will need more preparation. For a child of this age, try presenting the hospital stay as an adventure. All children know and like adventure stories. They dream about adventures of their own, where they meet with dangers, perhaps get hurt, but triumph in the end. They have slain the dragon! You can give your child a chance for his own high adventure, but first of all you will need to help him slay the dragon of fear in his own mind. And these dragons can be pretty terrible.

254

Why children fear hospitals

Some of a child's fear of hospitals stems from what he has heard. "Grandmother went to the hospital and died. Will I die too?" It is fairly easy to explain that grandmother was very old and it was time for her to die—or however you wish to put it. "Of course we all will miss her, but she is happy not to be old and sick any more." But a child's other fears are not so easily stated —or dealt with.

As grown-ups we enjoy talking about our hospital experiences. We tend to exaggerate the unpleasant aspects. We want to show how brave we were. Our children listen and remember.

Your child may know about hospitals only as a place where mothers go to get babies. You brought home a baby, didn't you? Will he get one there too?

Children talking among themselves or playing hospital can think up some pretty weird ideas, perhaps the result of half-understood remarks they have heard. Most children do not easily communicate their fears to adults. So you have to devise ways to find out what they are.

Playing hospital

Playing out a situation is the best way to help your child understand it. After all, children learn about life through play. Put on a paper nurse's cap and start to play hospital. Go through the important things: his admission, getting him into pajamas in the daytime, checking his temperature, and listening to his heart. Avoid the more frightening aspects, but be honest. "Now I have to pretend to give you a shot like Dr. Smith does. The real shot will hurt a little, so you can cry if you want to. . . . Now I'll take you to get [your throat, your eyes, or whatever] fixed up. It won't hurt because you will breathe something that will put you to sleep until you're all fixed up. . . . Now you're waking up, and here's Mommy right beside your bed. After you are all better, you and Mommy will go home." (It is probably better to say "fixed up" instead of "operated on." He understands what it means to fix things.)

Your child may want you to play hospital with him several

times until he feels secure. After that, he probably will play it out again with his toys or playmates.

Hand puppets. Using nurse and child-patient hand puppets often helps a child to express his thinking—and his fears. You can stick a cap on the girl puppet on your hand and discuss the experience with his child puppet. It is often easier for a child to ask questions for his puppet than to let them come from himself; it is more impersonal, and his sense of magic helps him to half-believe the puppet really is asking the questions.

Staging a real play. One school nurse staged a play about going to the hospital that went over big with 6- and 7-year-olds. It could be equally successful at home with children of 5 or 6 or over.

She made a crude hospital ward from a carton and peopled it with ten-cent-store dolls dressed as a nurse, doctor, mother, and child. As animator and narrator, she went through a hospital experience—that of having tonsils taken out. The children who had already had the experience were even more interested. It helped them re-live the experience, which is also an important thing to do.

ROOMING-IN

If you decide to room-in with your child, you will have a cot or convertible chair-bed in your child's room and will care for him as you do at home. Nurses will do the specialized treatment and will also take over ordinary care if you wish it.

Generally this arrangement provides great security for a child under 4, as well as contributing to your own peace of mind. It does not always work out well for the child over 4, and there are times when it is not good even for the young one. If you are so frightened by the hospital or by the child's illness that you cannot conceal your anxiety, you will only heighten your child's fear. This doesn't mean that you are not a good mother; it just means that rooming-in is not for you. Discuss your own fears ahead of time with your child's doctor.

Or you and your child may be at odds with each other at the

time of the hospitalization. In that case, it may be a relief for you both to separate for part of each day. Then the hours you spend together will be more pleasant for both of you. Some children become unusually trying at certain stages of growth, and their behavior does not necessarily become less inviting just because they are sick. So don't feel guilty about being irritated; just don't live in.

You may not be able to consider rooming-in because of your job. You may not be financially able to manage an absence from your employment, especially with the additional burden of medical expenses. You may also need to consider your other children; certainly they cannot be neglected. But it is worth a few sacrifices on the part of the rest of the family if you can contribute to the emotional well-being of your hospitalized child.

USING VISITING HOURS TO BEST ADVANTAGE

Don't be afraid to ask if you may hold your child. Unless moving him could hurt him, you will be allowed to do so, but ask first.

If the hospital rules allow you to go with him for X rays, to treatments, or to sit with him in the recovery room, this will help him feel confident; you are there. But go only if you can appear cool and confident yourself. If you are nervous and anxious, don't try to be too brave—it won't work. You will only make the child more fearful, and you may seriously hamper the work being done. The same can be said about staying with your child when he has medicines or treatments. Your presence may either provide assurance or promote disorder and resentment.

If, while you are visiting, the playroom opens and your child says, "Sorry, Mommy, I must go in the playroom now. I'll see you tomorrow," don't be resentful or jealous—rejoice! He is adjusting well.

EMERGENCY HOSPITALIZATION

In such situations there is little or no time for preparation. Stay as cool as you can (outwardly, at least) so that your child will be able to count on you to support him.

257

Accidents and emergencies can happen to anyone. Just make a determined effort to keep your head and act as a parent for your child's sake.

There are some things you can do beforehand to make such a situation easier to handle when or if it does come. Make sure your child learns about doctors and hospitals just as he learns about farms and farm animals and other aspects of living.

Let him look at picture books with nurses and hospital setups. Tell him stories about them. You can do your best to protect him from painful and unpleasant tales about hospital experiences. Tell him about nice things: hospital playrooms, friendly nurses, the fun of eating from trays or at a table with other children.

When you detect that wrong ideas have been given him, set him and his friends straight. At least he will not go to the hospital terrified by what he thinks to find there. You cannot protect him from the pain and discomfort, but you can be his comfort and support.

7

The Special Child

THE HANDICAPPED CHILD

THE HANDICAPPED CHILD

THE BLIND CHILD

A mother who learns that her child is blind is of course devastated. She sees all the beauty of color and light and mourns that her child will never experience these pleasures. Yet the child who has never seen may not miss those things he never had, and the child whose eyesight has failed later in life has many memory pictures in his mind. With proper teaching and stimulation, the blind child learns to "see" his environment through his senses of touch, hearing, and taste.

Most important in bringing up such a child is to teach him independence. It does not help any child to so protect him that he never learns to develop his own abilities.

It is better for the blind child, if home conditions permit, to have daily contact with sighted children. One little girl in a regular nursery school learned to slide on the playground slides, participate in games, and become one of the group—and impatiently pushed aside those who wanted to help her. Her twin sister, also blind, was more timid and required much patient teaching and help. Eventually, both girls took their place in the sighted world with confidence.

Intensive studies have shown that blind children have the potential to grow up into independent, confident people. But the parents must provide opportunities for them to do so. Give your child objects of different shapes, sizes, textures, and smells and describe them as he uses his sense of touch or taste. Let him pick a flower, feel it, and smell it. Take him to the children's zoo and let him run his hands over the tame animals. Let him feel wind, rain, snow, water. Some parents are shy about talking of "seeing" to a blind person, but the child does form a mental image and talks quite casually about seeing things.

THE DEAF CHILD

The child who was born deaf has no concept of language or of words. He has to be taught the words to express his ideas and concepts. The child who has once heard has the advantage of having learned to express his ideas.

People who work with deaf children emphasize the importance of talking to deaf babies. The mother whose infant is deaf often thinks there is no point in talking to him, since he cannot hear. But he can see. "Talk, talk, talk," the experts advise. The young infant watches his mother's face intently, the way she moves her mouth, her facial expression, the way she moves and acts.

Some cities have preschool classes for deaf children, where they learn to watch mouth movements. The instructor gives the child an object to hold, such as an apple, and at the same time names it distinctly: *ap*-ple.

There is much a parent can do at home before the child is of school age. Correspondence courses, such as those provided by the John Tracy Clinic for children of 5 and under, are available.* The child should be tested to see whether earphones can capture any residual hearing.

Most deaf children of school age profit by attending day school, particularly if they can participate in some activities with

* John Tracy Clinic, 806 West Adams Boulevard, Los Angeles, Cal. 90007.

hearing children. It will help them learn to lip-read. However, learning to speak is long-drawn-out and difficult for deaf children, and many children never become proficient. Most schools for the deaf do teach lip-reading and speech, since sign language alone may isolate the child from the community, but it is now believed that sign language as well should be taught.

It cannot be denied that the deaf person has a difficult adjustment to make. But early and persistent training, making use of all facilities for deaf children in the community, and treating him as a normal person will help him learn to live a normal life.

THE CHILD WITH MISSING OR DEFORMED LIMBS

A child with a major physical handicap arouses immense pity in his parents. It is difficult for mothers to learn to train and discipline such children. They are much more likely to protect them, excuse their faults, and show favoritism toward them. Actually this is the worst thing they can do. If the child is going to be accepted by other children, he must be treated as any normal child.

Children are very adept at compensating for the handicaps. A child who cannot use his arms can learn to use his feet and toes in their stead. Unless a child has been taught self-pity, he is not usually self-conscious or ashamed.

One little girl who had grotesquely deformed legs yearned to join in play with other children, and it was only her mother's sense of pity and shame that kept her isolated. When her mother was finally able to accept her daughter's handicap and permit her to meet other children, she discovered that after a preliminary "What's the matter with her?" the other children ignored the child's handicap and included her and her wheelchair in their play.

Will such a child receive stares, misplaced pity, and ridicule from some adults and children alike? Undoubtedly he will. But he will be able to accept these and continue to enjoy life if he has been treated at home as a normal person with a particular disability.

THE CHILD WITH CEREBRAL PALSY

Cerebral palsy is a broad term used for those forms of brain damage in which the parts of the nervous system controlling voluntary muscles are affected. It is one of the leading causes of crippling in children.

There are several forms of cerebral palsy, and sometimes a child has a mixture of forms. The spastic kind is the most common. Children who have this condition are unable to control movement of their muscles. Attempts to move arms, legs, and trunk result in poorly controlled jerky motions. They have difficulty eating, walking, or making coordinated movements. Frequently braces are necessary to help control muscle movements and to support weak muscles. At times, orthopedic surgery is needed to correct associated deformities.

Contrary to public belief, not all children with cerebral palsy are mentally retarded. A child may retain mental ability even when the physical disability is severe enough to make speech impossible or to impair sight or hearing. But unless ways can be found to help him make use of his mental powers, they will be of little use to him and will eventually deteriorate.

Cerebral palsy may be the result of interruption of oxygen supply prior to or during birth, or in some cases it may be of hereditary origin. A few cases result from infections of the nervous system, such as meningitis.

Home care and teaching

The most important support for the child comes from his knowledge that he is a loved and respected member of the family. His acceptance as a normal person with a disability is essential toward helping him accept and respect himself.

These children have to learn laboriously all the physical activities that unaffected children learn automatically. For the child who has difficulty maintaining balance, a high-backed chair with side pieces and a foot platform will be helpful. A safety strap to help hold him in place, and rollers or casters under the chair legs, will make moving about easier. Specially constructed toilet seats help these children achieve independence in toileting.

Self-feeding may be helped by the use of spoons with broad-

262

based handles for easy grasping. Plates with raised rims and suction devices to prevent slipping are useful. Cups with covers, with a hole to admit a drinking straw, prevent spilling.

Clothing easy to put on and manipulate will motivate the child to dress himself.* In fact, any household device that will help the child achieve some measure of independence will also go a long way to help him believe in his own worth.

There is no cure for cerebral palsy, but these children can be trained to make full use of whatever potential ability they have. A skilled therapist can frequently help in teaching them to use alternate unaffected nerve pathways to control muscles.

Many people with cerebral palsy have learned to care for their own needs, and some have been able to learn skills that enable them to find employment.

A great deal of supportive help is available to parents in most localities. Worthwhile source material may be had by writing to the United Cerebral Palsy Association, 321 West 44th Street, New York, N.Y. 10036.

THE CHRONICALLY ILL CHILD

A child's chronic disease creates unusual problems for both parents and child. True, children today are seldom kept in bed for long periods of time as they once were for rheumatic fever or nephritis. But their activity is bound to be restricted by the very nature of their illness—and that makes for difficult times.

Any child needs diversion to keep him from complete boredom and to prevent loss of interest. This becomes difficult if he is allowed only a minimum of activity and if visiting by his friends is restricted. It is true that "Time stretches out like a great desert for the patient who must spend a long conva-

* *Self-Help Clothing for Handicapped Children*, a pamphlet published and sold by the National Society for Crippled Children and Adults (2023 West Ogden Avenue, Chicago, Ill. 60612), offers a useful guide in the selection and adaptation of clothing for handicapped children.

lescence in bed." * He must have enough to do, geared to his condition, to keep him contented.

Another troublesome problem is that of discipline. Firmness, understanding, and imagination are needed on the part of the entire family. The child needs this support to help him build his own self-discipline. For the child's own good, he cannot be allowed to become spoiled or neurotic. He will be happier and more secure if he is treated the same as the other members of his family. Rules should be kept simple and adapted to his ability to keep them. Once they are made, however, they must be enforced, and violations dealt with kindly but firmly. This makes for happier relations for the entire family.

IF YOUR CHILD NEEDS LONG REST PERIODS

Probably the first consideration is to make the child's room easily accessible to the person caring for him. If you live in a two-story house, how about fixing up a downstairs room for his daytime rest?

A child who must rest but is allowed quiet play needs a back support. These can be bought in most department stores or can be made easily from a heavy packing case.

If you do not wish to buy a bed table, improvise one by placing a board across the bed and resting it on the ends of chair backs. Or take a sturdy carton, turn it upside down, and cut the sides out for leg room.

Suggestions for keeping a child occupied are endless. Crafts, puzzles, painting, reading are a few. Some books on activities for children who must be kept quiet are included in the references for further reading at the end of the book under the heading Activities and Recreation.

IF HE IS UNINTERESTED IN FOOD

Children with long chronic illnesses or long-drawn-out convalescences are apt to have very little interest in food. Yet you cannot adopt a take-it-or-leave-it attitude with such children.

---

* *Have Fun—Get Well!* an American Heart Association pamphlet obtainable from your local Heart Association branch.

How can a busy distracted mother stir up her child's interest in eating, especially if he is on a restricted diet?

The answer comes with a little ingenuity. Appetite is not stimulated by taste and variety of foods alone. Eating should be done in a congenial atmosphere, for it involves color and smell as well as taste. Try a colorful, gaily decorated table or tray. How about some homemade place mats? Shelf paper painted with gay scenes, or with brightly colored pictures of funny animals, clowns, or children pasted on it, makes an interesting setting. Bright-colored paper napkins with scenes or flowers help. If your child wishes, he can paint or color the flowers embossed on a paper nakpin for his next meal. Children love flowers, even dandelions or daisies. Just one at his place will brighten up his table. Candles are fun for him to watch burning (if you stay near at hand).

For social atmosphere, why not let your daughter dress up occasionally for a party? A purse, high heels, and hat set the scene. Stuffed animals make satisfactory guests. Toy tea sets or doll dishes complete the picture. The "hostess" may feel the compulsion to help her "guests" clean up their plates!

You can make foods more appealing by the use of vegetable coloring or of shapes and molds. It's certainly more fun to eat a sandwich in the shape of a lion or bear than an ordinary rectangle.

OTHER CONSIDERATIONS

A school child kept home for a long period feels very much out of things. How about having him correspond with his classmates, fellow scouts, or Sunday School friends? It will help him feel a part of his normal world.

Television and radio are great helps but are not complete solutions to the entertainment program. Don't rely on them too much.

One final word. If your child's illness seems endless and you can see little day-to-day progress, it is important that you get away every once in a while for a change of scene and a breath of fresh air. If you have no neighbors, relatives, or reliable baby-sitter to take your place for a few hours, check for homemaker services. Or call your local school of nursing; some student nurses like to earn money by baby-sitting. Or call your minister for suggestions.

Don't think you are running away from your responsibility. Both you and your child will greatly profit by a short absence from one another.

THE CHILD NOT EXPECTED TO RECOVER

One of the most difficult aspects of life occurs when parents have to face serious illness in their children. If this illness is one for which there is as yet no cure, the experience becomes nearly intolerable.

How do you handle it? If you know that some children *do* recover completely, you can pin your faith on the ability of doctors to see your child through. You quiet the anxiety in your heart as best you can, and you use all your energies toward providing the best possible atmosphere for your child. To a child, adults are all-powerful; they know all the answers. If his mother has doubts about his getting well, what use is there for him to try?

A sympathetic concern about the child's discomfort, together with a shining faith that it will pass, is the proper attitude. Bolstering the child's belief that he will eventually come through is the best gift you can give him.

Carrying on a normal way of life as much as possible is of equal importance. Overindulgence of a child because he is sick and might not get well is frightening to a child and undermines his morale. He becomes frightened, confused and suspicious. He reasons, "They never did these things for me before; they must want to make it up to me because they think I am going to die." Children are much more apt to try to reason things out for themselves than to ask questions.

Compassion, understanding, and sympathy are needed, yes. But the day-by-day strain tells on parents, takes a great toll of their patience and endurance. It is easy to slip into an irritable, nagging manner. Sometimes the problem looms so large in a mother's mind that she forgets the burden on the child. Later, she becomes overwhelmed with guilt. Getting away from the situation for a short time will help, even if this means only stealing a few hours to read a book or take up a hobby. She will come back to her problem with renewed courage.

But no one has found a cure for your child's disease, you say. How can you cope with this? When parents are first told that their child has leukemia, or some other condition for which there is no cure as yet, the shock is numbing. They think, This cannot be happening to my child. There must be some mistake. It is quite natural to ask for another opinion.

It is also inevitable that a parent will look back and wonder if this could have been avoided. It takes a strong spirit to rise above the regrets and thoughts of "if only things had been different." But you can do it. You can see to it that your child's remaining time with you is as pleasant and happy as possible. The months ahead are the ones you will cherish in your memory.

Encourage your child to live in a normal manner as far as possible. Special arrangements, such as celebration of Christmas in the summertime, or public dramatization of the child's illness, may cause him more anxiety than pleasure.

Occasionally, the pressure may become so great that you wish the ordeal were over. That is normal, so don't feel guilty about it. Just know that you are doing your best, that you must live from day to day. You will remember the sweet and tender moments of this experience and forget the anguish and fatigue.

What to tell your child about his illness? Most young children do not ask whether they are going to die. Just tell your child that he has an illness that may last for a long time. He will have times when he feels better, times when he will not. It certainly is no fun, you say, to be sick for so long. It's mighty discouraging. Everyone is working to help him feel as well as possible.

However, if he is hospitalized and a fellow patient dies, your child may start to wonder if this will happen to him as well. Even then, most people believe there is no kindness in telling him that he cannot recover from his illness. He no doubt will have periods, perhaps weeks or months at a time, when he will feel quite well. Why should he feel the threat of death hanging over him? You can say quite truthfully, "We are all working to get you well again," or, "We are all working together on this."

Sometimes an older child suspects that he has a fatal disease but clearly does not want to be told. Here again there seems no point in volunteering the information.

THE MENTALLY RETARDED CHILD

When a mother is told her child is mentally retarded, her natural instinct is to look for some area of escape to help her bear this seemingly unbearable knowledge. She may cling to the hope that just this once the doctor or psychologist is mistaken. She may be driven to seek other opinions, but eventually she must accept the reality and go on from there.

Nearly every mother in this situation goes through a period of guilt, of self-incrimination. Her mind goes back over her pregnancy. "If only I had not done so and so, this might not have happened." Even those who know better usually cannot help looking back. In fact, this may be nature's way of diverting a mother's mind from the fact until she had developed strength to face the impact of reality.

There are a few known causes of mental retardation. Heredi tary facts, biological accidents, certain medicines taken during pregnancy, and German measles during pregnancy are all on the list. Occasionally, a child suffers brain injury while being born. By far the largest number, however, are still due to unknown causes.

Whether or not the finger of suspicion can be pointed in any particular direction should not matter after the child is born, as far as the parents are concerned. After her initial period of grief and self-guilt, the mother must rise above it. "All right, we don't really know why this has happened, or even if we do, there's nothing we can do to change it now. But here is my baby who needs my love and care. How can I help him develop to the very limit of his capacity?"

Self-incrimination and guilt, if clung to, soon develop into self-pity and leave little room for compassion and love for the child.

Some parents find help talking with other parents who have gone through the same experience. There is a relief in the realization that one is not alone. The National Association for Retarded Children has sponsored parent groups in most localities.* But you may not be ready to enter a discussion group, yet you still need help. You need to be able to talk to someone who will listen and will understand your feelings. Ask your doctor for guidance. Perhaps he is the one to give you support. Or perhaps he will suggest someone whom he feels has even greater understanding and insight to offer you.

THE DOCTOR'S DIAGNOSIS

Sometimes the mother of a retarded child says, "My doctor did not tell me there was anything wrong. I found it out myself when my child didn't act like other children. Why couldn't he have told me right at the beginning?"

For one thing, it is quite likely that he couldn't tell for certain. It is seldom easy to diagnose mental retardation in a newborn baby. Even if some of the distinctive features of Down's Syndrome (mongolism) are present, they may also appear in a perfectly normal young infant. Nor does every true mongoloid child necessarily show all the features associated with the condition.

When a newborn baby *can* be definitely diagnosed as retarded, doctors today are generally in agreement that the parents should be told. It will be easier to accept the fact then than after the mother has had the heartbreak of seeing him fail to develop normally. But if a doctor merely suspects the possibility of retardation and has no real evidence, it can be quite cruel to speak at this time. He will watch the child carefully and ask for tests, if conditions seem to warrant, before making a decision.

* Check your phone book for the county or state branch in your community, or write the National Association for Retarded Children, 420 Lexington Avenue, New York, N.Y. 10017.

EACH CHILD HAS HIS OWN DISTINCTIVE PERSONALITY

Nurses working with children learn very quickly that every child's personality shines through regardless of his physical or mental deformity. If she did not have to give the special physical care his condition demanded, she would almost forget his deficiencies. In fact, it is not unusual to hear a children's nurse insist the child has more intelligence than he is credited with having. His unique personality has obscured his problems in her eyes. So it is also with mothers.

We have learned to understand retarded children in a number of ways. Perhaps the greatest understanding comes when we can see them as children, ordinary children, not as something different.

Just as a child may have diabetes or cystic fibrosis, so this child has a condition which affects his mental processes. That is the only difference. Retarded children are born, grow, and develop as other children do. Their particular handicap affects them in only one way: Their normal development stops at a lower level than that of an average child.

Think of a child's mental development as a ladder to be climbed. The unusually intelligent child climbs high on the ladder. The average child gets perhaps halfway up, while the retarded child may be able to reach the first or second rung. But it is the same ladder for all.

THE OTHER CHILDREN IN THE FAMILY

A slow or retarded child does not need to be a hindrance or embarrassment to his family. When the other members of the family have been brought up to see him as a child with a condition preventing him from full participation, he will be accepted for what he is. He is their brother; he is accepted at home; they will see no reason for being ashamed of him away from home. He is no more responsible for his condition than is a diabetic child for his inability to eat sweets.

MENTAL SLOWNESS IS NOT MENTAL ILLNESS

It is unfortunately true that many people still confuse retardation with mental illness. Retardation is not a sickness. It is possible for a retarded child to become mentally ill also. But a mental illness such as autism or schizophrenia is a psychotic disorder. Retardation is the inability of a child to learn and to adapt to the demands of society. It may be due to genetic causes, poor environment, or some damage to certain centers in the brain.

A child who is slow in a complicated setting may function perfectly in a more simple, less taxing environment. It is important to keep this in mind. Adapting the surroundings to his ability may be all the child needs. Others may simply need to have opportunities for learning, opportunities they have never had.

THE MEANING OF MENTAL RETARDATION

Once we used terms like *moron, imbecile,* and *idiot* which implied that the person was some sort of monster, different from other people and to be feared. Fortunately such terms have been discarded. Then we used *educable, trainable* and *dependent* in their stead to cover the various levels of mental deficiency. Unfortunately, these terms imply that a child reaches a certain limit, after which he can learn no more. But as we gain newer techniques and better understanding, some of these children surprise us. If we have to use labels at all, the newer terms *mildly, moderately, severely retarded* seem more acceptable. What does each category mean?

The mildly retarded child is one who is somewhat slower learning to walk, talk, and feed himself than are most children. His handicap is not especially apparent until he enters school. Then he may find keeping up with his class difficult and need special education methods.

He usually can achieve sufficient skills to make him eligible for employment as he grows older, and he may be indistinguishable from other persons in an average population.

The moderately retarded child has greater difficulty learning

271

to care for himself and to talk. He too can be taught health and safety habits as he grows older, as well as routine skills. He may show considerable manual ability in sheltered workshops.

A sheltered workshop allows a retarded person to work at his own pace, without competition or stress. The job may be simple repetitive work for the more severely retarded or more complicated assembly work for those moderately retarded. Workers are assigned daily jobs and work under supervision. Every attempt is made to make these workshops like other shops or factories, except for the lack of competition. The worker can take pride in himself as a productive person.

The severely retarded child shows marked delay in all areas, but with patience and special help he *can* be taught to feed himself and to learn acceptable toilet habits. With supervision he learns to conform to daily routines. As he grows to adulthood, he too may learn a routine manual skill and be able to function with self-respect under supervision in sheltered situations.

A very few children are so profoundly retarded as to be completely helpless. They appear to be completely unaware of their surroundings and need total care. We believe that such children should be put in institutions where trained personnel can look after their physical needs.

There has been national interest in the mentally retarded ever since the Kennedy administration stimulated it, and we have learned a great deal from the new programs that were started then. We have seen "hopelessly" retarded children taken out of the isolation of their rooms and placed in groups on blankets on the floor where bright-colored pictures, mobiles, and toys were put in their line of vision. Music, both soft and stirring, was played, and they were talked to all the while. Eventually, a child would turn his eyes or head toward the sound or sight. When he did he was immediately encouraged. It took endless patience, but the reward came in seeing some children learn to sit, some even to stand and walk and learn the meaning of simple words. It doesn't sound like much, but it shows the fallacy of saying, "Nothing can be done."

DOWN'S SYNDROME

In 1886, a British doctor named Langdon Down first described a condition found among the mentally retarded, a condition he called *mongolism* because of the slant-eyed appearance of the people who had it. The name is unfortunate because it seems to imply some connection with the Mongolian people of Asia and of course there is none. Many professional people prefer to call it Down's Syndrome, and that term will be used here. (The word *syndrome*, by the way, means simply a group of characteristics that make possible the recognition of a particular condition.)

There is a remarkable resemblance among all children with Down's Syndrome. They have the slant-eyed look, caused by a fold of tissue at the inner corner of the eye. Their faces are flat and broad, their noses short and with a flat bridge. Their tongues may protrude because their mouths are small. These children will be short.

Children with Down's Syndrome usually have a very lax muscle tone. They appear quite comfortable in positions that could not be assumed by a normal child. They have broad, short hands, a slightly curved fifth finger, and a straight line across the palm instead of the normal two lines. (Invariably when a class of nursing students is told of the straight line, one of them is sure to find that she has such a line on her palm.) Any one or two of these signs may be present in a normal person, and some of them are barely discernible in a child who does have Down's Syndrome.

Several other signs are looked for by the physician who suspects such a condition. They include skeletal abnormalities, distinctive spots in the iris of the eye, and certain unusual whorl patterns on the thumb and fingers. Congenital heart conditions are present in many. These children are also unusually susceptible to infections, particularly respiratory infections. However, the major feature of this condition is the mental retardation. Most of the children are moderately retarded, a few severely retarded. They are delayed in walking and in learning to talk. Most of these children can be cared for at home and can profit by training in special education classes, though some present special difficulties.

What causes Down's Syndrome?

We now know what happens to bring about this unfortunate condition, but we do not yet know why. In 1956 the discovery was made that people with Down's Syndrome have a chromosome abnormality in their body cells.

Chromosomes, the minute structures found in the nucleus of all living cells, carry the characteristics of the species and are passed on from parent to offspring at the time of conception. Each parent contributes 23 chromosomes to the new life. Those from one parent pair up with their counterparts from the other parent, making 23 pairs of chromosomes in each cell of the body.

With Down's Syndrome, there is an abnormality in the chromosomes, either in number or position. Chromosome 21 is most often affected: instead of there being a *pair* of number 21 chromosomes, there are *three*. (This condition is called Trisomy 21.) Why the presence of an extra chromosome at number 21 brings about mental retardation is not known. We do know, though, that Trisomy 21 appears most frequently in children born to older mothers: 65 percent of children with Down's Syndrome are born to mothers over the age of 30. In the United States, the disorder occurs about once in 600 births.

There appears to be no inherited tendency for Trisomy 21. Generally no previous case of Down's Syndrome can be found in the family background, but there is no absolute guarantee that the parents will not have a second child with this condition. There *is* a relatively rare type of Down's Syndrome which is inheritable. If more children are desired, chromosomal analysis may be carried out to determine which type the mother has. In any event, the parents should discuss the question of future pregnancies with their physician.

What are these children like?

Children with Down's Syndrome are generally good-natured and easy to get along with, but this must be said with reservations;

274

no child stays easy to get along with if he does not receive proper training and discipline, and a spoiled child with Down's Syndrome is just as spoiled as any other child. Children with Down's Syndrome are usually quite affectionate and are often fond of music.

Parents worry about their retarded children getting into difficulties when they reach the age of reproduction. The girls develop slowly but generally do menstruate and are capable of becoming pregnant. Boys with Down's Syndrome apparently are sterile; there is no record of any such male fathering a child.

These retarded children do need care and supervision throughout their lives. Because they usually deteriorate mentally later in life, many of them need to enter institutions at a later date, and it is well for parents to be aware of this possibility. But before that deterioration, these children get along as any other moderately retarded child does. They need to be taught self-help skills. They can attend classes for trainable children and learn to the limit of their ability. And they find their way into the hearts of their parents just as any other child will do.

PHENYLKETONURIA (PKU)

Phenylketonuria, popularly known as PKU, is a rare inherited disorder that appears in approximately 1 out of 10,000 births in the United States. This form of mental retardation is caused by a defect in body metabolism, as a result of which an essential amino acid, called phenylalanine, builds up to abnormal levels in the body tissues. It causes severe mental retardation in most of its victims. Untreated children have a musty body odor and are subject to eczema. Many of them become aggressive, destructive, and difficult to care for.

PKU can be managed with some degree of success if treatment is started before brain damage occurs. Damage cannot be reversed after it has occurred. Treatment is entirely dietary and must be started as soon after birth as possible.

Testing for PKU

The infant is normal at birth. It is not until he has taken protein into his system (e.g., any kind of milk) that the defect can be detected. A blood test performed 24 to 48 hours after the infant has started taking milk will show whether the phenylalanine level is abnormally high. The blood is obtained from the newborn by a simple heel prick and is sent to the laboratory for the Guthrie Inhibition Assay test. Most states in this country require that this test be done before the baby goes home from the hospital.

If positive results appear, follow-up studies of the blood chemistry are made to ensure that a possible false positive does not lead to unnecessary treatment.

Even when the baby's Guthrie is negative, one more precaution is taken in some states: They test the baby's urine when he is 4 to 6 weeks of age. On discharge from the hospital, the mother is given an addressed envelope with a piece of filter paper inside. She is to place the filter paper inside the 4- to 6-week-old infant's diaper. When it is wet with urine, she lets it dry, puts it in the return envelope, and mails it to the health department, where it is tested. In other states, the wet diaper is tested with a drop of ferric chloride on the baby's first visit to the doctor or clinic.

Dietary treatment

The baby who tests positive for excessive phenylalanine in his bloodstream is taken off milk feedings and put on a special formula. As he grows and is ready for solid foods, a very special low-phenylalanine diet is given him and is carefully adjusted to his needs as he grows older. This diet is quite restrictive—the child must be denied many attractive foods until at least his sixth year if brain damage is to be prevented—and is apt to become distasteful as the child sees others with a greater variety of food. He is likely to rebel and feel discriminated against. Helping him calls for fine teamwork between doctor, parents, dietitian, and other guidance help. But it is worth it, for some children who have been placed on this diet during the first weeks of life have developed well.

Older children who have already suffered brain damage cannot be helped by such a diet. It may tone down their aggressive and destructive behavior, but it is nearly impossible to keep an older child on such a diet if he has not grown up on it. Children who have never known any other can accept it better, although temptation has to be kept out of their way.

It is excellent practice to have any undiagnosed retarded child tested for PKU for the sake of other members of the family. If PKU turns out to be the cause, special care should be given to the testing of each newborn baby in the family. Any pregnant woman with a history of undiagnosed retardation in the family should mention it to her doctor.

OTHER CAUSES OF MENTAL RETARDATION

There are many other causes of mental retardation, though medical science is making great strides in discovering and eliminating them.

Rubella in a pregnant woman is sometimes a cause of retardation in her child but can be prevented by the use of the vaccine (see Chapter 1).

Brain injury can be caused by lack of oxygen before or during birth, but modern obstetric techniques are able to prevent many such cases.

Extreme malnutrition in infants and young children accounts for some cases, as does very premature birth. This means that the best prenatal and infant care must be available to every woman and child. It also means that the woman must take advantage of this service when it is available.

Illnesses and accidents during childhood lead to some cases of mental retardation: meningitis not detected early enough or not adequately treated; untreated and uncontrolled convulsive disorders, such as chronic lead poisoning. The ordinary fever convulsions of young children, however, do not result in mental retardation.

HOME CARE VERSUS INSTITUTIONAL CARE FOR THE RETARDED

If a child is not profoundly retarded, should he be cared for at home? We well know that no one can answer for the parent. Each family has its own individual problems, resources, strengths, and weaknesses. Parents can, and certainly should, seek information and guidance for their problem. But eventually the decision must be their own.

A mother who is employed may have difficulty supplying her retarded child's needs. Or, in a family with other children, the slow one may be overlooked in caring for the others. Sometimes the others are not given their fair opportunities because the slow one requires all the care and energy his mother has to give. No one answer can cover all situations.

When a family can love and accept its retarded child without reserve, and will seek out opportunities for his development, undoubtedly that child will be better off in his own home. But no one can state categorically, "Every retarded child is better off with his own family."

There is, though, general agreement that infants do better at home. Most institutions no longer accept babies, except in extraordinary circumstances where no other satisfactory care can be found. If an infant cannot be cared for in his own home, a foster home is substituted if at all possible.

Generally speaking, the care of a retarded infant differs very little from the care any baby requires. All young babies are dependent on adults for their basic needs. And all babies, regardless of their mental status, need loving. We know that every child, in order to develop mentally, needs to have opportunities to see, to hear, to play and to be talked to, held, and encouraged.

Superintendents of publicly supported residential homes are well aware of the need to supply emotional support to the retarded children in their care. They know that individual mothering is as important as training and education for these children —that their ability to improve is dependent on emotional security.

But however concerned the people in charge may be, they can function adequately only when the means for good care is available to them. They need funds sufficient for facilities and for training personnel, and people interested in preparing themselves for such service. Until we the public are concerned enough to do our part, progress will be slow.

The Foster Grandparent Program has proved successful in

working with the retarded. Retired men and women, after receiving some preliminary preparation, are finding satisfaction in providing the "parenting" these children lack. They hold and rock their charges, talk to them, love them. If advisable, they take them out for walks, perhaps to a lunch room for a treat. They usually work daily in 4-hour shifts and are paid at an hourly rate. They have made themselves indispensable.*

These foster grandparents work not only in institutions but may be available to help in the home as well.

A case history

Janet, a waif who had never known her mother, had been shunted from one foster home to another throughout her short life. Severely retarded, she gradually became completely unmanageable and landed eventually in a state-supported residential home.

When seen by those studying methods for helping such children, she seemed to deserve the label of "hopeless." She pinched and bit anyone who came near her. Food and dishes were sent flying. The only way she could be fed was by fastening her arms to her side and keeping out of the way of the food she blew out of her mouth. Even foster grandmothers could not give her care. She pinched them and smashed their eyeglasses before they could get started.

Then a program was started in a quiet room with no distractions. The student working with her removed her glasses and covered her own clothing. Janet was offered spoonfuls of food she liked. Patiently, time after time, spoons were retrieved, messes were cleaned up, and Janet was told firmly, "No, no." After several such private lessons, she was taken to the ward for a time, then brought back to the room for another try.

Within a few days, Janet kept her left arm at her side and grasped the spoon in her right, although still only to throw it. A few days later, though, she fed herself three or four mouthfuls before throwing. And the day finally arrived when the student felt real progress had been achieved. No, Janet had not

* For more information, contact your state or national Association for Retarded Children.

stopped throwing. But she did allow the student to hold her in her lap. Not only that, but she snuggled up closely. It was beginning to penetrate her emotionally starved mind that someone really cared for her. This was the most important step. The others would follow, given time and patience.

Helping your child at home

There are excellent books concerning the care and understanding of the retarded child in his own family. One of the best is Laura L. Dittmann's *The Mentally Retarded Child at Home.** This small book gives practical and sympathetic help for day-to-day problems. It includes guidance for toilet training and for teaching your child such basic skills as dressing and feeding himself. Other books are listed in the References.

Parents need frequent help as they try, often without apparent success, to guide their children along the road to independence. Special methods are needed, not special kinds of teaching methods but rather knowledge of how to break each step down into its simplest parts. As the child masters a simple movement, he builds on this until eventually all the movements involved in an action fit together. Few of us realize the complicated learning involved in the simple act of putting a button through a buttonhole.

Other sources of help can be found in your own community when you need them. Contact your state, city, or county health bureau or the local chapter of the Association for Retarded Children.

Discipline

In the sense of teaching acceptable and unacceptable behavior, discipline is as important for the retarded child as it is for any other. But it entails additional considerations because of the retarded child's limited ability to adapt his own behavior.

Discipline must always be consistent so the child will know what to expect. Language must be simple and direct; complicated explanation will only confuse him. Showing him what you want by example and demonstration—"Do it this way"—

* Children's Bureau Publication No. 374.

will bring better results than "Don't touch" or "Stop that."

The way to achieve best results without causing resentment and stubbornness is to set up a daily schedule and keep to it as closely as possible. Retarded children do well on routine. You will need to remind him, "After you put your blocks away, we'll have dinner," and at the same time give him a hand to get started.

Miss Dittmann tells about David, a mongoloid child.

Even at 3 he can be as stubborn as a ton of cement when it comes to leaving one thing and starting the next. He twinkles and smiles, but won't budge. . . . When his mother insists that he get out of the bathtub he . . . howls and hits at her arms as she reaches for him. . . . She lifts him out, singing a song about bedtime and slippers. And David gets absorbed in rubbing the soft fur of his slippers and forgets all his objections. If his mother became confused about her requests and let David win, bathtime the next night might be even more difficult. By the time David is 12, possibly no one can get him to do anything.*

Firmness and consistency are essential, but so are kindness, love, and understanding. Time out for a kiss for the hurt finger, for rocking a tired child, are important parts of the day.

When punishment is needed, it must follow the deed directly to be understood. The child may need to be taken away from the group, quietly but firmly, to help him gain self-control. If he is using "bad" behavior, perhaps more praise and approval whenever he behaves well may take away his need to misbehave.

Special classes

A child who experiences difficulty learning deserves a place where he can learn at his own speed. He may never learn if he sees his classmates easily grasping concepts that have no meaning to him.

City schools make provision for classes adapted to the needs of those who have difficulty learning. You will find these classes labeled as being for "trainable" or "educable" children. When a

* Dittmann, *The Mentally Retarded Child at Home*, p. 39.

child has difficulty learning but has normal sight and hearing, he is given intelligence tests before being placed in a special class. He will also be tested at intervals to evaluate any gains he has made. No one is interested in keeping a child in a certain group when he is capable of moving on.

Parents do their children a great wrong when they insist they be placed with others of greater learning ability. If they will examine themselves, they will find they are catering to their own wishes while ignoring the child's needs.

Community efforts

Some communities have united to provide preschool classes for retarded children. The classes are "preschool" in that they work to prepare the children for school. They are geared to the child's mental development, rather than his age. Here is one striking example.

In Tucson, Arizona, there was no provision made for retarded children in the public school system, and so a group of mothers of these children decided to do something rather than just talk about the need for a school. In 1962, with help from the Association for Retarded Children, they started a preschool for trainable retardates.* The community helped. Money for operations came from various sources. A church offered the use of its parish hall for five days a week.

Today this school has its own building. It has classes for retarded children from the age of 3. The only prerequisites for admission are that the child be trainable in self-care and be able to adapt to a group program. Classes are small, with a limit of 8 in a group. Parents are encouraged to help, and many do. Other volunteers are welcomed also. Financial needs are met by donations, memberships, and the maintenance of a thrift shop. A small tuition fee is charged, and scholarships are available. This group also provides a work activities center for severely retarded adults.

The program is aimed at providing opportunities for growth in self-care, physical coordination, language and speech development, and social adjustment. It has been eminently successful.

* Beacon Foundation for the Mentally Retarded, 25 East Drachman Street, Tucson, Arizona 85705.

PART TWO
Health Problems

8

A Doctor for Your Child

Some of you have no problem deciding what doctor is to help take care of your baby or older children. Perhaps you live in a small town and have a fine general practitioner who looks after all the children as they come along. Maybe he is even the doctor who took care of *you* as a child. But if you live in a city, particularly one of the larger ones, you may need advice. Don't worry; it is available.

If you are pregnant, ask the doctor who is giving you obstetric care. He knows pediatricians and general practitioners who do good children's work and can give you the names of several, especially those located conveniently for you.

If you are newly arrived in a strange city and need a doctor for an older child, call the local children's hospital and ask to speak to the chief resident. He is a man in the last year of extensive training, and he knows the whole staff. Ask him for the name of a doctor practicing in your area of the city. If there is no children's hospital, call the local general hospital and ask for the name of the head of the children's department. Then call him and ask if he can take your children as patients or refer you to a member of his staff who can. If you find your child's doctor this way, you are not likely to go wrong.

Asking your neighbors about a local doctor is another way,

but it is amazing how full of faults this method sometimes proves to be. It may work out beautifully, but it's chancy.

You may have asked yourself whether you want a pediatrician or a general practitioner. *Either may be perfectly satisfactory.* What you want is a doctor who has a real understanding of children and their problems.

General practitioners take care of 80 percent of the children in the United States. Why, then, should you consider a pediatrician? Because pediatricians are child specialists. They are really general practitioners who have confined their work to children. Their offices are geared to babies and children. They have received at least two extra years of training in the diseases and problems of childhood. They become adept at recognizing significant abnormalities in child growth and development; and, just as important, they understand clearly the wide variations in what is normal. Furthermore, pediatrics has been very important in the development of *preventive* medical care.

People sometimes have the impression that a pediatrician's care costs more. While fees vary in different parts of the country, pediatric office charges are usually about the same as general charges in the same area.

If you decide on a pediatrician for your children, he will want to see them at regular intervals, perhaps once a month for the first 4 months, every 3 or 4 months for older babies, and once a year after the second or third birthday. Some of the routine work in his office may be done by nurse assistants, but your doctor will be fully in charge and will know every important thing about your child.

Once you have selected a doctor for your child, give the arrangement a fair trial—but remember it is not irrevocable. You have a right to make a change if you find you do not get along with the doctor you have chosen. The doctor, too, has a right to discontinue with you if he senses a personality clash. A successful doctor-patient relationship is based on mutual respect and cooperation. Pediatricians rarely encounter a child with whom they have more than temporary difficulty, but how *parents* handle visits to the doctor is of some importance and deserves a bit more discussion.

285

If private office fees are beyond your means, ask about local hospital pediatric clinics or those run by city or county health departments. Charges are usually scaled to your income. Many pediatricians donate part of their time to service in such clinics.

THREE-WAY COMMUNICATION: THE DOCTOR, YOUR CHILD, AND YOU

Doctors, like everyone else, have their own individual personalities. At the extremes they range from the glad-hander to the quiet, noncommittal type. The man with whom you find it somewhat hard to communicate may get along with your child just fine. On the other hand, the man who socializes happily with you may make your son or daughter feel left out; the child may feel that the visit is really yours and that he has just been brought in for repairs like a broken appliance. Ideally, you want a doctor who is at ease with both you and your children, and fortunately that's the way it usually works out.

You should give your child a chance to establish his own rapport with the doctor, and let the physician establish contact without benefit of your explanations of your child's behavior. The majority of infants and children are very cooperative patients—most of the time. A few between the ages of 10 months and 3 years balk consistently. If they do carry on in the doctor's office despite their parents' reassurance, their behavior should be accepted without adult comment. The doctor will do what needs to be done with whatever firmness is necessary. Perhaps he'll remark, "It doesn't matter. He'll be better next time," but that's as far as it should go. To discuss it further is to give the matter undue importance in the child's eyes.

It is always best to take a young child's visit to the doctor's office as a matter of course. No big buildup is needed. When a mother comes through an examining room door with a 3- or 4-year-old and says, "Jimmy, this is Dr. Lee—he's a *nice* man," Dr. Lee knows he may be in for a rough time. That word *nice* plants suspicion in Jimmy right away. After all, she doesn't tell him that about other people. If she adds, "He won't hurt you," things are apt to be even worse. More than likely, the idea of *hurt* hadn't entered the child's mind until that moment.

Pediatricians bless the parent who takes a visit to the doctor in stride and handles it like any other routine part of daily living.

With older children the doctor often likes to direct questions to the patient himself before getting more information from the mother or father. The doctor might be examining the abdomen of a child who has been having stomachaches. He is doing fine gathering information by a few words between himself and the patient while he is probing carefully with his fingers. Suddenly the mother leans over and says, "It hurts right there." Putting words in a child's mouth is seldom helpful to the doctor.

Among the many reasons that children are usually wonderful patients is the fact that they do not ordinarily enlarge upon or minimize symptoms, except sometimes for their family's benefit. And when they do exaggerate or unduly minimize, it is usually obvious to the experienced physician.

Don't underestimate the doctor's ability to read many subtle signs, not all of them verbal. People who work with children often develop a sort of sixth sense that can yield phenomenal amounts of information with a minimum of talk. *Children sense this, and they know when their signals are being received.*

Doctors vary in the degree to which they can develop this ability to communicate with children, but if you sense a subtle communication between your child and his doctor, you should consider it a great asset.

It has, by the way, very little to do with whether or not the doctor seems sympathetic to your child's tears or tantrums. Indeed, oversympathy is not at all a part of what we have been describing and may even make it impossible. With children as well as with adults, the physician must be able to maintain objectivity. He cannot, after all, be swayed against taking a blood count because it will be momentarily unpleasant for the child! And he can be truly friendly with a sick child without being obviously affectionate. Children of all ages accept this limited relationship without resentment.

Again, though, parents sometimes make things more difficult by trying too hard to help. For example, say that the doctor is taking a blood-pressure reading as part of a physical examination. He will approach it matter-of-factly with a young child, probably without using the term *blood pressure*. After all, some children are likely to hear only the word *blood*. So the doctor will just pick up the cuff and say, "I'm going to measure how strong your arm is, and this is the gadget that will do it. Are you good and strong?" Usually there is no problem.

Unless, that is, he is dealing with a parent who is convinced that everything must be explained to a child in great detail. Then, all too often, as the doctor picks up the instrument and before he can say a word, the parent will say, "He's going to take your blood pressure. It won't hurt." The word *blood*, the word *hurt*—both are frightening to the child. Now there may be a problem getting a good pressure reading.

Don't misunderstand. Parents can provide valuable reassurance. There is a time and a place for lots of clinging—and that's most of the time and lots of places. But do be casual about things that must be done. Remember, too, that real trust and rapport with children is not built on promises, threats, or lollipops.

WHEN SHOULD YOU CALL THE DOCTOR?

Have you ever found yourself wondering whether or not to call your child's doctor? It is a recurring predicament. Many parents would like to avoid a doctor's bill but are perfectly willing to spend the money if necessary. They want to feel competent to make small decisions—and yet they do not want to be responsible for making a mistake.

Vivid accounts of unusual diseases in magazines and newspapers, on television and radio, and in numerous advertisements leave parents with the feeling that deadly illnesses await their children at every turn. As a result, some parents develop very real fears about even the simplest childhood ailment. Granted that an occasional child does develop a serious disease, you should always remember that the probabilities are strongly against it. Worry, instead, about the poisonous substances in the cupboard under the kitchen sink or in the family medicine cabinet, or about your child's safety in the family car. In terms of probability these are far more likely sources of injury or death than rheumatic fever, leukemia, meningitis, or all the other uncommon serious illnesses of childhood put together.

It is easy to decide to call when the child is obviously sick; the difficulty comes when a trivial complaint gradually builds up into a big worry in your mind. If that happens, call for the sake of having your doubts relieved. It will be better for the child, too, for a worried parent can unknowingly upset his child.

When you call the doctor about a child's illness, one of the things he will want to know is whether there is any fever. Underarm temperatures are very inaccurate. With older children who will cooperate you can take mouth temperatures by having them hold the tip of the thermometer under the tongue for a full minute (all thermometers will go nearly as high in one minute as in three, and the last fraction of a degree doesn't matter anyway). Depending on the time of day and the degree of activity, a child's normal temperature will vary from about 97.4 to 99.6. Usually it will be about 98.6.

For babies, the temperature is best taken rectally. The only difference between a mouth and a rectal thermometer is the size of the mercury bulb; a rectal thermometer's bulb is shorter and rounder. Rectal temperatures average about 1 degree higher than oral, but don't add or subtract anything when you report to the doctor.

Taking a rectal temperature is very simple. Lay the baby or young child on its stomach across your lap or on a bed or table.

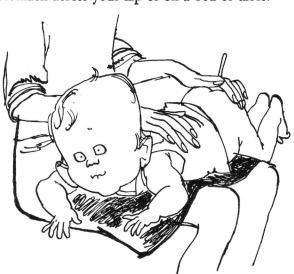

Lubricate the tip of the thermometer with petroleum jelly, cold cream, or salad oil, separate the buttocks with the thumb and finger of one hand, and with the other hand insert the tip of the thermometer into the rectum about 1 to 2 inches. Release the buttocks and hold the thermometer in place between your fingers with the hand flat on the buttocks. This will both steady the thermometer and keep the child from rolling. After a full minute, remove it. Roll the thermometer between your fingers until you can see the mercury column and the numbers. Wash the thermometer with cool water and soap and shake the mercury down so that it will be ready for use another time. Never wash it with hot water.

Parents may wonder how a doctor can give a definite answer after just a few questions or a brief examination. The answer is that what seems a complex problem to a parent is very often commonplace in a doctor's daily experience. People often say, "It must be very difficult to work with babies who can't talk." Quite the reverse is true. Children do not complicate the picture by an overlay of half-knowledge and opinion that might distort the answers they give. If the child is too young to talk, the experienced doctor goes by what he can see and hear and feel plus such symptoms as the parents describe. His ear is very sensitive to little shades of difference from the normal in descriptions of symptoms and to deviations from the average upon examination.

So call the doctor when you are in doubt. Call so that his knowledge and experience may relieve your concern.

WHEN YOU DO CALL THE DOCTOR

Once you have made up your mind to call the doctor, have your facts in order. A busy man may have fifty or more phone calls in a day and night. It is necessary that he keep them as brief as possible. Come right to the point. Be specific, and he will ask whatever else he needs to know. Listen to what he says and jot down any directions, doses, or appointment times. Something like the following pattern on the phone will serve both you and the doctor best.

1. Give your full name and address. (He may have several Mrs. Browns.)
2. Give your child's name and age.
3. Tell him why you have called—just the central fact. Don't try to give a detailed past history on the phone unless you are asked for it.
4. Mention when the trouble started, what came first, and what, if anything, you have done.
5. If you can, give the child's temperature.

Then let the doctor respond. He will know what questions to ask in relation to what you have told him. Let him lead the conversation, but don't hesitate to add anything you feel is important. If the next-door neighbors had scarlet fever last week, he obviously needs to know that.

Are you thinking, This is all so obvious? Let us show you by means of two recorded calls what a difference your phone technique can make.

"This is Mrs. Thomas Daly on Meade Street. My boy Charles—he's two and a half—threw up twice this morning, and now his temperature is a hundred and three."

"Does he have any diarrhea?"

"No."

"Any other symptoms at all?"

"It seems a little hard for him to swallow."

"Could be. Lots of strep throats around right now. Can you get him to the office at three forty-five?"

"Bring him out with a fever?"

"Under these circumstances it won't hurt him. We'll take a throat culture if we need it."

"All right. Three forty-five."

"Tell the girl at the desk to put you in one of the side rooms, not in the regular waiting room. See you there."

Everything necessary is included. Now listen to the following recording:

"This is Mrs. Allen. Is this Dr. Lee?"

"Yes, go ahead."

"Well, this is Mrs. Allen. How are you, Dr. Lee?"

"Fine, thanks."

"Remember when you filled out a camp form for Johnny last spring?"

"I did a lot of them."

"Well, he went to camp and he was O.K. when he got home in September—no, it was the last week in August, I guess—but now he has a stomachache all the time."

"All the time?"

"Well, sometimes it's all the time."

"When did it begin?"

"Well, when he got back from camp he was O.K. for three or four weeks, and then this stomachache started up. It started on the first day of Sunday School."

"How long ago was that?"

"Two weeks ago—no, it must have been three weeks, I guess, because my mother was here last week."

"Does the pain stop him from playing?"

"Are you kidding? Nothing stops him."

"How much of the time does he have the pain? Any special time of day? In the morning? After meals?"

"Sometimes he has it all the time. I think you should see him as soon as you can."

"All right. I'll transfer you to my secretary. Tell her I said to work him in this afternoon."

"How can I do that? He goes to school all day."

Sometimes you call merely to get the answer to what appears to you to be a simple question and are surprised that the doctor suggests that your child be examined. Perhaps you said, "My daughter, she's four now, complains of a full feeling in her ear and sometimes a popping sound. Could you prescribe something to clear it up?" He probably will not wish to do so without first examining her, because several different ear conditions can cause those symptoms. But by looking in the ear with the proper instrument, the doctor can tell whether the trouble is due to an infection, an obstructed eustachian tube, or an accumulation of fluid in the middle ear space—three conditions requiring different treatments.

A FEW DON'TS FOR THE TELEPHONE

Don't try to make an emergency out of some minor problem. You may get the doctor's immediate attention that way, but it may not work so well a second time. "Crying wolf" applies to adults as well as children.

Don't call repeatedly to ask the same thing. Some mothers call every time their baby has a fresh runny nose. Once you've learned what to do about a simple problem, handle it yourself unless you encounter something new.

And *don't* rush to the phone until you assess a situation.

"Doctor, please come quick. Bobby has a terrible cut."

"How bad? Where?"

"I don't know, he won't let me look."

"How fast can you get him to the hospital? I'll meet you there."

"I don't think it's *that* bad."

"Well, grab him and have a look. I'll hold the wire."

"O.K., wait a minute. . . . It's not so very big, Doctor."

"Where is the cut?"

"His hand."

"How big? I really need to know that."

"I guess not so big. It's at the tip end of his finger."

"*How* big?"

"It's really kind of little. Maybe I could just put a Band-Aid on it?"

9
General Health Questions

As a child grows, there are questions that come up about variations from the normal. Lacking experience of the range of normal conditions, you may find yourself in doubt. This chapter explains some of these variations and some broad aspects of health supervision.

IMMUNIZATIONS

You would not willingly let your child starve. You must not let him go without today's wonderful immunizations. You gave your child life—now give him protection against preventable diseases. The cost is trivial compared to the protection. The materials used have been steadily improved until now even mild reactions to vaccines are uncommon.

The following table gives a basic schedule. Your doctor may modify the timing somewhat, but none of these injections should be omitted.

Basic Schedule of Immunizations *

Usual Age	Material	Protects Against
1 to 2 months	D.P.T.	Diphtheria, whooping cough, and tetanus
	Oral polio vaccine	Paralytic polio
3 to 4 months	D.P.T.	As above
	Oral polio vaccine	
5 to 6 months	D.P.T.	As above
	Oral polio vaccine	
1 year †	Measles vaccine	Measles
	Tuberculin test	
18 months to 12 years	German measles and mumps vaccines ‡	German measles and mumps
18 months	D.P.T.	Diphtheria, whooping cough, and tetanus
	Oral polio vaccine	Paralytic polio
4 to 6 years	D.P.T.	Diphtheria, whooping cough and tetanus
	Oral polio vaccine	Paralytic polio
_2 to 16 years	D.T.	Diphtheria and tetanus

* There will be certain variations in program with various population groups, geographic areas, and epidemic conditions.

† Smallpox is disappearing throughout most of the civilized world; there have been no cases in the United States for several years. Smallpox vaccination will no longer be required in the United States except for special groups and travelers, to and from certain countries where cases still occur.

‡ Combined vaccines are available. German measles-mumps combination is in general use; others may be in use soon.

ANTIBIOTICS

Miracle drugs: we have seen the phrase so often that it has partly lost its meaning. Too bad, for in a sense that is what antibiotics are—or, at least, appear to be. Certainly they save countless lives, and their effect on serious infection often seems miraculous. But they are not cure-alls and they must not be used as such.

Penicillin was the first of these drugs. It was discovered as the result of an accidental laboratory happening, observed by a general practitioner named Alexander Fleming. Dr. Fleming's observation set off a search for additional substances that might kill germs without killing the patient. Other antibiotics were discovered in nature, and some have been prepared artificially in research laboratories.

Many types of dangerous infections are cured by the use of these drugs, *but diseases caused by viruses are not.* Unfortunately, the common cold and most upper respiratory infections are viral infections and are therefore not helped by any presently known antibiotic.

A considerable number of antibiotics are available to your doctor. The effectiveness and method of use varies from one antibiotic to another, the dose varies, and the occasional unpleasant side effects vary. It is a complex area of knowledge, and doctors have to study diligently to keep up with it.

Physicians are repeatedly amazed at the willingness of some patients to dose themselves or their children with these potent materials they know so little about. Every pediatrician sees the disgruntled parent who wants "a shot of penicillin" for anything wrong with her child.

When your doctor decides on an antibiotic for your baby or child, he has many things to consider: which one to use, in what dose, and by what method to give it. And he must weigh the risk of not using the antibiotic against the risk of unwanted, unpleasant, or dangerous side effects.

Don't urge the doctor to give a shot as opposed to medicine given by mouth because you feel it is quicker. It may be quicker, but it is sometimes dangerous. The injection route for antibiotics should be used only when the oral route is for some reason unavailable.

Don't pester your child's doctor for penicillin or other drugs just because you feel that "something must be done." Don't object if he does not want to prescribe such medicine without examining the child. If he does prescribe an antibiotic, don't cut his orders short. If an antibiotic is needed at all, it is needed for the full time for which it was prescribed. To stop beforehand may expose the child to complications of the disease for which the medicine was being used.

If you believe the child is having some allergic or other reaction, tell the doctor about it promptly.

Don't start an antibiotic without your doctor's advice.

Don't give your child an antibiotic that you have left over from some prior illness on the assumption that he has the same illness again.

Don't play doctor with antibiotics!

X RAYS

Parents frequently suggest that they would like to have some X rays taken. They seem to have the idea that X rays can solve almost any puzzling medical problem.

An X-ray picture is sometimes vitally important. The trouble is that X rays are often ordered when they are not actually needed.

Why not have the X ray? Why should this *not* be done? Because too much exposure to X rays in a lifetime can be harmful. The dose of radiation absorbed as a result of making an ordinary X ray of a bone or chest is quite small, but *it is the total in a lifetime that matters.* We receive a certain amount of background radiation from outer space every day. We should never add to the total by taking a single unnecessary X-ray picture.

Most pediatricians believe, for instance, that there is little justification for the repeated "full mouth survey" X rays used by some dentists in their search for an occasional tiny hidden cavity. A small cavity that can be filled when it becomes obvious is a lesser hazard, in our opinion, than frequently repeated X rays. An occasional dental film is certainly acceptable, but full mouth surveys on an annual or semiannual basis are not; they can add up to a total of 12 to 24 such surveys between the ages of 4 and 16. You have a perfect right to explain to your dentist that you prefer minimum use of X ray on your family.

Many minor injuries are X-rayed when they could be treated without such exposure. The doctors are not entirely at fault. Certain traditions have developed, supported by the law, about routine X rays when payment for accidents is involved. Thousands of skull X rays are taken after head injuries even though the patient is getting along perfectly well, because some lawyers may demand reports in such a way as to raise a question about the thoroughness of the doctor's care (despite the fact that an

X ray would have contributed no information of medical value).

Cases of vague abdominal pain are exceedingly common in childhood, but a careful history and physical examination may make the usual "G.I. series" X rays unnecessary. This particular examination rarely solves the child's problem and hardly ever produces useful information.

The point is this: No child should be exposed to *any* unnecessary X rays. You should not demand X-ray studies that your doctor may feel are actually not needed. You might better ask yourself and your doctor in each instance, "Is this particular X-ray exposure really necessary?" If it is necessary, fine; it should be done, and in sufficient detail to make certain that the maximum possible information is obtained. But whenever the child can be treated safely without it, avoid an X ray.

EYES AND SIGHT

When your baby was born his eyes were approximately three fourths of their adult size. Thus his eyes will grow by only 25 percent while the rest of his body doubles and redoubles until at maturity it is about 15 times birth weight. Considering their complexity, the eyes are remarkably free from trouble, but if you ever have doubts about your child's eyes at any age you should have them examined promptly.

Faulty vision

Blindness at birth is very rare indeed, for infection of eyes occurring during the birth of a baby is now prevented.

We cannot measure a newborn's vision immediately, but we can be sure that if the eye is structurally normal there is not likely to be any impairment of sight. By the end of 2 weeks it becomes obvious that babies do look at large objects, but it is not until they are between 7 and 10 weeks that they begin to follow movement. At this point you will know that your baby is really using his eyes.

A blind baby will not follow your movements and usually moves his eyes less than normal except, sometimes, for a peculiar flicking side-to-side movement called nystagmus.

It sometimes takes inexperienced parents a long time to

notice that their infant has a severe visual defect. Probably that is because a child with such a defect has never known anything different. There is no change in his behavior to call attention to the problem, as there is when a sighted child loses his sight.

It is quite difficult to detect minor degrees of visual defect in babies and very young children. Later, when they are able to take tests involving pictures, letters, or numbers, it becomes much simpler. But, fortunately, minor degrees of farsightedness, nearsightedness, or astigmatism do no harm to the eyes. They cause little or no trouble until the time comes for the close work of reading. Nevertheless, if you have doubts about your very young child's visual abilities, have him examined by an eye specialist. With special instruments there are ways of measuring vision indirectly.

The following things are reasons for a full examination:

> Turning in or turning out of an eye that has previously been straight.
> Holding objects or books closer than previously.
> Tipping the head when examining things closely.
> Any complaint of pain, aching, or tiredness in the eyes.
> Redness or watering that clears up with rest.
> Frequent headaches.
> Deteriorating schoolwork or a gradual discontinuance of reading and other activities requiring close eyework.
> Otherwise unexplained recurrent nausea.

The usual testing by means of letters on a chart is adequate for routine screening of the vision of older children. It is not sufficiently accurate for the testing of any child suspected of having a visual problem. Such a child will need more detailed examination.

Some pediatricians make rather complete eye testing a part of routine health supervision, using equipment productive of more detailed analysis than the simple test charts. If your doctor does not do this sort of testing, it will be a good idea to have your child's eyes checked by an eye specialist when school begins.

Other eye problems

Obstructed tear ducts. A little channel, the tear duct, drains tears from the eyes into the nose. Its opening is in the inner corner of the eye, about where the lids join. The fluid we call tears is constantly produced to keep the surface of the eye moist and clean. If it were not for the tear duct, this fluid would constantly overflow the eyelids and run down the face. When we cry, an excess of tears is produced and the overflow occurs.

In young babies the tear duct is very tiny and sometimes can't quite handle all the normal secretion. Then the baby seems to have a watery eye on one or both sides. The condition corrects itself as the tear duct grows larger, and by the time the baby is 3 to 6 months old the problem should be gone. If it persists beyond that age, call it to the doctor's attention.

Crossed eyes. During the first month or 6 weeks of life it is not at all uncommon for a baby's eyes to turn in too much *at times,* especially when the child is sleepy. It is not abnormal at this early age if it happens only sometimes. If it is constant or frequent it is not normal and you should ask the doctor about it. A crossed eye that is ignored too long will not develop normal vision. Either one or both eyes may be involved.

Occasionally an eye turns too far out instead of too far in. The time and type of treatment for these wandering eyes will depend on several factors that are quite technical. The decision will have to rest with the eye specialist.

Pink-eye (conjunctivitis). Children are quite susceptible to mild infections of the membranes which line the eyelids and cover the white of the eye. With conjunctivitis, or pink-eye, the eye appears reddened and there is often a yellowish discharge in the corners and along the lids. If there is enough discharge, the lids may stick together when the child is asleep. To unstick them, wet a piece of cotton or a soft cloth with warm water and gently apply it to the dried secretion. Sometimes there is moderate discomfort. The child's rubbing may further irritate the eyes and cause the lids to swell.

Pink-eye is quite contagious for other children, and it often spreads rapidly in schools, play groups, swimming pools, or other places where children are close together.

While these infections are seldom serious, it is best to call the doctor. There are highly effective medicines that he can order. In the meantime drugstores have soothing lotions that can be safely used. They are available under the general name *collyrium* or under various brand names.

The slight redness that occurs with colds and the itchy, watery, and sometimes reddened eyes that go with hay fever are not at all the same as pink-eye and do not have the same thick, sticky discharge.

Swollen eyelids. There are quite a few causes of swollen lids, but insect bites are the most frequent and the most likely to produce swelling of only one lid.

Any infection or irritation such as pink-eye, a stye (described farther on under the heading of Lumps), or any foreign material that causes the child to rub his eyes may result in some swelling.

Puffy lids often occur with allergies (see Chapter 12). Hay fever is the commonest offender, but food allergies may also be the cause.

Sinus infections occurring with or after colds may cause marked swelling. In such cases the child usually feels sick and has pain or headache. Sinus infections accompanied by swelling of eyelids need medical attention promptly (see Chapter 11).

Certain kidney diseases may cause great swelling of the lids, but these diseases are quite uncommon. (They are described in Chapter 15.)

EARS AND HEARING

It is rare for a baby to be born deaf. If one is, this should be discovered as soon as possible so that special training can be started early.

It is not very difficult to discover *total* deafness in newborn babies, but despite the articles in popular magazines it is not a simple matter to determine partially defective hearing. Total deafness is indicated by the baby's lack of reaction to an unexpected loud sound. For testing, the baby should be lying quietly,

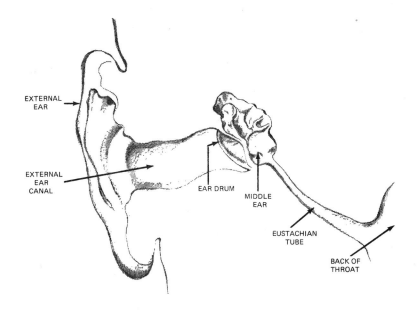

EXTERNAL
EAR

EXTERNAL
EAR
CANAL

EAR DRUM

MIDDLE
EAR

EUSTACHIAN
TUBE

BACK OF
THROAT

placed so that he cannot see the person testing him. In order to avoid a response to jarring or vibration, the tester should be careful not to touch the crib. When all is ready, the tester sounds a noisemaker or bangs two pans together. If the baby appears startled, he hears.

It is hard to be sure the baby hears softer sounds until a bit later when, at about 3 months, he responds to spoken words. Parents do not often fail to notice total deafness in their child, but they are often unaware of hearing that is far below normal. Delay in the beginning use of words by a baby who is otherwise obviously intelligent suggests at least partial deafness, and a careful professional testing of the hearing should be done. No child should be considered slow or backward until it is certain that his hearing is normal.

The majority of doctors' offices are not well equipped to test hearing in babies and very young children. If you have any doubts you will need the help of an ear specialist or a special hearing clinic.

LEGS, FEET, AND JOINTS

Before birth, babies are folded up quite tightly. In the last weeks of pregnancy there is not much room for them to move around and they may lie in one position for many weeks, unable to stretch arms or legs. After birth the legs may appear quite bowed at first, or the feet turned in. This is normal.

One of the many things checked by the doctor on the very first examination is the range of motion of the hips, knees, ankles, and joints of the feet. If these are normal, the appearance of bowlegs and turned-in or turned-out feet is unimportant.

When your infant has regular health checkups you will notice that the doctor continues to watch his legs, feet, and joints for the normal pattern of change. Those doctors who are most experienced with babies and young children usually recommend little in the way of corrective shoes, braces, and other apparatus because they know nature's patterns of self-correction. Some shoe stores and some less experienced physicians tend to use corrective measures which are unnecessary.

Grandparents, friends, and neighbors may upset you with remarks about your child's legs and feet. That's because old myths are persistent. For example, rickets used to be prevalent. This is a nutritional disease causing soft bones that once badly deformed the legs of toddlers. Good diet and vitamins totally prevent rickets now. It is rare except in extreme poverty areas.

Bowlegs. As we said, almost all young babies are bowlegged. Unless the condition is extreme, it requires no treatment. Contrary to popular belief standing and walking do not make bowleg worse; standing is the beginning of self-correction. The legs straighten as they bear weight and walking begins. During the child's second and third years the doctor will check on the progress of the straightening. Only if it fails to proceed normally will corrective measures be needed.

Knock-knee. Between the ages of 1 and 4 many children appear knock-kneed. The condition is often more obvious in boys than in girls. A child standing with his knees just touching may have as much as a 4-inch gap between his ankles.

Again, this is a condition that tends to correct itself. Occasionally, if there is also marked toeing-in and the doctor finds things not improving at a normal rate, he may decide to add little wedges or supports in the shoes. But only a trained person should make this decision and prescribe any necessary corrective shoes. Ill-advised or too much correction may do more harm than good.

Flatfoot. All babies and very young children appear flatfooted. You cannot see the arch in their feet; what there is of it, and that's not much, is filled in by fat pads. Not until a child is past 4 will the beginnings of the arch be apparent.

Nearly every mother asks about her child's flat feet—and most of the time what she is questioning is the chubby, perfectly normal infant foot.

The doctor checks a child's feet at every health examination—or he should. He can tell a great deal at a glance as the child walks and still more by looking at the soles of the shoes. So when you take your child for a checkup, it's fine to have him clean and wearing his best, but if he has on new shoes be sure to take the old ones along too. A great deal of information about your child's feet is written on the soles of the old shoes.

Once in a while a child has flat feet along with an excessive toeing out and a tendency for the foot to roll outward at the ankle. Then corrective exercises or special shoes may be needed.

Under no circumstances should you add arch supports to your child's shoes before having his feet examined by an expert. The arch of the foot is supported, at least in part, by muscles. Arch supports, by relieving the developing muscles of part of their job, sometimes make matters worse in the long run.

But if you feel your older child's feet are excessively flat, ask his doctor about it—and don't forget to take along those old shoes.

Toeing out. Many babies toe out when they are learning to walk. It gives them a steadier base. Gradually the toeing out becomes less and less noticeable. Toeing out usually requires no treatment. If it does not improve with time or appears really excessive to you, ask the doctor about it.

Toeing in (pigeon toe). Many cases of pigeon toe will correct themselves—many, but not all. The reason is that there are three types of toeing in, and the three require different management.

In the first and commonest kind, the front half of the foot is turned inward but the rest of the foot and leg are normal in position. What's to be done depends on how severe the in-turning is. When it is mild, the parent can be taught how to stretch and straighten the foot a little bit every day so that by the time the baby is ready to walk the foot will straighten easily to its normal position. Then the mere act of walking will complete the correction. If the turning in of the forefoot is more severe, correcting it may require that the baby wear special shoes long before he is ready to walk. A few cases require temporary casts on the lower legs and feet. But no matter what its severity, it is correctable—as long as those needing treatment are treated early.

The second type of pigeon toe results when the main leg bone below the knee (tibia) is turned or rotated inward. Often there is rather marked bowleg with this type. Provided the foot itself is normal (let the doctor decide), this kind of pigeon toe will correct itself with growth and walking. Yet all too often we see casts, braces, or special shoes on these babies. The result is unnecessary expense and effort for the parents and sometimes discomfort for the child. But parents or grandparents can be very persistent if they think a child's feet do not look right. And even if their doctor tells them otherwise, they may shop around until they find someone who agrees with them—often to his own profit.

The third type of pigeon toe results from inward rotation of the thighbone (femur). You'll need the doctor's help to determine this. Fortunately, it is another self-correcting condition.

Again we say: Beware the expense of special shoes and apparatus unless they are ordered by your doctor. Though many shoe stores are perfectly reliable, others employ self-styled "experts" who seem to have little grasp of what really needs correcting and what will correct itself.

Clubfoot. Real clubfoot is a rare defect. The foot is pointed down, turned in, and firmly fixed in this position. The condition is caused by the absence of certain bones or muscles or, in some cases, by the fusing together of bones in the ankle and foot. Its correction requires highly skilled treatment by a bone specialist. One or more operations are often required.

Congenital dislocation of the hip. This condition, a faulty development of the socket of the hip joint, can be detected only by careful physical examination of the baby, and it is therefore seldom noticed by the parents. It is *not* always possible to find it immediately after birth. Most often it is discovered between the ages of 1 and 3 months. Results of corrective treatment are excellent, provided the condition is found early. If not corrected before a child is older, the child will walk with a strange waddle for which the treatment will be very difficult and the results less satisfactory. Most cases can be treated without operation by simple splints to hold the legs in a corrective position. Strangely enough, babies do not mind the splints. Early discovery of this problem is still another reason for health checkups.

Other hip conditions. A limp that develops in the absence of any obvious injury to leg or foot should not be taken lightly. Somehow parents do not seem to pay as much attention to a limp as they do to many less important things. If a limp persists for more than two or three days, you should have the child examined. Limping is often a sign of trouble in the hip joint, even though the pain often occurs in the region of the knee. The child should have a careful examination; sometimes X rays are needed.

Most problems of the hip joint require treatment. It may be nothing more than a few days' rest without weight-bearing, but that rest may be very important. In other cases, prolonged treatment may be needed to avoid permanent damage. Do not ignore a persistent limp in any child of any age.

LUMPS

From time to time you may be frightened by the discovery of a little lump on your child. Most such lumps are quite harmless, but without special training and experience you cannot know by their location and feel just what they are. Therefore you are perfectly right to call the attention of the doctor to any lump that you can't identify. Let him decide whether anything needs to be done. To relieve your mind, we will identify here some of the commonest of the lumps.

Enlarged lymph glands. The lymph glands are scattered about the body as part of the defense system. Generally they are so small and soft that they cannot be felt or seen. But when there is an infection in a particular area, the lymph glands in that area may enlarge. You are particularly likely to notice them in the groin, in the armpit, on the sides of the neck, and at the back of the skull under the scalp. Even an insect bite may cause local lymph glands to swell. So may a scratch, tiny cut, pimple, or any other injury. If they are tender, are accompanied by fever, or are getting bigger rather than smaller after a day or two, let the doctor know. Once enlarged, they may sometimes take weeks or even months to return to their previous size.

LUMPS UNDER THE SCALP. With some families it is quite common to have small cysts in various locations under the scalp. These usually do not become apparent until late childhood. They are harmless, though sometimes they become quite large.

LUMPS UNDER THE NIPPLE. Almond-size lumps often appear under one or both nipples in boys and girls between the ages of 9 and 13, and these little swellings are often slightly tender. Don't be concerned about this; it is a normal development. Sometimes one side will start months before the other. In the boys it subsides. In the girls it is the beginning of breast development.

LUMPS IN THE EYELIDS. Sometimes little cysts or infections of hair sockets or mucous glands occur in the eyelids. They may or may not be tender. If they are painful or very noticeable, ask the doctor about it. Such infections are not serious and are readily corrected.

Sties are little pimples occurring right on the edge of the eyelid. It is a rare child who grows up without having had an occasional sty. While they are uncomfortable for a few days, they do no harm to the eye itself. They are caused by bacteria getting into a hair follicle at the edge of the lid. Usually they come to a head and break open. After that, healing is rapid. The doctor may suggest warm compresses to hasten the process and perhaps some eyedrops to help check the infection. If a child has many sties, the doctor will want to check him over to make sure no underlying problem is lowering his resistance to infection.

BED-WETTING
Bed-wetting by a child after the age of 3 or 4 is sometimes a problem for parents—and it becomes a problem for the doctor, because the importance of bed-wetting tends to grow out of all proportion in their minds. Admittedly it is annoying to have your child's bed wet night after night while his friends' go dry. You will be worried, sometimes angry, and often frustrated. The longer it goes on, the more frustrated you will feel.

Some children are very unhappy about their bed-wetting. Others seem quite unconcerned or, if the truth were known, are subconsciously unwilling to give it up.

We must be clear about two things. First, we are not talking about occasional accidents. We are talking about children who have gained control during the day but who continue to be wet at night. Second, we are not talking about those occasional children who have trouble keeping dry both day and night. Such children may have some structural problem in the urinary tract and should be studied thoroughly. Finding and correcting any physical abnormality is very important.

We will assume, then, that your child of 3 or more is dry during the day but wets the bed regularly at night. Why does he do so?

The majority of bed wetters are simply very deep sleepers. So soundly do they sleep that the signals from a full bladder are not received. These children have no physical abnormality, no deep psychological block, no psychiatric problem. This type of bed wetter gets over it all by himself as he grows older. The main thing is for you to be patient. If you make a big issue of it, you may convert a simple thing into a long-lasting psychological hurdle for the child. This youngster needs understanding, support, and encouragement—and that's the *only* treatment he needs.

There is a smaller group of bed wetters whose problem goes back to the fact that too much emphasis was put on early toilet training. This group learned early that they got more attention by being wet than by being dry. Once this feeling becomes deeply set in a child's mind, it takes a long time to eradicate it. The whole thing is often at a subconscious level, so that as the child grows older he may make all sorts of statements about wanting to be dry when in fact he deeply desires the attention that went with being wet. That is one important reason for avoiding efforts at toilet training until a child is ready and able to understand it—and, when training begins, for praising success but restraining criticism of failures.

There are a few cases of bed-wetting in older children which seem to revolve around stress and anxiety. These children are more apt to be intermittent wetters. Emotional tension during the day resulting from constant nagging or unreasonable demands for perfection may be followed by periods of bed-wetting. School anxieties often play a part too. Shaming should be avoided. You may need help from the doctor in evaluating your own feelings and finding ways to reduce tension for such a child.

You will get all sorts of advice, such as not to give the child fluids after 6 in the evening or to wake him several times during the night; to make him wash his own bedding; to use an alarm clock or buzzer that goes off when the bed is wet; to give him drugs to make him sleep less deeply or to relax the bladder muscles. None of these works very well except, possibly, when the child is about ready to correct the problem himself. Don't use any of them without medical advice, except perhaps to cut down on fluids late in the day until you find out *why* the child is a bed wetter. The doctor can help you with this and may be able to bolster your wavering patience. Talk it over with him. It is important that you do nothing that might interfere with the natural tendency of this problem to correct itself.

Sometimes a child who really wants to get over wetting his bed may be helped by learning to hold back for a while when he has to urinate during the day. His bladder capacity can be measured and he can be coaxed, with much praise, to increase it gradually. After a while he may reach the point where his capacity is such that he can go all night without voiding. But even this simple approach should be dropped if the child shows any resistance to it.

Failure of any method of treatment is sometimes more than just a failure of method. It may in fact set back any progress toward improvement. Be patient. Nowhere is patience more important.

CONSTIPATION

We cannot discuss this subject unless we understand the meaning of the word *constipation*. Real constipation is the inability of the lower bowel to perform its evacuative function normally.

One mother rightly ignores the fact that her breast-fed infant has a bowel movement only every third or fourth day. Another mother, under the same circumstances, is on the phone twice a day about it. (No doubt these attitudes go back to the home where she grew up.) We believe that more than 90 percent of all constipation in children is really a problem only in the minds of the parents—at least to start with. That leaves only 10 percent or less to represent real constipation initially.

CONSTIPATION IN INFANTS. Babies vary tremendously in their bowel habits. Some have only a couple of movements a week and are perfectly healthy. Some have four or five very soft movements every day, and they, too, are perfectly healthy. Some have semiliquid movements; others pass what mothers usually call "marbles." Some have a movement and no one is the wiser until the odor is noticed; others grunt and fuss and get red in the face because their various muscles are not yet too well coordinated. All are normal. If your baby is doing well otherwise, the less attention you pay to the character and frequency of his movements the better.

Nor is there cause for concern just because a given baby's movements vary from very loose to very hard, unless passing the stool is actually painful.

Sometimes a baby may make a really big fuss about moving his bowels. If he does and has marblelike results, try adding 1 or 2 tablespoonsful of molasses to his milk or formula each day; 2 or 3 teaspoons of prune juice or strained prunes can be given for the same purpose. If that does not help, double the amount every few days. Should this fail, check with the doctor but listen to what he says and don't keep worrying about it. It is very important that your child not become aware of your concern in this matter.

In general, avoid enemas and suppositories. They never really solve any but the most temporary problems.

If a very young baby has only occasional movements and his stomach seems distended or if he is persistently uncomfortable, talk to the doctor about it. He will check the opening of the rectum to make sure it is normal in size. And he can offer safe changes in formula or medication for occasional use.

OBSTINATE CONSTIPATION IN THE OLDER CHILD. With older children constipation may temporarily follow an illness, a trip that upsets routines, or a new step in life such as school. Once in a while a dose of milk of magnesia will do no harm, but, again, too much attention or too frequent use of laxatives should be avoided.

If an older child has pain or blood with his movements, have him examined. There may be a small tear or fissure which needs treatment.

Chronic constipation in children past 3 who had little or no difficulty during the first year is almost always a psychological problem. Sometimes it goes back to overemphasis on toilet training at too early an age. In other cases there is just too much concern on the family's part about bowel function in general. At some point the child senses that more attention is to be had by *not* having a bowel movement than by having one. This leads to withholding. After a while the normal urge to defecate subsides. Gradually the rectum becomes less and less

311

sensitive and the normal reflex no longer functions. The occasional passage of a very large hard stool may then be somewhat painful, and so the child holds back for still another reason and a vicious circle is established.

This type of constipation is very difficult to correct. Much patience and understanding are required. Nothing under the sun will succeed with these children as long as there is intense and obvious family concern. This concern must be switched to emphasis on the child's successes in daily living, all his good points and the little triumphs. Only such change of emphasis and great patience will succeed. Meanwhile the doctor may prescribe an initial cathartic followed by the use of mineral oil as a lubricant over quite a long period.

MILD OR OCCASIONAL CONSTIPATION. Mild cases of constipation may respond to a few simple steps that you can safely carry out yourself. But while using the following suggestions, try not to connect any of them in the child's mind with the constipation. In other words, do these things *without* talking about why you are doing them.

1. Increase the total fluid intake by about two full glasses a day, using fruit juices or plain water but *not* additional milk.
2. Add raisins, dates, prunes, and figs to the diet. Canned figs in syrup are especially helpful.
3. Use fruits and vegetables wherever you can—raw, if possible.
4. Encourage more exercise if the older child is the quiet, inactive type—jump ropes, swings, riding toys, anything to give real muscular exertion.

If, despite these simple things, you feel that your child has problem constipation, take him to your doctor rather than trying any treatment involving laxatives or other medications.

OBESITY

Parents tend to worry most about a thin child. The doctor is much more likely to be concerned about the one who is overweight.

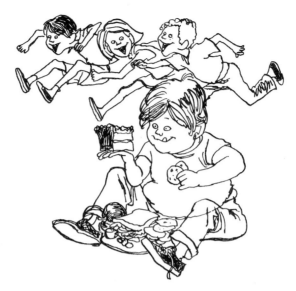

We all know that obesity is caused by overeating. Everyone—infant, child, or adult—needs a certain number of calories in order to have energy and stay healthy. It is the taking in of more calories than are needed that leads directly to gaining weight. Calories *do* count. When there is a weight problem, it is essential to count them.

With their constant activity, children tend to burn off carbohydrates—starches and sugars—quite effectively. On the other hand, they utilize fats and oils at a slower rate and store these as body fat whenever there is any excess of calories. So the first step in helping a fat child is to cut out all visible fats and oils from his diet. Butter, bacon, cream, fried foods, peanut butter, whole milk—such things have no place in the diet of an overweight child.

The control of obesity is more difficult in children than in adults because children need a different number of calories at different ages. Their intake must be adjusted to their normal expected weight at any given stage of growth. Thus for the first several months a baby needs about 50 calories per pound of body weight, but the child in his middle teens needs only 20 to 25. All figuring is done on the basis of the expected weight range.

There is no single precisely correct weight for a child at a given moment, but there very definitely is a range of normal weights. This range depends on the child's age, height, and body build. Your doctor has tables available for reference and can quickly tell, after weighing and measuring your child, whether he falls within the range of normal. Of course, for really fat children no consulting of tables is necessary; the overload is obvious.

In many ways fat children have a tough time. Their playmates make fun of them. Adults look at them with pity, dismay, or outright disapproval. Knowing they are not popular, they retreat into themselves, becoming loners. They have difficulty taking part in games, social activities, and sports. They are slow or awkward, their muscle tone is poor, and the excess weight makes them tire quickly. Since they cannot compete, they choose quiet pleasures, one of which is eating. They tell you that they don't care about being fat, but inside they care terribly.

Causes of obesity

If you have an obese child, you will soon realize that there is much more to the problem than occasional dieting. There is a whole complex group of interlocking factors involving age, environment, heredity, body build and temperament, motivation, and psychological needs. Some or all of them will have a bearing on your efforts to help him slim down. Let's look more closely at some of these factors.

AGE. Babies from 5 months to 1 year, and some children from about the age of 6 to 11, are normally quite chubby. These periods of relative plumpness are temporary. The standards for children of all ages take this into account. Your doctor will know whether your child is beyond the normal range.

ENVIRONMENT. If the family is full of hearty eaters who don't mind being fat themselves, no one can expect the child to accept having his own food severely limited. In such a setting everyone will have to be part of the program if the child's weight is to be controlled. Sometimes this makes things very difficult. Family patterns are usually stubbornly resistant to change.

314

HEREDITY. The tendency to become fat can be inherited. This accounts for the fact that there are occasional fat children who really do not eat more than their slimmer friends. They develop more fat per unit of food taken in. The difference lies in the efficiency with which they utilize their food and store part of it as fat. Restriction of calories will limit their body fat, but for them the restriction must be more severe than for other individuals.

BODY BUILD AND TEMPERAMENT. We must distinguish between the fat child and the stocky child. The doctor uses measurements of hip bones and ribs in addition to height and age in determining normal weight. A child can be built "four square"—broad, chunky, solid—and yet not be overweight. After all, many fine athletes are heavy-boned and well muscled but not fat. To attempt to make a stocky child lose weight is unreasonable and may even be unhealthy for him.

Temperament also affects weight. Children who have placid, relaxed personalities expend less muscular energy. A tense, tight person burns more fuel even while doing nothing and has less left over to store as fat.

MOTIVATION. Here we have a critical factor in controlling a fat child's weight. Most fat young children are not easily motivated to give up the pleasure of eating. No amount of threats, pleading, or shaming will help. Not until children are in their teens does real motivation usually become a controlling factor. At that point many truly begin to care about their appearance. Provided the child has not already withdrawn too far into a protective shell, he may now begin to reduce with a vengeance, so much so that we must watch to be sure he does not overdo it—especially if *he* happens to be a *she*. If this teen-age motivation develops, the solution to overweight is usually in sight. Unfortunately, such motivation does not come to every fat adolescent. Some still find it impossible to do what they would very much like to do.

PSYCHOLOGICAL NEEDS. The most difficult fat children to control are those whose overeating is the result of some deep psychological need. This is the group most likely to fail to im-

315

prove with the coming of adolescence. They are the ones who frequently adopt something of a clowning attitude, though they are *not* happy children; the jolly fat person is found more in literature than in real life.

Deep unhappiness or insecurity can lead a child into compulsive eating, a seeking for pleasure in food. Here is one of those vicious circles. The more deprived, unloved, or dissatisfied the youngster feels, the more he eats. The more he eats and fattens, the more he is teased and excluded from the games of other children. The more he is excluded, the more unhappy he is with his daily life and the less active he becomes. So he eats. He continues to be fat despite protestations that he really is not eating very much. He will protest but will sneak and steal food almost while protesting.

Such compulsive eaters and their parents usually need some psychiatric help in getting at the root of their problem. No program of weight control will work for very long unless the basic emotional reason for the compulsion is uncovered and corrected.

Glandular Problems and Obesity. Nowhere in this discussion have glandular conditions been mentioned as a cause of obesity. Nearly every parent with a fat child wonders whether there is an underactive thyroid or some other internal malfunction. It might be easier if there were, but this almost never happens.

Helping the obese child

For the control of fatness in a growing child, it is often sufficient just to hold the line rather than to demand actual weight loss. If weight gain stops while other growth continues, the net result is decreased obesity. Only when the child is very much overweight or his growth period nearly ended will actual loss of pounds be needed.

Long experience has taught us that casual efforts at weight control seldom work. A definite program is necessary, and as a rule you will need the doctor's help in establishing and maintaining it. But even before you consult the doctor, there are certain things you can do.

316

First of all buy a calorie counter and find out, over a period of 10 days, just what the child's daily intake of calories actually is.* Keep a record day by day. Omit nothing that he eats or drinks. If you do this honestly and completely, you will establish a valuable base line from which to work.

Next remove every bit of visible fat and oil from the diet. If food will make a grease spot on paper, avoid it. This means no cream, butter, margarine, bacon, peanut butter, potato chips, fried foods, or any other greasy or oily food. It also means skim milk instead of whole milk. Fats are very high in calorie value, and removing them is an important part of calorie control for children.

Have plenty of carrot sticks, celery, apples, oranges, or other fruits for snacks. Do not have cakes, cookies, and candy readily available, but don't try to exclude them completely. Children burn sugars and starches quite efficiently and will need a reasonable amount for energy.

While you are taking these simple steps, you can be teaching the child to count his own calories. Make a game of it. Your son or daughter will soon have memorized the calorie value of all the common foods and may take great pride in this new knowledge.

At this point, if weight gain is arrested, you may have the battle half won, but it is likely to be a long fight and you will need staying power.

If weight gain continues, have the doctor give the child a physical checkup. Let the doctor know in advance that the visit is in relation to overweight. Take your calorie records along. You will learn from the doctor what your particular child's basic calorie requirement is at his particular stage of development.

There are two schools of thought about how the child's diet should be set up. Some doctors prefer simply to establish the total calories permitted per day and to allow the child free choice of foods within those limits. Other physicians prefer rather carefully planned meals and will give you printed food lists and

* The Vest Pocket Calorie Counter, distributed by Doubleday & Company, may be bought at book counters. It gives the caloric value of ordinary household measures of all foods.

sample menus. A vitamin supplement may be ordered with either system. All doctors will agree to the restriction of food fats and an emphasis on fruits, leafy vegetables, eggs, whole-grained cereals, lean meats, and skim milk.

Whatever system your doctor prefers, it is important that there be a sense of program and that you stick to it. This will usually involve a monthly visit to the doctor, at which time the child will be weighed and his progress discussed. In the early months, at least, these visits are a necessary factor for success. Knowing that he must face up to rechecking by an outsider will be a great help to the child in staying on the track. If the youngster is 10 or older, it may help to have him keep some of his appointments with the doctor by himself. You can take him, but let him have his own conference; it will give him a much greater sense of his own responsibility. This works surprisingly well in some cases.

Do not nag, shame, or threaten. If you find your efforts are leading to anger or frequent unpleasantness or bickering, ease up a bit—and discuss the situation further with the doctor. Success is most likely when the child sees his diet as a co-operative project and not as something that is thrust upon him without any real effort to make him a partner. Be sure to praise him for any success. Let him know you are proud of his effort and his improved appearance. Kindle his own pride in what he is doing; it will be your greatest asset.

A mother told us some years ago that the biggest discovery she had made while trying to help her fat child was that "dieting starts in the market." She was absolutely right. The potato chips, cake, and peanut butter that are not available can't be eaten.

HEADACHE

It doesn't seem right that a child should have headaches, but some of them do. If your child has headaches, try to remember that for every headache with a serious underlying cause there are thousands with no threatening implications at all.

The causes of headaches are many. Nearly every illness with fever is likely to produce a temporary headache; the common cold is the number one offender. Eyestrain is another frequent cause; every child with recurrent headaches deserves an eye examination. Anxiety and situations producing prolonged nervous tension yield their share of headaches, but less commonly in children than in adults.

Food allergy is a cause that is often unrecognized. Its discovery offers instant cure; have the child avoid the offending food. Some foods are more commonly troublemakers than others. Chocolate, for instance, is near the top of the list. A small boy announced to Dr. Lee one day that he had a "chocolate headache." It made the doctor laugh, but the boy was right; he and his mother had discovered that eating candy bars was followed by a headache, and later they had narrowed the cause down to chocolate. Dr. Lee was able to clear up the remaining pieces of the puzzle when he told them that cola drinks generally contain chocolate too. When those were also eliminated, it was the end of the child's headaches. With a little detective work you may be able to track down the particular food at fault for your own child (see also Food Allergy in Chapter 12).

Migraine—the vicious, sick headaches that are all too familiar to some adults—are distinctly uncommon in children. When they do occur there is almost always a family history. Usually the headache is sudden, severe, accompanied by nausea, and followed by a period of deep sleep after which everything is fine. A child with such a pattern should be carefully examined by the doctor to eliminate other causes of severe headache, and you should get the doctor's help for any bad headache that comes with high fever, stiff neck, recurrent vomiting, unusual clumsiness, or personality changes.

Headaches that come very frequently will also need study. You may find the cause of milder ones by yourself; look for patterns related to daily living and eating. For instance, there is no disease that causes headache before school in the morning and at no other time.

NOSEBLEED

The most effective way to stop a nosebleed is to have the child sit up while you hold his nostrils between your thumb and forefinger. Squeeze the two sides together. Hold firmly for 3 to 4 minutes and then release the pressure slowly. Repeat if necessary.

The nosebleeds that children have when struck on the nose are usually soon over and need cause no great concern. On the partition between the two sides of the nose there is a small area where multitudes of tiny blood vessels are right under the surface. It is believed they are there to help warm the cold air as it flows in. In any event, it only takes a superficial scratch to make this area bleed. Other nosebleeds need a bit of explanation.

Nighttime nosebleeds. The most frequent cause of nighttime or naptime nosebleeds is a child's putting a fingernail in the nose when he is asleep or half asleep. It is especially apt to happen during head colds. Blowing the nose the following day may start it up again. If your child has nosebleeds when he is in bed, and without unexplained fever or other symptoms, cut his fingernails short, file them down so that there is no available cutting edge, and keep them that way for two or three weeks.

Nosebleeds in childhood are common and usually do not signify any serious condition. But if, after you have filed his fingernails, your child continues to have nosebleeds frequently, you should call them to the doctor's attention. Sometimes a simple office treatment directed at the little capillaries inside the nose is all that is needed.

Nosebleeds associated with blood clotting defects. If you have a family history of individuals who bleed more than normally from cuts, tooth extractions, or other minor injuries, it is possible that your child's nosebleeds are related to a blood clotting defect. You should ask your doctor about this.

Nosebleeds associated with rheumatic fever. Certain cases of nosebleeds are associated with rheumatic fever. If, along with nosebleeds, there is unexplained fever or joint soreness or pain, be sure to call it to the doctor's attention. This is not common, for the treatment of streptococcic infections is sharply reducing the frequency of rheumatic fever. (See also Rheumatic Fever in Chapter 16.)

STIFF NECK

Stiff neck occasionally frightens parents because of its well-known association with meningitis (discussed in Chapter 13), so it is important to realize that stiff neck all by itself is *not* a sign of meningitis. Sleeping in a queer position, turning a somersault, or doing some other unusual exercise may cause severe stiff neck. Then it is muscular and the child is not otherwise sick. There is no fever, no vomiting, no headache—no complaints at all except for the pain and soreness in the neck.

Occasionally, a stiff neck begins very suddenly while a child is asleep. He goes to bed feeling fine and wakens unable to move his head without severe pain. He will hold his head in a cocked-to-one-side position. Most often this occurs just as a child is getting over a cold or sore throat. *Wry neck* is another name for this problem. It has a lot in common with the lumbago or sudden stiff back that troubles grown-ups from time to time. With or without the doctor's help, these sudden stiff necks get well, but if the condition is very painful, a sedative may be needed to help the child rest.

ABDOMINAL PAIN

One of the commonest complaints of childhood is stomachache, but the stomach itself is seldom at fault. So we will use the phrase *abdominal pain*.

Not every little passing pain in the middle requires the doctor's attention, but parents are frequently undecided about calling him, because they are aware of the danger of appendicitis. If the pain is very severe or is constant you will, of course, call for advice immediately. But most abdominal aches and pains are mild or moderate and tend to come and go. What then?

There are no fixed rules, but here are a few helpful suggestions. Except after injuries, the majority of abdominal complaints come on rather gradually. Nothing catastrophic is likely to happen if you take a little time to observe the child. Then, if you do have to call, you will be in a better position to give the doctor a good description. He will want to know several things. Try to have these answers ready when you call.

1. When and how did it start?
2. Is the pain constant or does it come and go?
3. Is it related to going to the toilet?
4. Is the child up and running around?
5. Any vomiting or diarrhea?
6. Any fever?
7. Any loss of appetite?

Given that much information, the doctor can usually decide whether the child needs to be seen immediately or can wait for a later examination.

For every case of appendicitis or of the rare and more serious causes of abdominal pain there are dozens of pains caused by less threatening things. Some children have vague abdominal pain with almost every sore throat or other upper respiratory infection. In very young children ear infections are very commonly accompanied by "stomachache." Many vague recurrent complaints are due to food allergy, tension, or anxiety. The common, repetitive, just-before-schooltime pain is usually recognized for what it is by parents (but see also Appendicitis in Chapter 16).

TONSILS AND ADENOIDS

Most parents are aware that fewer tonsil operations are done now than in the past. What has changed medical attitudes? Are there ever good and proper reasons for removal of a child's tonsils or adenoids or both?

The greatest single reason for the reduction in "T and A's," as the removal operation is called, has been an increasing awareness that the operation frequently falls short of producing many of the benefits that were once credited to it. Then, too, there is considerable new knowledge about the function of these parts of the body. When everything is considered, it becomes quite obvious that the place for most tonsils and adenoids is right where they are in the back of throats and noses.

You should have some knowledge of these much-maligned little structures in order to understand the questions that arise concerning them. And if you are ever told that your child should have tonsils or adenoids removed, you have every right to a careful explanation as to why their removal is necessary.

Both the adenoids and the tonsils are part of the body's lymphatic system, a widely dispersed but interconnected complex of lymph glands which ultimately connects with the bloodstream. A principal function of this system is production of the antibodies that help to defend us against infection. Most of the lymphatic system lies deep in the body, but the tonsils and adenoids are an exception; they are located right at the surface in the back of the mouth and nose. From infancy to 7 or 8 years of age they are normally quite large. Then they become progressively smaller in relation to the size of the child.

Because of their deeply folded structure, they have a very large surface area. This surface is strategically located for contact with the myriads of germs that constantly enter the mouth and nose. Immediately under their folded surface are swarms of cells called *lymphocytes* that produce infection-fighting antibodies. These lymphocytes are highly mobile. Some of them, in response to infection, travel through the lymph passages to the lymph glands, taking with them exact information as to precisely what kind of antibody is needed, and antibody production starts. Eventually enough antibody is made and released into the blood to overcome the kind of infection located in the tonsil area. It is clear to us now that the tonsils and adenoids serve as sentry stations from which originate signals for the production of needed anti-infection antibodies. Fortunately, they are not alone in this function, and if they have to be removed, the whole antibody defense system is not crippled.

There was a time when many children had T and A's for what would now be considered very inadequate reasons. Even today, many pediatricians believe that 75 percent or more of tonsil operations are done without sufficient cause.

The operation, like all surgery, carries certain risks. The dangers range from death during or after the procedure to post-

323

operative hemorrhage and to later psychological repercussions related to intense anxiety and fear at the time of operation. Admittedly these complications are not common when the operation is done under the best of modern conditions. Nevertheless, every conscientious physician constantly balances the risk inherent in any operation against the danger to his patient if the operation is *not* performed. When this is done, it turns out that remarkably few T and A's are needed.

No longer should it be suggested that a child's tonsils be removed in the hope that he will have fewer colds. He will not. Simple enlargement is not a sufficient reason, and snoring, poor appetite, fidgeting, or lack of pep are no more valid.

Is the operation ever really necessary?

Valid reasons for tonsil and adenoid surgery. Following are the medical reasons for surgery. But even they are not considered sufficient unless proper treatment has failed to clear up the problem.

1. Frequently recurrent or chronic middle ear infections (see also Earache in Chapter 11).
2. Hearing impairment directly related to diseased or greatly enlarged adenoids.
3. Recurrent or chronic nasal sinus infections (see Sinusitis in Chapter 11).
4. Persistent day and night mouth breathing if the adenoids are actually causing nasal obstruction.
5. Recurrent or chronic streptococcal tonsillitis (see Chapter 11).

There are a few additional rare reasons for tonsil removal that must be left to your doctor's judgment.

It is not always necessary to remove both the tonsils *and* the adenoids. Either structure alone may be chronically infected or causing a mechanical problem, and only the offender need be removed. Removal of the adenoids is a simpler procedure than the combined operation and usually causes the child less postoperative discomfort.

If you have doubts about the need for recommended tonsil surgery, remember that you have a right to seek another opinion.

10
Ailments of Infancy

BIRTHMARKS

Often a mother's first question about a new baby is "Are there any birthmarks?" Usually the answer is *no*. If there are any, they are quite harmless. Just how they got their name is a mystery, for they have nothing to do with anything that happens during birth. A birthmark is simply a mark present at birth.

There are all sorts of legends about birthmarks, all of them rubbish. Birthmarks are not caused by anything that mothers do or fail to do during pregnancy, and fortunately most of them go away without any treatment at all.

The commonest of all birthmarks is a reddish blotching over the bridge of the nose, the upper eyelids, and sometimes across the forehead. There is often a similar area of color on the back of the neck at the hairline. These are smooth and level with the skin. Stretching the skin between two fingers makes them disappear momentarily. This type is not permanent. Somewhere between the ages of 4 months and 4 years they disappear completely. No treatment of any sort is needed.

Next commonest is the kind called a "strawberry mark," which may be located anywhere on the body. It is bright red, slightly raised, and often has a rather nubbly surface. It may be present at birth or may appear during the first few months of life. Strawberry marks grow slowly for a while and sometimes reach a considerable size. Later they slowly begin to lose color, shrink, and finally disappear completely, leaving no trace. Almost never do they require treatment. Removing them by any method always leaves at least some scarring. They are never malignant. Very rarely, one grows in a sort of mushroom shape and is bothersome because of protrusion from the surface. If it is sufficiently annoying, it can be removed surgically, but this is seldom called for. Too much unnecessary treatment of this kind of birthmark is still going on.

A more unsightly and far less common kind is called a "port wine stain." This type of birthmark most often occurs on the face. It is usually dark red or purplish-red in color and may be of considerable size, unsightly but otherwise harmless. It does not go away and, unfortunately, there is no really satisfactory method of treatment or removal.

THRUSH

Occasionally, 3 to 6 days after birth, the lining of the infant's mouth may appear speckled with small white areas that do not rub off. The infection is caused by a yeast. This yeast lives in the mother's vagina, and the baby acquires it during birth. There are many old wives' tales about thrush. Ignore them.

Thrush seldom causes any real trouble, but the baby's mouth may be slightly sore. There are medicines that get rid of thrush simply and quickly. The doctor will order what is necessary.

CRADLE CAP

Cradle cap is a condition that affects the scalp of young infants, an accumulation of little yellowish flakes or crusts on the scalp and sometimes on the eyebrows. Often it is associated with some soreness and redness behind the ears and in the diaper area. Mothers hate it because they feel that it makes the baby appear unwashed. If your baby has this problem, you need feel no guilt; it has nothing to do with dirt. It seems to afflict babies who have oily skin and usually clears up between 8 and 12 months of age. In occasional cases, if cradle cap is severe, a considerable amount of hair may fall out, but it is temporary and need cause no alarm.

If the cradle cap bothers you, rub a little plain mineral oil or petroleum jelly into your baby's scalp in the evening and wash it out with soap or shampoo in the morning. Most of the crusting will be removed. It may be necessary to do this every few days. If this method fails, consult your doctor.

DIAPER RASH

Almost every baby has some diaper rash at times. Some babies, despite their mother's best efforts, have severe diaper rash almost all the time. If you have an infant with a bad rash, you probably feel embarrassed and guilty about it, but it may not be your fault at all.

Diaper rash is not a single condition. It is a group of rashes of different causes, occurring on an area where local conditions vary greatly and on babies whose skin sensitivity runs the gamut from relatively tough to very tender. Small wonder no single treatment works for all babies—or even for one baby at different times. It is not hard to understand your frustration when, after doing your best to keep the baby dry and clean, he still has bright-red, angry-looking, and very sore skin all over his bottom.

Because there are so many factors involved, you may need the doctor's help in dealing with a severe or persistent diaper rash. But the majority of cases respond to treatment that you can safely try before calling for help.

A newborn baby's skin is very soft and tender; he has been literally living under water up to the time of birth. The diaper rashes that occur in the first few days are usually just a matter of the skin adjusting to a new environment and will disappear without treatment as the skin toughens up.

Occasional infants, blonds and redheads especially, continue to have very sensitive skin long after the newborn period. For these babies it is important that the diaper area be kept as clean and dry as possible, but without your becoming obsessive about it. There are mothers who wash and rewash their babies until the soap removes all the natural oils from the skin, depriving the skin of part of its own natural defense. A baby's bottom should be cleaned gently with plain water most of the time. You can do a thorough cleaning once a day with any good soap. A little baby lotion can be used after this washing.

Diapers should be changed often enough so that a baby is dry and clean at least most of the time. This usually means at least six dozen diapers a week for the first few months.

If you launder your own diapers, give them a final rinse with a mild antiseptic solution. Ordinary liquid laundry bleach is all right, or use one of the products specially made for diaper rinsing. Lacking these, use a cup of vinegar for each 3 or 4 gallons of final rinse water.

If, despite these simple measures, your baby still has a problem with diaper rash, leave the diaper area exposed to air as much as possible. Put the baby in a warm place with no diapers at all, except at mealtimes, until the rash clears up, and change the bedding frequently. It looks unattractive, but this is the greatest single way to treat diaper rash.

When the baby *is* wearing a diaper, try a protective ointment. There are many useful products in the drugstores and baby departments. Plain white petroleum jelly is often as good as more expensive products. Whichever you use, carefully wash and dry the skin before applying the ointment.

One common type of rash is associated with a strong smell of ammonia in the diaper, most noticeable when the baby has been wet for a good while. The ammonia is *not* in the urine when the baby voids it. In other words, the urine is not "too strong." The ammonia develops in the diaper as the result of the action of bacteria after the urine is passed. Since there is almost universal misunderstanding about this, we repeat: *There is nothing wrong with the baby or his urine.* Special diaper rinses often help with this problem. Many diaper laundry services will supply specially rinsed diapers if you ask for them.

If your baby continues to have more than a slight diaper rash in spite of your doing the simple things, call it to the attention of the doctor. Occasionally, skin infections develop that do require special treatment. But try not to let it worry you, for even the worst diaper problems are sooner or later a thing of the past.

COLIC

Perhaps no other condition of otherwise normal infants is so worrisome and tedious for parents as "3-month colic." Colic usually begins in the first 2 weeks of life. Despite the name, not all cases last a full 3 months, while some last much longer.

In simplest terms, colic is an overactivity of the muscles of the baby's gastrointestinal tract. The contractions of these muscles produce crampy pain. The baby cries. The harder he cries and the more excited he gets, the worse the pains seem to be.

It is a frustrating experience for a mother, for it often seems that nothing she can do is of very much help to her baby; he just continues to cry and squirm. But it doesn't take much pain to make a baby cry. It is an all-or-nothing sort of reaction, and things often appear much worse than they really are.

Experienced pediatricians know that colic may be the expression of many different things. Occasionally it is caused by an allergy to milk. In that small and fortunate percentage of cases, the cure is quick: a switch to a milk substitute.

Sometimes it reveals a tense, nervous personality in the child who later proves to be a constantly active person with a low sleep requirement and often a very high I.Q.

Occasionally there is a curious feedback mechanism between an overly anxious mother and a hyperactive baby. The mother's tenseness somehow rubs off on the baby, and a vicious cycle is started. This is the origin of the trite and superficial statement that "to treat colic, give the mother a sedative." But many a mother, suffering through long bouts of screaming on the part of her colicky baby, has been accused of causing the colic by her nervousness when, in fact, she is simply reacting to it.

The pattern varies, but usually a colicky infant will take feedings ravenously, seem satisfied for just a short time, and then pull up his legs, begin to squirm about, and cry lustily. It may happen only at a certain time of day or night for an hour or two, or it may be nearly constant.

Every baby with this trouble should be thoroughly examined

329

just to rule out other possible causes of discomfort. Once the doctor has determined that the baby does in fact have colic, he will offer suggestions and perhaps medication. Be patient. It takes a bit of doing to find the best combinations for a particular baby. Remember that it's harder on you than it is on the baby; that he will thrive and gain in spite of it; that it will not be permanent; that most colicky babies develop into smart, competitive, successful people. Colic is a time of trial for parents, but it *is* temporary.

FEVER CONVULSIONS

A convulsion results when, with sudden fever, the brain cells which control the muscles begin to fire off intense, random, uncoordinated impulses. The child may be just twitching or he may have sudden violent contractions of the muscles of his face, eyes, arms, and legs. His breathing may be temporarily interrupted and his skin color changed to dusky red or slightly blue. His eyes roll up, and he is likely to be unconscious for a brief period. He looks as though he is dying but he is not.

Every doctor knows that nothing in the whole range of childhood sickness causes such naked fear for parents. He also knows that convulsions that come with the onset of many simple infections or with a sudden rise in temperature are not really dangerous. In a few seconds to a few minutes the convulsion will stop, normal breathing will begin again, and the crisis will be over. But the appearances *are* frightening. The important thing to remember is not to panic. Your child is *not* dying.

Force yourself to take these steps to reduce the fever:

1. Uncover the child.
2. Get his clothes off. Do not worry about his catching cold.
3. Moisten his skin all over with *cool*, not cold, water. Keep applying the water. If the weather is hot, fan the child also. The convulsion will stop in a few minutes and the child will be better.
4. Have someone call the doctor.

By the time the doctor can get to you the convulsion will probably be all over, and you will wonder whether he can believe how awful it was!

Most fever convulsions occur in children from several months to 4 years old. You should call the doctor, even though the seizure will probably be over before he arrives; he will want to check to be sure no serious infection is present, and he will probably give an injection or order some medication to prevent another seizure from occurring. He may have you keep some medicine on hand to be given to this particular child any time there is fever that might trigger a fever convulsion. It is the rapidity with which the fever rises that counts. A gradual rise to 105 degrees may make no trouble at all, while a sudden rise to 102 may result in a seizure—*if the child is prone to seizures.*

Parents often ask us whether the occurrence of one or more of these convulsions means the child will have epilepsy. The answer in most cases is *no.* The child who has many such seizures over a period of years may be an exception. So may the child whose convulsions occur with almost no fever. If your child has seizures that are not accompanied by fever, certain tests will be in order. (See also Epilepsy in Chapter 16.)

HYDROCELE

Occasionally a boy baby will have a firm lump in the groin or scrotum at birth which is simply a sac of clear liquid in the passage between the abdomen and scrotum. Such a swelling is called a *hydrocele.* It is absolutely harmless and will probably disappear without treatment. Sometimes a hydrocele is associated with an inguinal hernia. Your doctor will be able to distinguish between the two.

HERNIA

There's a great deal of misunderstanding about hernias. The word *rupture* seems to be used interchangeably with hernia, and that's unfortunate, for rupture implies something burst or torn while hernias are not that at all.

There are two common types of hernia: umbilical hernia, which rarely requires surgical correction, and inguinal hernia, which almost always does require operation.

UMBILICAL HERNIA. Before a baby is born, it is nourished by blood vessels of considerable size that run through the umbilical cord and into the baby's abdomen at the navel. At birth when the umbilical cord is tied off, the blood vessels shrivel up and the opening into the abdomen closes. But sometimes this closure in the tough ligament of the abdominal wall is incomplete. The skin promptly heals over the surface, but the defect in the abdominal wall persists. This permits the abdominal contents, the intestines, to push out against the covering skin. You then discover that when the baby cries, raising the pressure inside, the navel bulges. Depending on the size of the underlying opening, the bulge may be pea size or plum size. Crying simply makes the defect visible; it does not cause it. Nor does this condition have anything to do with the umbilical cord or how it was tied or cut off.

Umbilical hernias are harmless, and in most cases no treatment is needed; nature tends to close the gap. Strapping or taping is unnecessary and often results in sore and infected skin. If the defect is large and has not closed by the time the child is 7 or 8 years old, closure by operation may be needed. This is highly successful and recurrences are rare. But in our experience not one umbilical hernia in fifty ever needs surgery.

INGUINAL HERNIA (HERNIA AT THE GROIN). Strange as it may seem, the testicles in boy babies originate far up in the abdomen beneath the kidney on each side. During the embryo's development, they move down, pass through a passage or canal in the groin where the leg attaches to the body, and remain thereafter in the external pouch of skin called the *scrotum*. The final descent into the scrotum takes place quite late in prenatal development.

Sometimes the passageway does not close completely after the migration of the testicles. Then anything that raises the pressure in the abdominal area may force a small loop of intestine through that same passage. When this happens a bulge or lump appears in the groin. Crying, coughing, sneezing, or, later, lifting—any of these may be accompanied by the appearance of the bulge. Note that they do not *cause* the defect;

they merely make it apparent. The cause is the failure of the passage to have closed off.

Because the passage is rather long and turns a corner on the way, it is possible for the loop of intestine to get caught and not be able to slip back into the abdomen. When this happens there is apt to be pain, nausea, and sometimes vomiting. When a loop of intestine gets caught like this it is said to be "incarcerated." Prompt surgical operation is required or serious damage to the intestine may occur. Such an operation is more difficult than the repair of the hernia before incarceration occurs. For this reason all inguinal hernias should be repaired soon after they are discovered.

The same potential passage at the groin is present in baby girls, but it is small and much less likely to be the site of a hernia. In our experience there are over ten times as many inguinal hernias in boys. But in both boys and girls, such hernias should be surgically corrected. While all operations carry some risk, for this operation the risk is minimal—and is greater without the operation than with it. For an incarcerated inguinal hernia, if left alone, can lead to obstruction and gangrene of the intestine, a hazardous situation indeed.

UNDESCENDED TESTICLE

As has been explained, the testicles develop in the abdomen, just below the kidneys, early in a boy's prenatal life. Later, but still before birth, they migrate down along the back wall and through an oblique passage in the groin into the external sack of skin called the scrotum. But if the migration of the testicles gets behind schedule, the baby will be born without apparent testicles.

This delayed descent is not in any way harmful. Usually the missing testicles are present but still inside the abdomen. One or both of the glands gets as far as the inner opening of the inguinal canal and gets stuck there. A careful medical examination is needed to determine just what the situation is and what should be done about it.

A testicle that remains in the abdomen will produce normal male hormones but because of the slightly higher temperature inside the body it will not produce sperm. Therefore, if both testicles remain inside, the child will grow up to be sterile.

If one gland is in its normal location, there is no problem of sterility. One functions as well as two, although there is then no margin of safety if that one should be seriously injured.

Undescended testicles can be corrected surgically in almost every case, but considerable judgment is needed to decide on the timing. No one wants to operate on a child if there is a chance that the testicle will complete its migration without help. The doctor will base his decision on the present location of the missing part, its degree of motility, the age of the child, the size of the scrotum, and whether one or both glands are absent.

When both are absent and spontaneous descent is not likely, there is general agreement that surgery should not be delayed beyond the child's fourth year. If one testicle has descended, some doctors believe it best to wait until the boy is 8 to 11 years old before operating to bring down the other.

Even if there were no other reason to operate, boys of that age are apt to be quite cruel in their jokes about anatomical deficiencies. A boy on the receiving end of such jokes can be badly hurt.

Sometimes a partly descended testicle that is on the way down responds to an old-fashioned test. It's worth a try. Have your child sit in a tub of very warm water for 10 minutes. If, when he stands up, the missing testicle is *definitely* present in the scrotum, no surgery will be needed.

CONGENITAL HEART DISEASE

No one needs to be told that the heart is a complicated piece of equipment. With its myriads of muscle bundles, its sturdy yet delicate valves, and its precise electric controls, it is a great wonder that so few hearts have any defects.

The general anatomy of the heart has been known for a long time, but only recently has medical science found ways to see the inside of the living heart. These techniques have truly revolutionized the whole outlook for babies born with defective hearts. Not every abnormal heart can be fixed, but the day is long gone when a "blue baby" or any other baby with an abnormal heart was automatically faced with a very short or restricted life.

Every baby born with a heart defect should have a complete diagnostic study in a medical center especially equipped for this kind of work. It is not always necessary or wise to have such a study done immediately. The timing depends on many factors which your doctor will have to sort out for you, but only by doing these studies can it be determined whether the defect is correctable.

It is unfortunately true that some infants are born with a heart so badly deformed that the condition is obviously incompatible with life and no surgery can possibly succeed. We can only be grateful that for these children there is no pain.

The heart develops very early in prenatal life. By the tenth week of pregnancy the miniature heart is complete in all its complexity and takes up the ceaseless rhythm of work and rest that will continue uninterrupted throughout life.

It is not always clear what interferes with the orderly processes of prenatal development. We do know that some virus infections in the early months of pregnancy can damage the developing heart. Fortunately, German measles, perhaps the greatest threat of all, is coming under control. (See German Measles in Chapter 13 and Immunizations in Chapter 9.)

If you have a baby with a heart defect, it is important for you to realize that it is not the result of anything that you did or did not do during your pregnancy. All those old stories about frights, falls, too little work, too much work, or thinking the wrong thoughts are, as far as we know, just folklore.

Instead of dwelling on what went wrong, you must pick yourself up and do what is now best for your baby under the circumstances. Of the many, many different anatomical defects, the most common ones can now be corrected or at least improved.

While we are talking about hearts, there is one thing that needs to be emphasized: Heart *murmurs* are not always a sign of trouble. Nearly a third of all children have what is called an *innocent murmur* at least part of the time. (The old term "functional murmur" is misleading.) These murmurs have no significance. They do not mean trouble. The doctor can recognize them for what they are. He may not want to tell you that your child has a murmur, even an innocent murmur, because he knows how hard it is to convince you that it is harmless. But he *should* tell you because your child may be ill at some time when your doctor is not available, and another doctor, hearing a murmur while examining the *sick* child, will not know whether the murmur is part of the present illness. If you can tell him that the murmur was there when the child was well, it will be a great help. Remember, *innocent murmurs do not mean disease or defect. They do not require treatment or restriction of activity of any sort.*

11

Upper and Lower Respiratory Infections

Strictly speaking, any infection of the nose, ear, and throat area is called an upper respiratory infection (U.R.I.). A common cold is one; so is a sore throat, tonsillitis, laryngitis, or a sinus infection. While we can sometimes specify just what structure is most involved, more frequently several are infected at once. It is to these more generalized infections that the term U.R.I. is usually applied. When infection passes down into the windpipe (trachea), the bronchial tubes, or the lungs, it becomes a lower respiratory infection.

The covering or lining of all parts of our respiratory system is continuous, providing an interconnected pathway for the spread of infection from one part to the next.

The great majority of U.R.I.'s are caused by viruses. There are over 30 known viruses capable of causing the symptoms collectively known as the common cold. In addition, there is a whole group of viruses that can cause more severe coldlike infections of the "grippe" or "flu" types. Bacteria, when they play a part, are usually secondary invaders—except for infections caused by streptococci, which are likely to be primary invaders.

At present all we can do for virus colds is to treat the symptoms: the stuffy nose, sore throat, cough, fever, and general discomfort. Medications simply relieve these symptoms to some degree while the body marshals its defenses and finally over-comes the invading virus. Most uncomplicated colds last from 7 to 14 days. In young infants and children symptoms such as runny nose and cough may last much longer.

Remember, antibiotics do not help the common cold and should not be used. Parents are often disappointed that the doctor will not order an antibiotic for their child's cold. And if, as sometimes does happen, the child later develops an ear infection or some other complication, they feel that it could have been prevented. Unfortunately, it is not that simple. The use of antibiotics as a preventive in the early stages of upper respiratory infections has not proved worthwhile. Indeed, it is not without hazard, for antibiotic-resistant infections may result that are very difficult to treat.

You should respect your doctor every bit as much for re-fraining from the indiscriminate use of antibiotics as you do for his skill in using them properly when they are really needed —when, for example, late-arriving bacteria cause complications. Then, and only then, antibiotics can play an important part.

The common cold, its complications, and other infections of the respiratory system are discussed in the pages that follow. Considerable space has been given to ear troubles because of the major role they play in childhood.

COMMON COLD

Incubation:	Usually 3 to 5 days
Symptoms:	Young children may have fever at first; otherwise (as for adults) scratchy throat and runny nose
Cause:	Any of many cold viruses
Treatment:	Warmth, humidity, aspirin, deconges-tants, cough syrups
Prevention:	None at present; avoid excess fatigue and exposure to infected persons

---

The common cold presents many paradoxes and questions. We think of colds as a single disease yet, as we said, the symptoms may be caused by literally dozens of different viruses. We are really talking about many different infections with similar symptoms. The body can develop a temporary immunity to any of them individually but not to the whole group by having one or two. That's why children so often have one cold after another. This is particularly true of young children as they start group activities such as nursery school; they are exposed to many cold viruses and, as yet, have immunity to almost none.

The development of a cold requires the presence of a virus (usually via another person) and a state of susceptibility in the patient. The dose and virulence of the virus may vary greatly, and so may the individual's resistance or immunity. It is the changing balance of these variables that makes it so hard to understand why a person gets a bad cold at a certain time and under a given set of circumstances, but not at another time under seemingly identical conditions.

In daily life, most of these variables are quite beyond practical control. Our state of resistance, however, is influenced by excessive fatigue and by such matters as severe chilling or long-term faulty nutrition.

Colds in children are no different from those in adults except for the tendency of infants and the very young to have a higher temperature. The onset of a fresh cold is one of the commonest causes of fever in younger children and in infants. Sometimes the fever precedes the other symptoms of the cold by 12 to 24 hours. After a day or two the fever subsides but the cold continues. If a young child has a fever and an obviously fresh cold, you can safely wait awhile to call the doctor.

It is quite a different thing when a child begins to run a fever in the *later* stages of a cold. Usually this indicates that some secondary infection is taking place. At this point there is the well-known paradox of the common cold: The doctor can do more for the complications than he can for the primary cold itself. It is with the complications that antibiotics come into use. Therefore call him when fever comes late in a cold.

There are many nonprescription medicines for the symptoms of colds: nose drops and oral decongestants for stuffiness, analgesics like aspirin for discomfort and headache, antihistamines (supposedly to help dry things up), cough suppressants, and various combinations of these. Such medicines do help to some degree, but they do not cure the cold or even shorten its duration. The cold will still last its 10 days or 2 weeks.

Nose drops should not be continued for more than 3 to 5 days because they may cause irritation and secondary swelling. Three or four times a day is a reasonable limit for aspirin; the total daily dose should not exceed ½ grain per pound of body weight. Larger doses will not be more helpful.

When it comes to the complications of colds there are few, if any, nonprescription medicines that are effective. Most complications result from bacteria gaining a foothold in a localized area of the respiratory system. In this situation the doctor can definitely help. First he must decide upon the principal location of the infection. In some cases he may take cultures or do other tests to pinpoint what kind of germ is causing the trouble. Secondary sore throats, earaches, sinus infections, and bronchitis can all be helped by judicious use of proper antibiotics. Once located and identified, secondary cold germs are up against a tough situation nowadays.

Small babies with head colds have some special problems. Under 2 or 3 months of age they sometimes don't seem to be able to breathe through their mouths when their noses are stuffy, and so breathing becomes a struggle for them. Breast or nipple feeding is difficult because they have to stop after every two or three swallows to get air. They cannot blow their noses, and they do not clear their throats effectively. They do sneeze and cough, which helps temporarily. But a bad cold can be frustrating and tiresome for both mother and infant.

The use of decongestant nose drops helps to some degree. Keeping the baby in a warm, well-humidified room most of the time is worthwhile. (Very dry air will thicken and dry nasal mucus and thereby compound the problem.) There are good vaporizers available, many of which generate large volumes of water vapor without heat.

If you use a vaporizer that depends on boiling water and steam, *keep it out of reach where it can't be knocked over* onto a baby or child. Many burns come from hot steam vaporizers.

We think it is best to consult your doctor if you have a very young baby with anything more than a slight cold, especially if this is his first. Don't give medications to infants unless you know the proper doses and timing.

If you have a child age 2 to 6 who has one cold after another, try to tell yourself that things will get better as he grows older. The 5-year-old who has seven or eight bad colds a year (that amounts to something like 16 weeks of symptoms) will probably have only two or three by the age of 10.

To summarize: Your child is going to have colds. They will last 10 days to 2 weeks. Medications like aspirin, decongestants, antihistamines, cough syrups, and various mixtures do not cure or shorten colds, though they do help to minimize the symptoms. There is no reliable preventive. Cold shots, vaccines, excess vitamins have not stood the test of time. Excessively hot dry air in living quarters and excessive fatigue are two factors that may make catching cold more likely. Hothouse people, like hothouse plants, are apt to be less hardy.

SINUSITIS

The nasal sinuses are air-filled spaces in the bones surrounding the nasal passages. All are connected to the nose by small openings, and their lining is continuous with that of the nose. These hollow spaces add resonance to our voice. When their openings are shut off by swelling or when they are filled with fluid, the normal resonance is prevented. Every cold involves the sinuses to some degree.

When infection is trapped inside, a good bit of pain and fever may result. Sometimes, in young children, it causes swelling of the eyelids. Sinus infections are not usually much of a problem in children up to the age of 5 or 6. Even older children have far less sinus disease than adults. In children the infection usually clears up right along with the cold that caused it. In the occasional instance that it fails to do so, decongestants and antibiotics, as ordered by the doctor, usually do the trick quite promptly.

When chronic or recurrent sinus infection does occur in children, there should be a careful appraisal of the tonsils and adenoids. Enlarged and infected adenoids may be the basic problem. Relief of the sinus disease may necessitate the removal of the adenoids.

CROUP
(*Laryngitis*)

Incubation:	Not usually transmitted to others
Symptoms:	Harsh, barking cough; hoarse voice; IF DIFFICULTY IN BREATHING DEVELOPS, CALL DOCTOR
Cause:	Viruses or bacteria of certain kinds
Treatment:	Steam or water vapor inhalation; antihistamine; very rarely, operation to install artificial airway (tracheotomy)
Prevention:	None

If your young child wakes up unexpectedly with a seallike barking cough and difficulty breathing in, you should do two things promptly:

1. Call your doctor. Describe the symptoms. Answer his questions. Listen carefully to what he tells you to do. Then do it promptly.
2. Get started on providing moist warm air for the child to breathe. Running a hot shower in a closed bathroom is quickest. Take the child into this steamy room. Hold him on your lap. Let him find the position where he breathes most easily. If you can't steam up a room with a shower, improvise something in the way of a tent to confine steam or water vapor from a vaporizer, croup kettle, or simply a pot of very hot water. Then let the child breathe the vapor in the tent. *Beware of burns.* Don't leave the child for a moment if he can touch the container of hot water or if other children can reach it.

When croup occurs in the middle of the night, it seems something of an emergency. It is common enough, and troublesome enough, that parents should learn about it.

Some children never have croup. Others have it repeatedly. It may come at the beginning of a cold or when there has been no sign of a cold at all. Croup is really laryngitis occurring in an infant or young child. It is quite uncommon after the age of 6.

Laryngitis is an inflammation of the larynx or voice box, the structure at the top of the windpipe just below the mouth. The larynx is the point of entry for air on its way to the lungs. Stretched across its opening are the vocal cords. Attached muscles can increase or decrease the tautness of the cords and widen or narrow the space between them. Inflammation of these cords and the surrounding structures causes what we know as laryngitis, with its loss or change of voice and discomfort.

In adults the space between the cords is large and the cartilage of the larynx is firm, and so swelling does not usually reduce the breathing space dangerously. But in babies and very young children the space is rather small. If swelling reduces it to the point where the child can no longer separate the edges of the cords, the cords vibrate as he breathes in and the curious crowing sound of croup begins.

There are two common types of croup, but they are not always sharply delineated; they resemble each other more than they differ.

Spasmodic croup is most common. The child wakens with a harsh barking cough and a raspy harsh sound on breathing in. There is little or no fever and few signs of a cold or sore throat. As the name implies, this kind of croup is caused by spasm of the muscles of the larynx. When the spasm relaxes, the attack is over. Usually spasmodic croup responds well to simple treatment: steam, and antihistamine or ipecac given in such dose as your doctor may order. The morning after, the child may show no sign of the episode, but another attack may occur in the middle of the following one or two nights. Medication usually can prevent these subsequent attacks. With experience, and always providing the child is having no real trouble breathing, many parents learn to treat mild spasmodic croup.

Croup with fever usually comes on more gradually, is more resistant to treatment, and takes much longer to clear up. *Always call your doctor if your child has croup and is feverish.*

343

The steam and ipecac or antihistamine may help, but an antibiotic and other treatment may also be needed.

In either type of croup, with or without fever, the appearance of labored breathing is a cause for concern, and you should confer with your doctor promptly. If you cannot reach him, take the child to the nearest medical facility—a hospital emergency room, if possible. Hospitals have special croup tents and other equipment for the rare case that needs it. If in doubt, play safe.

SORE THROAT
(Pharyngitis)

Incubation:	2 to 5 days or more
Symptoms:	Sore throat, fever
Cause:	Various viruses; occasionally streptococcus
Treatment:	Penicillin when due to streptococcus
Prevention:	None

Everyone has an occasional sore throat. The symptom is always the same, but the cause may be any of several kinds of infection.

Careful studies of large numbers of people have revealed that the great majority of sore throats are caused by viruses. Most viral sore throats are mild and soon over. Except for the discomfort they cause, these infections are not of great importance, for complications are few and far between. Therefore you need not call the doctor each time your child has a scratchy throat. But do call him if it lasts for several days or is accompanied by fever.

The sore throat that so often occurs with a fresh head cold is usually of short duration and seldom needs any special treatment. Children whose stuffy noses force them to breathe through the mouth often have a sore throat in the morning that is gone by noon.

Streptococcal sore throat

The real problem lies with those sore throats that are caused by streptococcal infection. Such sore throats can be very severe and make the patient very ill and, if untreated, may occasionally be followed by troublesome complications. Certain kinds of strep throats when accompanied by a rash are called scarlet fever (see Chapter 13). So whenever a sore throat persists more than 2 or 3 days or is accompanied by fever, call your doctor.

Even an experienced doctor cannot always distinguish between a strep infection and other less threatening kinds just by examining the throat. To make sure, he needs to take a throat culture. This laboratory aid is being used more and more to help make a precise diagnosis and avoid the use of penicillin when it is not needed.

Some doctors feel they need not take cultures on a routine basis. True, a doctor can often recognize a strep throat for what it is without a culture if the condition is very severe, and then, of course, the use of penicillin is justified without the culture. Also, if a culture is not available, experienced medical judgment is far better than guesswork. *Nevertheless, the day is here when cultures should be used for accurate diagnosis of most sore throats.*

It has been clearly proved that the prevention of rheumatic fever (see Chapter 16) depends on the identification and antibiotic treatment of streptococcal infections. Rheumatic fever, with its threat of severe heart disease, was a great crippler of children in the past. The coming of penicillin and its substitutes has changed all that. But to be effective in preventing rheumatic fever, the penicillin must be given for a full 10 days or more. Often the child with a strep throat seems well after 2 or 3 days of penicillin, and parents are then tempted to stop the medication. *If penicillin is needed at all, it is needed for a full 10 days.* To do less is to possibly expose your child to the ravages of rheumatic fever.

TONSILLITIS

Incubation:	2 to 5 days
Symptoms:	Fever, headache, more or less sore throat, vomiting
Cause:	Streptococcus; various viruses
Treatment:	Penicillin when caused by streptococcus
Prevention:	None

Tonsillitis is an acute infection and inflammation of the tonsils. The child usually becomes ill quite abruptly with high fever (104 or 105 degrees is not uncommon), sore throat, headache, and vomiting. The younger the child, the less severe the sore throat tends to be. Babies under 1 year of age seldom get this disease.

There are two principal types.

Streptococcal tonsillitis is by far the most important because its occasional complications include rheumatic fever and nephritis (kidney inflammation). If your doctor thinks your child has the strep form of tonsillitis, he will use penicillin for treatment for a period of 10 days. (In proper doses penicillin by mouth is fully effective. Injections are not usually necessary.) Not only does this bring about prompt improvement but it also prevents such complications as rheumatic fever, *if* the treatment is continued for the full 10 days. The usual case of strep tonsillitis will result in the loss of about 3 to 4 days of school, and the child will return to school *still taking his penicillin.*

Viral tonsillitis produces just about the same symptoms but in rather milder form. It tends to be more prevalent in summer months. Children recover in 4 to 7 days with only aspirin for treatment and without complications. If your doctor sees a lot of children he soon becomes adept at recognizing this type. Sometimes he will see epidemic patterns developing in limited populations of children—a neighborhood, a camp, a nursery.

Despite this, there can be real difficulty in distinguishing the two kinds of tonsillitis. Don't try to sort out these two similar diseases by yourself. The only reasonably sure way of doing it is by means of a throat culture. The importance of cultures lies in the fact that strep tonsillitis requires penicillin while viral tonsillitis requires no special treatment at all. If cultures are not available to your doctor, he will depend on his experience and judgment in deciding when to use penicillin.

We are often asked whether an attack of tonsillitis means the tonsils should be removed. The answer, in general, is *no*. Only when infection becomes chronic and cannot be eradicated would the question of removal legitimately arise. (See also Tonsils and Adenoids in Chapter 9.)

EARACHE

Because of the great frequency of ear infections in children and because of their importance in relation to hearing, we want to give you a detailed account of the problem.

The accompanying diagram of the ear is slightly distorted and flattened for clarity but shows the basic relationships that are so important in understanding how infection gets to the middle ear and how it may spread to important surrounding structures.

The eardrum is a sensitive but tough translucent membrane separating the outer ear from the middle ear. In health, the pressure on the outside and inside of the drum is kept quite constant. When you swallow, the eustachian tube opens momentarily to allow the pressure in the middle ear to equalize with that in the back of the throat and thus with outside atmospheric pressure. Without this pressure equalizing, the eardrum cannot move back and forth freely in response to sound waves and the sharpness of hearing is reduced.

The in-and-out motion of the eardrum in response to sound waves is transferred across the space of the middle ear through three tiny hinged bones and thence to a very small opening in the inner ear. At this opening in the inner ear, a coiled fluid column is set in motion. Fine sensory nerve endings pick up the motions, which are at the same rate or frequency as the initial sound waves that struck the outer eardrum. These sensory nerve endings relay to the brain (by tiny electrical impulses)

347

the rapidity and amount of motion in the fluid column. The rate and amplitude of the electrical impulses is interpreted in the brain as sound. Anything that interferes with this chain of events, from the initial impact of sound upon the eardrum to the final interpretation in the brain, causes a hearing loss of greater or lesser degree.

In the colder climates, where colds and sore throats are frequent, ear problems are among the most common illnesses of childhood. Indeed, apart from those related to swimming and diving, most earaches are a complication of colds and sore throats. The ear is a highly complex organ, and infection of its various parts may take several different forms. There may be a virus infection of the eardrum itself (myringitis) or a collection of pus in the middle ear caused by any of a number of kinds of bacteria (otitis media). There are also mechanical problems due to improper pressure balances and faulty drainage of fluids. The list of abnormalities is considerable.

Parents often feel that an earache is an earache and that all can be treated alike. That is not so. Examination of the ear requires the use of a magnifying instrument called an *otoscope*, and the correct interpretation of what is revealed through its lens requires knowledge, experience, and judgment. The eardrum is translucent in health. With proper illumination, certain of the structures in the middle ear may be seen right through it. The appearance varies with the problem, but the drum is a sensitive index of what is going on.

The price of improper management of ear infections may be deafness. Some slight loss of hearing occasionally occurs even under the best management if severe infection is present.

In the era before antibiotics, many an ear infection was followed by a serious infection of the honeycomb bone called the *mastoid*, which lies in the skull behind and below the ear. So frequent was this complication of ear infections that many hospitals had special beds assigned for the care of "mastoid cases." Surgery was required to save the hearing, a delicate operation that required at least 10 days in the hospital. Today, with proper management of ear problems, deafness due to infection can largely be avoided and mastoid surgery is seldom needed.

OTITIS MEDIA
(*Infection in Middle Ear Space*)

Incubation:	Usually follows cold or sore throat; interval varies
Symptoms:	Pain in ear (temporary), partial hearing loss
Cause:	Viruses or bacteria
Treatment:	Varies with type
Prevention:	Avoid swimming when any upper respiratory infection is present

When a child has an earache, the most frequent cause is an infection in the middle ear that comes in the course of a cold (see diagram of the ear on p. 302). Because of the swelling and congestion of the air passages, the eustachian tube, which connects the back of the throat and the middle ear space, becomes partly or completely closed off and pressure increases in the middle ear space. The pressure stretches the eardrum and causes pain. The lining membrane of the middle ear is infected, and, because the eustachian tube is closed off, secretions and pus accumulate and have no route of escape.

A mild earache will often subside with simple remedies such as the use of heat, aspirin, filling the ear canal with clean warm salad oil or ear drops, and using nose drops or an oral decongestant. But if an earache, even a mild one, persists several hours in spite of these simple measures, or if it is accompanied by fever, or if the pain is severe, the doctor's help will be needed.

How he treats the problem will depend on what he finds when he examines the ear. If he orders an antibiotic, give it for the full length of time he prescribes. Do *not* discontinue it because the pain is gone, or the infection may not completely clear up.

With certain kinds of infection, the doctor may find the eardrum bulging and under considerable pressure from an accumulation of pus. If this is the case, he may need to make a small incision in the eardrum (myringotomy). It will relieve the pain almost immediately and reduce the chance of hearing loss caused by the continuing presence of pus.

Whether or not an incision is necessary, the doctor will probably want to reexamine the ear again after a few days, and in certain cases he may want to arrange for a hearing test after treatment is completed.

SEROUS OTITIS (FLUID IN THE MIDDLE EAR)

In this condition there is an accumulation of uninfected (sterile) fluid trapped in the middle ear. The child's hearing is somewhat below normal. As a rule there is no pain, but an older child may complain that the ear feels full or stuffy. The cause of the trouble is not absolutely certain: Sometimes it follows an ordinary middle ear infection; in other children it may be related to hay fever or other allergies.

Usually the parent or the teacher notices some loss of hearing. Sometimes, serous otitis is discovered by the doctor in the course of a routine physical examination. Having determined its presence, he will probably first try to clear it up by using decongestants and antiallergy medications. Usually this treatment succeeds. The help of an ear, nose, and throat specialist may be needed in exceptionally stubborn cases.

Sometimes it is necessary to place tiny plastic tubes through the eardrum to establish good drainage and ventilation. It is a highly successful procedure, and full hearing is usually restored. After several weeks or months the tubes are removed.

Never ignore a seeming loss of hearing in a child. The cause must be precisely determined if treatment is to succeed.

SWIMMER'S EAR
(*External Otitis*)

Incubation:	Variable after swimming
Symptoms:	Pain, swelling, itching of external ear canal
Cause:	Bacterial or fungus infection in damp external ear canal
Treatment:	Requires proper instruments — sometimes special antibiotics
Prevention:	Shaking water from ears after swimming

When water remains too long in the external ear canal after swimming, the skin lining the canal may become softened and infected. (The same thing occasionally happens in very humid hot climates even without the swimming.) Because the skin of the ear canal adheres tightly to the underlying bone, the swelling that comes with infection causes a good bit of pain. Just moving the outside ear hurts (this is not usually the case with the more common middle ear infections).

Infections of the external canal, while very annoying, are not dangerous and do not lead to impaired hearing. They may, however, be stubborn and difficult to eradicate.

The trouble with home remedies for this condition—such as putting vinegar in the ear—lies in the possibility of mistaken diagnosis. Vinegar may be helpful for swimmer's ear but wrong for a ruptured eardrum or a draining middle ear infection. As a rule you will need your doctor's help both for accurate diagnosis and for treatment to avoid a prolonged infection.

The earplugs sometimes used by swimmers are *not* helpful in preventing swimmer's ear. It is our opinion that they are worthless and sometimes harmful.

Once the condition is completely cleared up, there are drops which can be used after swimming that may prevent recurrence.

EAR WAX

Some people sweat more than others—and some produce more ear wax than others. The wax that is produced varies from semifluid to semisolid. In those children who produce firm wax, there is a tendency for it to accumulate in the external ear canal, sometimes to the point of complete obstruction. Misguided attempts by mothers to clean a young child's ears with cotton-tip applicators may *cause* obstruction; with each use of the cotton tip a little wax is pushed deep into the canal where it cannot be reached by ordinary means. When the ear canal becomes tightly plugged, it affects hearing to a moderate degree.

Wax can be removed by several methods. The least objectionable, from a child's point of view, is by putting a few drops of special wax softener in each ear at bedtime. It may be necessary to do this every evening for a month, but finally the wax softens and works its way out.

Since plugged ear canals are in no sense an emergency, it has always seemed unwise to us to insist on immediate mechanical removal of wax. It is an unpleasant experience for a young child to be held down while someone digs and scrapes in the ears. Even warm-water irrigation is unpleasant and actually frightening for some children. Unless it is essential that the doctor see the hidden eardrum because of infection or some other acute problem, it is better to take the slow way.

SWOLLEN GLANDS IN THE NECK

When children have colds, sore throats, or tonsillitis, it is not unusual for them to have some swelling of the lymph glands below the jaw and in the sides of the neck. These glands are, after all, part of the body's defense mechanism. They are packed with lymphocytes, those tiny blood cells that produce antibodies against infection.

Most cases of swollen glands subside after a few days without any treatment. If, after 2 or 3 days, the swelling is still increasing or if there is much fever, check with the doctor. Some cases do require antibiotics to help get rid of the infection.

It is not always easy to tell swollen glands from mumps

(see Chapter 13). The swelling of mumps usually spreads up onto the face, while that of swollen glands usually does not. In the days before antibiotics, abscesses sometimes formed in severe cases of swollen glands and necessitated surgical drainage. This is almost never necessary now.

BRONCHITIS

Incubation:	Usually follows a cold
Symptoms:	Cough; sometimes fever
Cause:	Most often viruses; sometimes bacteria
Treatment:	Humidity, rest, cough syrups, antibiotics
Prevention:	None

Cough is the outstanding symptom of bronchitis: persistent, annoying cough. There may be fever as well. Most often bronchitis occurs as part of a cold or grippe or any of the influenza-like virus infections. Indeed, any cold really worth the name is accompanied by some degree of bronchitis.

The bronchial tubes begin at the lower end of the windpipe, or trachea, and are the passages by which air ultimately reaches all the tiny air spaces in the lungs. The two largest bronchi, one going to the right lung and one to the left, are about the size of a pencil. They divide and subdivide until the smallest, the bronchioles, are but the diameter of a pin.

Since their lining is continuous with that of the windpipe, voice box, throat, mouth, and nose, it is easy to see how infection up above spreads down to cause inflammation. In terms of anatomy there is no sharp dividing line between bronchitis and pneumonia. If infection continues to spread down through the bronchial tubes, it eventually reaches the lung itself and what was a bronchitis becomes pneumonia.

The infection of the lining of the bronchi produces irritation and an excess production of mucus. The irritation and mucus cause the cough, which is in a sense a defense mechanism; without the cough the chest would simply fill with secretions. A further help in moving secretions away from the chest are the cilia, those untiring little hairlike structures in the bronchial tubes; they beat in such a fashion as to aid the cough in cleaning the passages of mucus. Fortunately, children do not ordinarily suffer the paralyzing effect of smoking upon the cilia.

Sometimes the bronchial irritation is so severe that the cough becomes almost constant and is exceedingly fatiguing. Then good cough syrups play their part in treatment. If they are properly used, they should provide *partial* relief of cough. As we have just seen, the abrupt elimination of the cough may be harmful, so large doses of cough medicine are not in order.

Humidity or the inhalation of water vapor or steam is helpful in thinning the secretions and thereby aiding in their expulsion. Antibiotics are helpful in some types of bronchitis. Since exercise, by increasing breathing, may further aggravate the cough, it is best to try to keep the child relatively quiet. Mild sedation may be helpful.

If the cough arrives in the late stages of a cold and is accompanied by a rise in temperature, or if the cough gets worse instead of better after a day or two, the child should be seen by his doctor, who can order antibiotics and other medications if they are needed. Not only can the bronchitis be helped but occasionally a subsequent pneumonia may be prevented.

However, most cases of bronchitis clear up without special treatment. Bronchitis can be an annoying, persistent, and fatiguing infection, but the outlook in children is almost uniformly excellent.

Very young infants are an exception. You should always consult the doctor if a baby's cough is severe or if fever is present in the later stages of a cold.

Asthmatic bronchitis

A few children have a particular kind of bronchitis whenever they have a bad cold (see also Asthma in Chapter 12). It is like any other case of bronchitis except that it includes wheezing and difficult breathing. Essentially, it is an allergic response to an infection.

Doctors who specialize in allergy are apt to think of it as asthma complicated by infection. Pediatricians usually think of it as bronchitis complicated by asthmatic breathing. From a practical point of view it doesn't make much difference.

Parents are apt to become discouraged by the frequency of recurrent attacks and concerned that some permanent damage will be done to the child. They can be comforted by the fact that children tend to outgrow the problem, though it is true that children with asthmatic bronchitis are more likely than others to have various allergic symptoms later in life. The episodes of wheezing with colds can be greatly helped by special medications: usually both an antibiotic and something to relieve the difficult breathing and wheezing. Antihistamines do *not* help and may even make matters worse.

If your child has had repeated attacks, the doctor may ask you to keep something on hand to be given at the very first sign of a wheeze. Response is best when medication is started at the beginning of a recurrence. Some physicians have a fair degree of success in reducing the frequency of attack by giving a series of injections of a bacterial vaccine. While this may reduce the episodes of wheezing, it does not prevent colds and is by no means a cure.

Sometimes there are other factors that contribute to these attacks. If a child is even slightly allergic to some inhaled dust, it may add to the severity of the attack of asthmatic bronchitis. The doctor can help you to track down and perhaps eliminate some of these troublesome additional substances.

PNEUMONIA

Incubation:	Most often a complication of a cold
Symptoms:	Rapid breathing, cough, fever
Cause:	Infection of the lung by virus or bacteria
Treatment:	Antibiotics when due to bacteria
Prevention:	None

Pneumonia occurs when infection is established in the tiny air sacs of the lungs (alveoli). Most pneumonia in young children comes as a complication of some sort of a cold or other virus infection. But it may occasionally come quite suddenly without any recognizable preceding infection.

The onset is usually accompanied by rising fever, increasing cough, and a mounting rate of breathing. Rapid breathing beyond what is expected from fever should always make you suspect pneumonia. The following table gives the expected resting breathing rates for children of various ages. (In counting the rate of breathing, count only the inhale or breathing-in phase.)

Resting Breathing Rates at Various Ages

(Count Only Inspiration)

Age	Rate per minute
6 months	28–38
1 year	24–34
2 years	20–30
4 years	20–26
6 years	18–24
10 years	16–22
15–20 years	15–18

Crying or exercise raises rate promptly.
Fever raises rates about 2 to 4 per degree.

Although bacteria cause many cases of pneumonia, certain of the viruses may also be responsible. Babies and very young children are especially prone to infection by a type known as *respiratory syncytial virus.* Antibiotics are effective in curing pneumonia caused by bacteria. The child's own resistance usually wins out over the viral types.

Patients are aware that there are various kinds of pneumonia, but the descriptive medical terms, so precise in their meaning, can be confusing. If only a limited area of lung is involved, doctors often call it *pneumonitis.* When there are many small scattered areas involved, it is called *bronchopneumonia*—and that is the type that infants and very small children are most apt to have. If a whole lobe of the lung is affected, then it is *lobar pneumonia;* if more than one lobe, it used to be spoken of as *double pneumonia.* If only the central part of the lung (the hilum) is involved, it is *hilar pneumonia,* the type most often caused by viruses. All these names are simply descriptive.

The basic problem is the same: infection of the lung tissue. The severity of each case depends on the virulence of the infection, the total amount of lung involved, and the resistance of the patient.

The principal function of the lungs is to transfer oxygen to blood. Pneumonia interferes. As soon as the infection has spread enough to cut down on the transfer of oxygen, the patient begins to feel short of breath and the rate of breathing increases. The usual cough and fever may be absent in very young infants, but rapid breathing is always present.

It was only a short while ago that the word pneumonia struck terror into the hearts of parents, and rightly so. The mortality from pneumonias of childhood was high, and recovery in every case was doubtful. All that has changed. Physicians no longer apply mustard plasters, hope, and fresh air while awaiting the dreaded "crisis." Today we have a whole arsenal of potent antibiotics. They are so effective that death from pneumonia in childhood is now very unlikely indeed. Automobile accidents have long since taken the place of pneumonia on the causes-of-death list.

Your doctor will need only his stethoscope to confirm the diagnosis of pneumonia. There are times, however, when he may need additional information to find out what kind of pneumonia is present. If he orders a chest X ray, blood count, or culture, it will be in an effort to refine the diagnosis. The antibiotic he chooses may depend, at least in part, upon this information.

Give the medication he orders for the full duration of time specified. In the home treatment of pneumonia, the most frequent mistake parents make is to stop the medication the moment the child feels better. Carry out the doctor's orders fully, no matter how well your child feels. If the diagnosis is made with reasonable promptness, most children with the common types of pneumonia will be up and about after just 2 or 3 days of treatment. Usually they can be treated at home. The conquest of pneumonia is one of the brilliant chapters of accomplishment in medicine.

12
Allergy

At least 15 percent of the babies and children who are brought to the doctor's office have allergies of one sort or another; they are hypersensitive to something which makes them sneeze, wheeze, itch, or have a variety of other symptoms. Many of these cases are recognized for what they are by parents. Other cases masquerade as a variety of other conditions. Food allergy, hiding under the guise of recurrent stomachache, is in our experience the commonest of these unrecognized allergies.

Babies are not usually born allergic. What, then, causes some of them to develop allergic symptoms?

The role of protein in allergy
Proteins are fundamental parts of the structure of all living material. A great variety of them make up an essential part of the food we eat. Our digestive apparatus breaks the proteins in our food into their basic structural units, simpler substances called *amino acids*. These amino acids are then absorbed into our blood, carried around the body, and reassembled into our own individual body protein. It is as if you took a brick wall apart down to its individual bricks, transported them to a new location, and then put them together to form a different wall.

358

Each person's individual proteins are different from any other person's. We may call them self-proteins. They are basic to making you yourself. They are very different, too, from bumble-bee protein, or mouse protein, or the protein of corn or egg white or cow's milk or, indeed, any other protein.

Nevertheless, all these proteins are built of amino acids, just as all brick walls are built of bricks. All living tissue needs about twenty kinds of amino acids from which to build its own kinds of protein.

If, instead of amino acids, some undigested protein is absorbed or injected into the blood, the body recognizes it as a non-self, or foreign, protein and wants no part of it. Let's say you had white of egg, a common food protein, injected into your vein. At first nothing would happen. Why should it? You can eat egg white without harm. But remember that when you eat it, you digest it; you break it down to amino acids which are then absorbed into the bloodstream. Now it has been injected undigested, and certain types of cells in the blood, like sentries of an army, will recognize it as a foreigner, an invader, called an *antigen*, and spread the message to millions of other similar blood cells.

Your body's cells will then begin to form substances that will react with, neutralize, and get rid of the invader. The substances they manufacture in response to the invasion are called *antibodies*. It takes time for them to be made, but once started the buildup becomes more and more rapid. As the antibodies increase in numbers, the foreign protein is gradually neutralized and eliminated.

The soldiers are still available after the initial invader is overcome; your body now has a sort of standing army of antibodies ready to fight that particular foreign protein whenever it appears again. A renewed appearance of the same material will result in a far faster buildup of antibodies than was the case with the initial invasion—and a far more intense reaction on your part. You may have had no reaction to the first injection. But you will to the second. For now you have become *allergic* to egg white.

These, then, are three of the most basic facts about allergy:

1. A foreign protein gaining access to the body is recognized as non-self protein (called an antigen).
2. The presence of an antigen in the body results in the formation of neutralizing substances (called antibodies).
3. When antigens and antibodies come together, a reaction occurs. As a result of producing antibodies to destroy a foreign protein, a person is said to have become *sensitized*. When a sensitized person again encounters the foreign protein that caused sensitization the body will react, in one way or another, and the person is said to be *allergic*.

Normally, a person does not have a foreign protein injected directly into his bloodstream. How then does a person become sensitized under natural conditions? Two examples will serve to reveal the mechanism as it occurs in everyday life, one involving hay fever and the other a food allergy.

Heredity's part in allergy

Some people are more likely than others to become sensitized, or allergic, under natural conditions, for the tendency to develop allergies is inherited. We are not saying that some individuals are *born* allergic but rather that there is a great likelihood of their becoming allergic under a given set of circumstances. Let's look at a typical case history.

Mr. Benton decides to take his 8-year-old son Bob out of the city on a short camping trip. Bob's mother does not join them because grass pollen gives her asthma. Bob invites Sam, a boy his own age, to go along. Sam's parents have never had any allergy problems.

It is late August, an ideal time for such a trip. Mr. Benton selects a meadow as their campsite. Here the three of them camp and fish for a few days. The weather is clear and windy. Ragweed is plentiful and in full bloom. Its pollen is invisible, but countless billions of the tiny grains float freely in the air. The three campers inhale millions of these tiny particles. They return home in good health and high spirits. The trip was a great success, and the boys go back to their city pattern of living with the hope of taking another trip the next summer.

Twelve months later Mr. Benton takes the two boys camping again. Everything is fine—except that in the early morning hours of the very first day Bob begins to sneeze repeatedly. His nose is stuffed up. His eyes itch and are watery. He does not feel sick and feverish, as he might with a fresh head cold, but the symptoms are very annoying. What is the matter with him? He has hay fever.

What, exactly, has happened? Why has this boy suddenly developed this annoying allergic disease when neither his father nor Sam is troubled?

Remember that Bob's mother, who has asthma, is an allergic individual, so the boy came into the world with more than an average tendency to become allergic under certain conditions. During the first camping trip Bob inhaled a great deal of ragweed pollen. Most of it was deposited on the moist membrane of the lining of his nose, and some of the pollen, foreign to his body, was dissolved in secretions and managed to pass into the cells of this lining membrane. Right under the surface of the lining are numerous capillary blood vessels. Some of that foreign protein, which was whole and undigested, came into contact with the blood cells that form antibodies. Because the dose of protein was relatively small, it took a while for a large amount of antibodies to be formed, but by the time Bob returned the second year those antibodies were ready and waiting. Bob was sensitized to ragweed protein. He had become allergic to this frequently inhaled pollen. And not until frost killed off the ragweed that fall was he free of the symptoms of hay fever.

FOOD ALLERGY

The function of our digestive tract is to digest food and to absorb into the body such of the products as are needed. As we said, digestion breaks proteins down into amino acids. These acids do not cause allergies. For allergy to food proteins to develop, it is necessary for some undigested protein to get past the barrier of the lining of the digestive tract.

Think of the lining of the small intestine as a sieve with microscopically small openings. These openings allow small particles (molecules) to pass through to the blood. Amino acid molecules are small enough to go through, whereas protein molecules are, in general, very much larger. Thus whole proteins capable of stimulating the production of antibodies do not normally pass through the sieve. The protein molecules are kept where they can do no harm until the digestive juices, or enzymes, split them up. Under certain conditions, however, the sieve is temporarily damaged and some of the protein molecules slip through.

For a second example let's take the case of a 2-year-old child who has one of those temporary but unpleasant upsets with nausea, vomiting, and diarrhea. The lining of her small intestine is irritated and inflamed by the virus that caused the upset. Her mother, feeling that she needs extra nourishment, mixes part of a raw egg with a little cereal and feeds it to her. Normally the egg-white protein would be broken down to its amino acid building blocks before being absorbed. But now, because of the irritation of her intestine, some of the egg-white protein molecules slip through the slightly damaged sieve and enter her blood. (As proteins go, egg white, or albumin, has a very small molecule which makes it a likely troublemaker.)

You already know the rest. Foreign protein in the blood means the development of antibodies—in this case antibodies to the egg-white protein. After a while the child begins to have symptoms every time she eats egg-white. The symptoms may vary but most often consist of vague recurrent stomachache, or a little diarrhea, or possibly hives. She has become allergic to egg white. Her antibodies now meet the egg albumin right beneath the lining cells in her intestine. The resulting reaction causes the symptoms.

The allergic reaction occurs and produces symptoms in whatever part of the body is most involved. When this reaction occurs in the lining of the upper respiratory tract, the patient has hay fever; when in the skin, hives; when in the intestinal tract, diarrhea or abdominal pain.

FINDING THE FOOD TROUBLEMAKERS. In young babies, cow's milk is by far the most frequent cause of food allergy. The symptoms are usually crampy stomachache and mild diarrhea. Occasionally a milk-sensitive baby will have recurrent vomiting.

Other infants with milk allergy appear to have a chronic cold or bronchitis. All these babies are likely to fuss and cry a lot. They seem generally uncomfortable and miserable.

Most modern infant feeding formulas are based on cow's milk, so it will not help the milk-allergic baby to switch from one kind of cow's milk feeding to another. Fortunately, though, there are now excellent substitutes, most of them made from soy beans. A trial of one of these milk-substitute products will usually relieve milk-allergy symptoms within 48 hours. After several months on a no-milk routine, some infants develop a tolerance for milk and are then able to take at least small amounts without symptoms.

As an allergic child grows older, other foods enter the picture more often. Egg white, seafoods, nuts, and chocolate are all rather likely causes of trouble.

The commonest symptom in the older child is a stomach-ache that comes anywhere from 30 minutes to 2 hours after eating. It is a persistent, nagging pain or discomfort. It can vary in severity within a few minutes. Usually it is not located in any one spot but seems to spread over the whole abdominal area. After 3 to 6 hours it fades away, only to recur when the same food is eaten again. The pain is often what doctors call dose-related. If, for instance, chocolate is at fault, the child may be able to take a little without trouble, but the pain returns on any day when a large amount is eaten.

Cooking is another factor that sometimes makes it difficult to see the relationship between a food and the symptoms. A child who is egg-allergic may have no symptoms after eating an egg that has been thoroughly baked or boiled for 30 minutes or more. Let that same child eat a 2½-minute egg and he may be uncomfortable for hours. Prolonged cooking alters the structure of some proteins so that they are incapable of taking part in the allergic reaction.

Apart from abdominal pain, children may have a variety of other symptoms related to food allergies. Headaches, hives, dizziness, fatigue and lassitude, achy pain in muscles, stuffy nose, chronic cough, and asthmatic attacks are all on the list.

You will need the doctor's help in tracking symptoms to their

363

source. It is sometimes a time-consuming and difficult project, and the doctor may turn for help to a specialist in allergies when the task proves unusually difficult. The well-known allergy skin tests are not very reliable where foods are concerned. They should be used only after careful watching and eliminating of test foods from the diet have failed to give the needed information. Selective restriction of suspect foods gives highly accurate information and costs nothing. You simply eliminate a particular food for a few days and then begin to give it again. If symptoms disappear and reappear, the answer is obvious. It's not as simple when several foods are involved, but even then it can often be worked out.

Antihistamines usually give relief from the symptoms of food allergy, but long-range treatment should involve discovering what foods are at fault and avoiding them.

Treatment of allergy

The allergic reaction is due in part to the release of an irritating substance called *histamine* from special cells that seem to congregate wherever an antigen-antibody reaction is occurring. The drugs called *antihistamines* help by neutralizing histamine.

Sometimes the allergic reaction produces spasm in certain fine muscle fibers such as those in the walls of the bronchial tubes. Drugs such as adrenaline and ephedrine that relax this spasm give relief.

So-called allergy shots are accurately graduated doses of the whole protein to which the patient is allergic. When given in exactly the right doses, at proper intervals, and over a long period of time, these shots serve to neutralize the patient's antibodies. For example, ragweed shots neutralize ragweed antibodies. When there are no ragweed antibodies left to react with actual ragweed pollen in the nose, the hay fever is better—but only as long as the patient keeps taking the injections.

ASTHMA

Asthma is an illness in which difficult breathing is accompanied by wheezing. The wheezing is caused by spasm of the many tiny muscles in the walls of the small bronchial tubes that carry air to the lungs. The contraction of these tiny muscles, plus the accumulation of thick, stringy mucus, partly closes off the tubes. The wheezy sound is produced as air is forced through these narrowed air passages. The greater the narrowing, the more difficult the breathing.

The most frequent underlying cause of asthma is an allergic reaction to some form of inhaled foreign protein: pollens, dusts of many kinds, mold spores, and sometimes chemical air pollutants.

One child's asthma may be due to ragweed pollen only, another to cat hair only, a third to dust from a mattress. Often a careful study is needed to find out what is causing a child's allergic reaction.

You will hear some people say that asthma is all psychological and others that it is all allergy. One becomes less certain as he becomes more experienced; asthma is a complex disease with multiple and interwoven causes. But we do know that the bronchial muscles are responsive to signals from the nervous system. Sometimes they contract in response to an emotional upset or anxiety. A frightening experience, problems in school, concern about family relationships that appear to the child to be falling apart—such things may trigger and sustain asthmatic attacks.

Parents of asthmatic children may notice other particular things that trigger attacks: exposure to very cold dry air, the beginning of an ordinary head cold (see Asthmatic Bronchitis), or the announcement that Mother will be away for the weekend. Sometimes several factors are at work at the same time. An observant mother will often come to realize which things or combinations of things are followed by asthmatic attacks, and she will try to help her child avoid them as much as possible.

Parents whose children react to dust (which is a mixture of many things) may find it necessary to prepare a "dust-free" room in which the young patient can sleep (see following sections). The presence of furred or feathered household pets is so often a factor that many allergists refuse to treat an asthmatic child unless such pets are removed. Cats are especially apt to be offenders; fish and turtles are safest.

Treatment of asthma

Even a moderate attack of asthma may frighten both mother and child the first time it happens. Remember that, despite the child's obvious discomfort, things will be better after a while. If you panic, you are likely to communicate your fear to your child, and his anxiety may make the attack worse. So put on as good a front as you can. Reassure your child. Meanwhile, call the doctor, because there are helpful drugs which can be given. If your child has had previous attacks, you probably have something on hand for treatment. Use it at the first sign of wheezing. Proper medication is quite effective in asthma, but it works best when given promptly.

Avoid the natural tendency to try one medicine after another, or several in combination, without the specific approval of the doctor. Overdosing and certain combinations of medicines can be dangerous.

If your doctor finds it very difficult to find the cause of repeated attacks of asthma, he may wish to get the help of an allergy specialist to find the source of the trouble.

If you have a very young child with asthma, take comfort in the fact that there is a tendency for him to improve as he gets older, particularly as he gets into his teens.

Setting up a "dust-free" bedroom. Some allergic children, especially those with year-round hay fever or those with asthma, do better when they sleep in a "dust-free" bedroom. The air in all living spaces is swarming with unseen dust particles, no matter how good the housekeeping. But it is possible to reduce this air-borne dust, and it is worth the trouble to see symptoms improve after the child sleeps in such a bedroom for a few nights.

First, wash the walls, woodwork, ceiling, and all other surfaces, including radiators and the insides of closets. Plug holes or gaps around pipes or windows. Wax the floors.

Woven materials should be eliminated. Leave no curtains, draperies, rugs, or upholstery, and remove pictures and pennants from the walls. No furry or stuffed toys should stay. Venetian blinds are dust traps, as are bookcases and books which are not

366

in use. Closets should be emptied and clothing kept elsewhere. This one room is for sleeping, reading, or study, not for any other activities. Scrub the bed frame. Vacuum the mattress and springs. If possible, buy allergy-proof casings for these. Use no mattress pad. If a pillow is necessary, it should have an allergy-proof cover. An alternative would be to use an inflatable pillow with a washed cotton cover.

Washable cotton blankets are best. If you are certain the child is not wool-sensitive, you may use 100 percent wool covers which have been washed. Any blankets should be washed at least once a month, and no quilts or puffs should be considered unless they are cotton filled with dacron. A dacron sleeping bag may be helpful in very cold weather, but it must be vacuumed regularly inside and out.

Keep the windows and doors closed. Allow no animals in this room. Do not use sprays, powders, deodorants, air fresheners, or insecticides. If you have a forced hot-air furnace, keep the filters clean by changing them often. Install filter material over the room hot-air inlets.

Vacuum the room completely at least once a week when the child is not present. Use a new vacuum bag. Damp-wipe the walls and ceiling occasionally.

In the summer an air conditioner is a great help.

HAY FEVER

Hay fever, with its stuffy nose, sneezing, and sometimes itchy eyes, is the commonest of the allergic troubles. As we saw, it develops when a child of any age is exposed to pollens and dusts in the air and becomes sensitized to one or more of those substances.

Most often it is exposure to ragweed pollen or grass pollen that causes hay fever. That's why it is so often seasonal. You can get a good lead as to the cause of your child's hay fever just by knowing the dates it begins and ends each year.

Some children are less fortunate and have symptoms all year around. Then it is called *perennial rhinitis*. Mold spores, cat dander, feather dust from pillows, and a host of other substances may be at fault.

Treatment starts with trying to avoid the offending substance. Often that's not possible, but medicines do help. There are antihistamines that may make the difference between misery and reasonable comfort. If these medications are not sufficiently effective, allergy shots are used. This is a long and tedious process, but it can help greatly with the constant stuffy nose and sneezing that interferes with sleep night after night.

Some fairly effective medicines for hay fever can be bought at the drugstore without prescription, but if a young child has symptoms be sure to check with the doctor. Do not use nose drops or sprays without a doctor's advice.

HIVES

Hives are swellings in the skin that itch intensely. They look much like mosquito bites. Their size varies from very tiny to that of a silver dollar. An attack of hives may last from a few hours to several days or more. Until a few years ago there was really no good relief from the itching. Now antihistamines usually work promptly and effectively.

Most often hives are an allergic reaction to something in the diet, but sometimes they are caused by other things in the environment. Once the particular cause is determined, most future attacks can be avoided. It will take a bit of detective work.

Seafoods and nuts are more commonly the cause than other foods, so watch out for those first. If these don't seem to be involved, use a small notebook to keep a record of the child's diet. Write everything down that he had to eat or drink for 24 hours before the hives appeared. If another attack comes, get out the notebook again. You may have to do this several times before you see what particular food or drink was taken each time. But once you know, you've solved the problem.

Occasionally hives follow skin contact with some outside substance. Bubble bath has been at fault many times. The cause in such cases is usually obvious.

If your child does get hives, don't belittle the itching. It can make him miserable. If you can't get the prescription you need right away, place him in a cool (but not cold) bath to which two cupfuls of bicarbonate of soda have been added. Cold wet cloths applied to the skin may also give temporary relief.

Prolonged anxiety is occasionally followed by hives in children. This is not common among younger ones but does seem to happen to adolescent girls. Medications are less helpful with this kind of hives. They tend to recur until the cause of the emotional tension blows over or is straightened out.

Work with children has its little moments of humor, even with so prosaic a thing as hives. Dr. Lee once had a younger child with very persistent hives. She was about 5. Talking about it with the mother in the child's presence, at one point he remarked, "Remember, it'll all blow over in time."

His little patient burst into tears. Surprised, he asked what had made her cry. "I don't *want* to blow over," she said, and started to cry hard all over again. Turned out her nickname was Ittle!

ECZEMA (ATOPIC DERMATITIS)

Eczema is a troublesome skin condition that occurs occasionally in a baby who has allergic tendencies. The trouble may be precipitated by reaction to something in the diet or by an external substance like wool, soap, or detergent. Sometimes several things contribute, and so it is difficult to determine all of them.

Usually eczema begins on the face as patches of reddened, rough skin that itch severely and then get sore as a result of rubbing. When large areas of skin are involved, the baby may not get much rest because of the itching.

The doctor will consider the many factors that may be playing a part and will help you eliminate things that may be causing the trouble. You may have to give milk substitutes, to use special ointments or lotions, and to pay close attention to many things in the environment. It takes time. Do not expect your doctor to bring about a rapid cure, because that is impossible in many cases. Be patient. Treatment will minimize the discomfort, and the baby will thrive despite the eczema. If you get discouraged, remember that even the most severe cases eventually do get better.

369

USEFUL ALLERGIES

So far we have discussed the allergic reaction as a cause of illness, which it very often is. At times, however, it serves another purpose: This same basic reaction is one of our best defenses against infection. When the invading foreign protein happens to be part of a bacterium or virus, the body manufactures antibodies in the same way. Then, if that kind of germ comes along again, the antibodies are waiting and destroy the germ, making it unable to invade to any degree. When that happens, we say the person is *immune* to that particular invader. We could as rightly say he is allergic to it. But this time the allergic reaction serves a useful purpose.

Immunity and allergy are closely intertwined and are fascinating to study. Allergy, in a sense, is a miscarriage of the purposeful process of immunity.

13
Contagious Diseases

GRIPPE

The word *grippe* is a bit of a wanderer. Unlike most medical terms, it has a broad and sometimes vague meaning. Because it is not a precisely defined word, its use varies from place to place, time to time, and doctor to doctor. To make things even more confusing it is used more or less interchangeably with the abbreviated word *flu*, even though influenza is actually a separate disease caused by distinct viruses. Pinned down, doctors will admit that grippe is a sort of catch-all, a term used to cover a whole group of infections caused by several kinds of viruses.

The words *common cold* are used in the same loose fashion to cover infections by at least 30 separate viruses. Usually there is sneezing, stuffy nose, scratchy throat, and moderate cough. If in addition the particular virus involved causes a lot of headache, muscular aches, chills, fever, and perhaps a severe cough, it is more likely to be called a "grippy" cold or just grippe.

These more severe infections are usually accompanied by much fever and are caused by viruses other than the common cold viruses. There are adenoviruses, rhinoviruses, Coxsackie viruses, echo viruses, parainfluenza, and others. Some produce more cough, some more severe headache, some brief skin rashes, some very sore muscles. With any of them the doctor may say your child has grippe. Since there is no separate and specific treatment for each kind, it does not matter much that they are lumped together.

The day may come when there will be more specific medicines for particular viruses. Until then you will continue to get the old advice: rest, plenty of fluids, aspirin, and patience. Mother Nature will get your child well. The doctor's principal function is to make sure the illness is nothing other than grippe and to treat occasional complications such as ear infections.

Is it possible to be more definite about the exact diagnosis? Yes, it is possible for the knowledgeable doctor who has special laboratory facilities available. But it does not have much practical value. Virus diagnostic work is time-consuming and expensive. By the time necessary specimens from the patient can be delivered to the lab, the virus cultured, isolated, and identified, your child will be recovered and back at school.

Instead of going through all that work and expense and being told, perhaps, that your child had an infection with Coxsackie virus Type 17, you are simply told that he had the grippe. It is often not possible for your doctor to distinguish a good hard case of "grippe," caused by any of the viruses mentioned, and real influenza.

INFLUENZA

Incubation:	2 to 3 days
Symptoms:	Chills, high fever, and aching, as for a severe cold
Cause:	Influenza virus (several types)
Treatment:	No specific medicines
Prevention:	Vaccines give some protection, but see text

There are several flu viruses, but all of them produce just about the same symptoms. Usually the patient has chills, high fever, headache, sore throat, achy muscles, runny and stuffy nose, and cough. Except for the cough the whole thing lasts only 4 to 7 days. The cough clears up more slowly.

Flu tends to be seasonal, occurring in large epidemics during winter and spring. Because it is a virus infection there are, as yet, no drugs that are really effective in its treatment. Antibiotics are useless in all viral infections, and flu is no exception. Aspirin does help the child to feel better, and staying in the house may help to prevent complications.

After an attack of flu, many patients feel under par for quite a long time. Recurrence of fever after a period of normal temperature may mean a complication. Most of the complicating secondary infections can be cured with antibiotics. Therefore the doctor should be notified if fever recurs.

Flu vaccine, widely heralded in the past few years, is *not* recommended for healthy children, for youngsters sometimes have rather severe reactions to it. The protection it gives is far from perfect, and the disease itself is not dangerous in otherwise healthy children. Your doctor may decide to give the vaccine if your child suffers from asthma or certain other troubles that make the complications of influenza more likely. Immunity from an attack of flu is variable but seldom lasts more than 4 years. There is little or no cross-immunity between the various strains of virus. If three varieties of flu hit a community successively, it is perfectly possible for a person to get flu three times. Fortunately, the interval between separate waves of different types of flu in any one geographic area is usually several months at least.

GASTROENTERITIS
(*Nausea, Vomiting, Diarrhea*)

Incubation:	Variable; usually 2 to 4 days
Symptoms:	Nausea, vomiting, cramps, diarrhea
Duration:	Variable
Cause:	Most often viruses; occasionally bacteria such as salmonella; sometimes spoiled food (food poisoning)
Prevention:	None

There are few among us who have not been through the unpleasantness of an attack of vomiting and diarrhea. It is common enough everywhere, but city populations are particularly exposed because close contact enables it to jump easily from one person to another.

Gastroenteritis is caused by several kinds of viruses and occasionally by bacteria such as the group called salmonella. To our misfortune, an attack of one kind confers no immunity against any other sort. Thus it is possible to have several episodes in a year's time, all presenting the same unpleasant symptoms but each caused by a different kind of infection, passed around by direct or indirect contact with other people. It is a miserable thing, and when children get it they are every bit as unhappy as grown-ups.

Luckily it *usually* does not last long, about 12 to 36 hours. No medicines are needed in cases of short duration. There are, in fact, none that make much difference in the first few hours.

Offer the child cracked ice, *sips* of water, weak tea, or soft drinks in small but frequent amounts. After the vomiting has stopped completely for 3 or 4 hours, you can try more fluid and let him gradually work up to drinking all he wants. If the diarrhea continues in severe form, the doctor may order paregoric or some other medication to help control it.

The only danger, particularly for very young or very small children, lies in the loss of so much body fluid that the child gets out of chemical balance and becomes dehydrated. If the vomiting is frequent and persistent over several hours, the diarrhea severe and lasting over 24 hours, call the doctor. Occasionally a baby or very young child needs to go to a hospital to receive fluids by vein if they cannot be retained by mouth. Intravenous fluids make a great difference. Recovery is usually quite prompt.

Children bounce back fast. As soon as they feel a little better they usually want to eat. You will do well to make them go slowly. Restrict them to small portions of soft foods like Junket, Jell-O, custards, and soups to start with. Too big a meal too soon may cause a setback. If, after eating, vomiting starts again, go back to the cracked ice and clear fluids. It pays to make haste slowly in adding foods.

374

DIARRHEA

Diarrhea can be a nuisance for a mother—and a serious matter for very young babies. Mostly it's a nuisance. Taking care of an infant or young child who has messed himself, his bed, and everything in it is not a pleasant chore. Small wonder that mothers run for the phone at the first sign of a really loose bowel movement.

Mothers tend to misuse the term *diarrhea* more often than almost any other. It is important in our present discussion to be precise. Many very young babies, especially if breast-fed, will have from three to five soft, sometimes quite runny, movements every day. That's normal. The baby is fine, eats well, and is thriving. There are fewer movements as the days and weeks go by. This is not diarrhea; it is not abnormal. On the other hand, an older baby who usually has one or two formed stools a day and then suddenly has several liquid movements in succession does have diarrhea. He will probably have cramps and not feel too well.

If your baby is under 2, call the doctor promptly when diarrhea develops. Infants lose fluid and body salts much faster in proportion to their size than do older children. This in turn causes dehydration and chemical imbalances which are very difficult to correct if they go too far. If your small baby's mouth begins to seem dry and his eyes to look sunken—and he is listless and lethargic—waste no time in calling the doctor. These are dangerous symptoms and hospital care may be urgently needed. At the hospital it is possible to supply fluid, salts, and sugar by vein, usually with rapid improvement and recovery.

There are many causes of diarrhea, ranging from simple digestive upsets to severe intestinal infections by bacteria or viruses. When diarrhea proves to be resistant to ordinary treatment, your doctor may want to take cultures or do other laboratory tests before trying other treatment.

Many mild cases can be handled simply by cutting back to a bland diet and nonfruit liquids. Give such fluids as plain water, sweetened weak tea, soft drinks, chicken broth, beef bouillon, and skimmed or nonfat milk until the diarrhea begins to subside. Then *gradually* add foods like Junket, Jell-O, custards, cooked cereals, crackers, bread, and lean meat. Save fruits and vegetables for last.

There are medicines that can be bought in the drugstore without a prescription that are helpful for mild cases. Plain old paregoric—which does require a prescription in many areas— is still one of the most effective remedies. If you use it, be sure you ask about the proper dose for your child.

When such measures are ineffective, do not persist with them too long without getting medical help, particularly if there is repeated vomiting, fever, or blood in the bowel movements.

MEASLES	
Incubation:	10 to 14 days
Symptoms:	Fever, cough, reddened watery eyes, blotchy red rash
Cause:	Measles virus
Treatment:	Nothing specific; something to relieve cough and to control fever if very high
Prevention:	Measles vaccine is very effective at any age, preferably at about 1 year

Measles begins like an ordinary cold that keeps getting worse. The cough becomes more and more severe, the fever rises irregularly, the eyes become bleary and reddened.

The most troublesome symptom is cough. If there is no cough, it is not measles! The cough is harsh, frequent, persistent, and tiresome.

About the third or fourth day a blotchy, red rash appears. When first noticed the rash is on the face and neck, but it spreads slowly down until the entire body is covered except for the palms and soles. During this stage the child may seem very ill. Severe measles is no picnic. You will need the doctor's help.

Two or three days after the rash starts, about the time it reaches the ankles, the patient begins to improve. If, after some improvement, the child seems to be getting worse, you should call the doctor again. Most complications are caused by bacteria and can be controlled by proper use of antibiotics. Because the complications of measles are sometimes more serious than the disease itself, you should not try to see it through on your own.

The old idea that light damages the eyes during measles is not true. The disease does, however, cause some irritation of the eyes, and the child may be more comfortable in a partly darkened room. Watching television or reading will not be harmful. As a rule the child will miss 7 to 10 days of school.

Fortunately, measles is rapidly disappearing wherever the vaccine is being used. If you have a child who has been exposed to measles and who has not been vaccinated, a dose of gamma globulin given by the doctor will assure a milder case.

GERMAN MEASLES
(*Rubella*)

Incubation:	14 to 21 days
Symptoms:	Slight to moderate fever; variable pale-pink blotchy rash; slightly swollen lymph glands; sometimes, in older children, achy joints
Cause:	German measles virus
Treatment:	No specific medicines
Prevention:	Vaccine, best given in childhood

Despite frequent confusion, there is no relationship between German measles (3-day measles) and "real" or "regular" measles. The two diseases are caused by different viruses. German measles is a very mild disease, sometimes so mild as to go all but unnoticed. It has few complications except when it occurs during the first 6 months of a pregnancy. Then it is capable of causing serious defects in 15 to 25 percent of the babies. (See also Chapter 1.)

German measles produces slight to moderate fever and sometimes mild malaise, headache, and aching joints. A mottled pink rash appears more or less over the whole body in one day. By the fourth day most of the symptoms are over and the patient feels well again. Without experience it is difficult to distinguish mild scarlet fever, mild "regular" measles, certain echo virus infections, and German measles itself. Better let your doctor do the sorting.

An effective vaccine for preventing German measles became available in 1969. Children should be vaccinated between the first and third years, or any time later in childhood if they have not received it previously. By immunizing children, the source of infection for adult women is largely removed.

It is not yet certain whether it is safe to use the vaccine for women during pregnancy. For this reason it is usually not given to women in the child-bearing age group unless there is certainty that pregnancy will not occur in the ensuing 3 to 4 months. A pregnant woman cannot become harmfully infected from a recently vaccinated child.

The last great epidemic of German measles in the United States in 1964 was followed by at least 8,000 stillbirths and more than 20,000 defective babies. The children born with these defects, largely of heart and eyes, represent a tragedy that could have been prevented had the present vaccine then been available. It has been estimated that the total care and education of a child damaged before birth by German measles may average as high as $9,000 per year. Apart from the personal anguish to parents and children, this is a burden that society as a whole can ill afford. The answer to this terrible problem is now at hand. Every child should receive the vaccine.

ROSEOLA	
Incubation:	Uncertain
Symptoms:	High fever, occasionally fever convulsions, sometimes puffy eyelids
Cause:	Probably a virus
Treatment:	Aspirin; tepid water sponging to reduce fever if very high
Prevention:	None

Roseola, sometimes miscalled "baby measles," occurs once in nearly every child below the age of 3. It causes worry out of all proportion to its importance because it often produces fever up to 105 degrees or more. There are few other symptoms until, on the fourth or fifth day, a pink mottled rash appears on the chest and abdomen.

Despite the high temperatures, most babies with roseola do not seem very sick. By the time the rash appears, the fever is nearly gone and the child is rapidly improving. The whole thing lasts only 4 to 6 days. Second attacks are almost unknown.

Because the temperature reaches such high levels, occasionally a child has a fever convulsion during roseola. (See Fever Convulsions in Chapter 10.) Such convulsions are frightening for parents, but they are not dangerous. Lowering the child's temperature by sponging usually stops them promptly. Rub him down with slightly cool water and keep him uncovered so the water can evaporate freely. Do not worry about chilling the child; there is a lot of heat to be dissipated. The doctor can give a sedative medication that will prevent a recurrence of the convulsion.

Remember, almost every baby has roseola once, and they all get well in just a few days.

CHICKEN POX

Incubation:	11 to 21 days
Symptoms:	Variable fever, pimply skin rash, moderate to severe itching
Cause:	Chicken pox virus
Treatment:	No specific medicines; anti-itch preparations, aspirin, mild sedatives
Prevention:	None

Chicken pox varies greatly from one case to the next, but it is certainly one of the least serious of childhood infectious diseases. On the average, younger children are apt to have milder cases than older people, but there are exceptions.

Fever is extremely variable as to time of onset, height and duration. The rash begins by looking very much like a crop of mosquito bites. Then a clear water blister forms at the top of each spot. The blister becomes cloudy, breaks, and a little crust forms. Some children itch a good bit; others not at all. Cut and file your child's fingernails very short to prevent damage from scratching, the pocks do not permanently scar unless deeply scratched and infected.

Bathing in tub or shower at least twice a day with plain tepid water, followed by *patting* dry with a towel, tends to minimize the itching. The various lotions that are available for the treatment of poison ivy rashes are also helpful for the itching of chicken pox. If, in spite of these measures, itching is still a problem, the doctor can order medicine to be taken internally that will help.

Chicken pox spots appear in the mouth and throat, around the rectum, in the vaginal area, and on the eyelids. In all these places they may lead to moderate discomfort. If any appear on the eyeball the doctor should be promptly consulted.

Sometimes children are frightened by their appearance in a mirror and need to be reassured that the pocks are going to go away.

School-age children usually miss about a week.

SCARLET FEVER	
Incubation:	3 to 7 days
Symptoms:	Fever, very sore throat, headache, vomiting, red sandpaperlike rash
Duration:	2 to 5 days, but 10 days' treatment is essential
Cause:	Particular kind of streptococcus
Treatment:	Penicillin or a substitute for 10 days
Prevention:	Penicillin may be used for close contacts

Scarlet fever, once greatly dreaded, is now easily and very successfully treated. The disease is really a special kind of strep throat that is accompanied by a reddish skin rash with a surface that suggests sandpaper.

Symptoms usually begin 3 to 7 days after exposure to someone who has the disease or to someone who is just carrying the particular strep germ. The onset may be quite sudden, with sore throat, headache, fever, and often vomiting. A few hours to a day or so later the rash appears on face and body. The severity of scarlet fever varies greatly from place to place, from year to year, and from one child to the next. Some are very sick indeed.

If you suspect scarlet fever, talk to your doctor, for you will need his help in getting the best of modern treatment. Penicillin or a substitute antibiotic brings about rapid improvement and prevents most of the complications which were once so feared: ear and mastoid infections, pneumonia, rheumatic fever, and heart damage. The penicillin can usually be given by mouth; occasionally, when vomiting is a problem, the first dose may have to be injected.

After 2 or 3 days of treatment the child becomes noninfectious and the chain of contagion is broken. That is why the big epidemics of the past are now uncommon.

It is very important that the antibiotic be given for 10 days and *not* just until the child seems better. If treatment is stopped in less than 10 days, the infection may not be completely eliminated. Mild cases, sometimes called *scarletina*, should also be treated for the full 10 days.

Despite proper treatment, there are occasional kidney complications. For this reason the doctor may want a urine examination about 2 weeks after the beginning of a case of scarlet fever.

School absence is 4 to 10 days. The doctor may permit the child to return to school while still taking penicillin.

Remember: Don't cut corners with scarlet fever—or, for that matter, with any strep throat.

MUMPS

Incubation:	14 to 21 days
Symptoms:	Fever, headache, swelling and tenderness below and in front of ear
Cause:	Mumps virus
Treatment:	No specific medications
Prevention:	Mumps vaccine, at any age after 1 year; most important after 10 years

---

The onset of mumps is so variable that parents are often misled. Only when the swelling of the face comes right at the beginning—which it by no means always does—is the diagnosis certain at the onset. Often the disease starts with fever, loss of appetite, headache, nausea, and irritability, a combination common to many of the infections of childhood. When the swelling does appear, it begins in front of and below the ear. Sometimes only one side of the face is swollen; sometimes the opposite side follows a few days after the first. Mumps involves the salivary glands. Most often it is the parotid, which is located inside the lower half of the face. The swelling is soft and smooth to the touch, always tender, and sometimes quite painful. It varies from very slight to the classic puffed-up moon face that most parents expect to see. Whether or not both sides are involved, the disease is followed by immunity.

It is sometimes difficult to distinguish the swelling in a mild case of mumps from the swollen lymph glands in the side of the neck that often accompany or follow sore throats. An abscessed tooth may also give a good imitation of mumps, sometimes with no pain at all in the tooth. Experience helps. Mumps *feels* different to the fingertips. This fact often enables the doctor to be certain in a moment.

The pancreas, a digestive gland in the upper abdomen, is often involved to some extent, which accounts for the abdominal pain, nausea, and vomiting.

Occasional complications occur which involve the testicles, ovaries, hearing nerves, or the membranes around the brain, as in mumps encephalitis. Though that complication sounds terrifying, it usually means only very severe headaches and then full recovery. The involvement of testicles and ovaries is *not* common in childhood and, despite the talk and fear, very rarely produces sterility.

Many an old wives' tale swirls around the subject of mumps. There is no evidence that ointments, flannel wrappers, ice bags, hot packs, or any internal medication have the slightest influence on its course, duration, severity, or complications. It seems to make little difference whether the child is confined to bed or given the run of the house. A light diet that is low in fats and oils may minimize the stomachache, and aspirin helps the other aches and pains.

Because it is less contagious than many other infections, a good many individuals reach adult life without having had mumps. It may be decidedly more troublesome in the adult, and complications are much more frequent. Fortunately mumps vaccine protects adults as well as children. It should be used before exposure occurs.

For an average case of mumps, about 1 week of school time is lost.

WHOOPING COUGH

Incubation:	7 to 14 days
Symptoms:	Very severe cough in long paroxysms
Cause:	A special kind of bacteria
Treatment:	Even temperature, high humidity, special antibiotics under doctor's supervision, antiserum for small babies
Prevention:	Vaccine, given in early infancy

Whooping cough is a dangerous disease for babies under 1 year. In older children it is not life-threatening, but it can be a severe trial. It is ordinarily transmitted only by close contact with a case.

It starts like a mild cold with a troublesome cough, but the cough gets rapidly worse and does not respond to cough remedies.

During the more and more severe paroxysms, the child gets red in the face and appears about to strangle. These protracted spasms of coughing are followed by the long inspiratory gasp or whoop. Vomiting frequently follows. In a mild case the cough may come only 3 or 4 times a day; when severe, the paroxysms are frequent enough to exhaust the child. Little children are frequently quite frightened by the cough and the subsequent feeling of struggling for air.

Home remedies are not of much help, but the child should be kept in a warm, humidified room as much of the time as possible. A vaporizer of some sort can be used to keep the humidity high. If you use a boiling water vaporizer, be careful to avoid accidental burns of the patient or other children in the household. So-called cold steam vaporizers are much to be preferred.

You will need your doctor's help. He has no medicine that will promptly cure whooping cough, but he can prescribe drugs to ease the coughing and allow the child to rest and sleep. Certain antibiotics help to some degree. There is a serum made from the blood of specially immunized adult donors (pertussis immune globulin), but it is more helpful for very young babies than it is for older children.

Whooping cough is preventable. The vaccine should be started in early infancy and injected in three doses about a month apart. Whenever a case does occur, everything possible should be done to isolate the patient from other children, especially infants.

A case seldom lasts less than 5 to 8 weeks or more. It is an exhausting experience for the child and his family. Prevention is the only really satisfactory answer to this trying disease.

DIPHTHERIA

Incubation:	Variable, usually 4 to 6 days
Symptoms:	Fever, sore throat, headache, and very marked prostration
Cause:	The diphtheria bacillus
Treatment:	Special serum and antibiotics
Prevention:	Diphtheria toxoid

Diphtheria is another dangerous but preventable disease. A child with diphtheria is very obviously ill. He has a sore throat covered by a yellowish white coating, often a very hoarse voice, croupy cough, and difficult breathing. But these same symptoms can be caused by much less dangerous infections. So if your child does have such symptoms and has had his diphtheria shots, you can rest easy.

If he has *not* been immunized, do not delay in getting medical help. Be sure to tell the doctor that your child has not had the preventive.

MENINGITIS

Incubation:	Variable, usually 5 to 7 days; only the type caused by meningococcus is readily transmissable
Symptoms:	Fever, severe headache, stiff neck, stiff back, vomiting
Cause:	Several kinds of bacteria
Treatment:	Intravenous antibiotics *in hospital*
Prevention:	None

Fortunately meningitis is not very common, for it is always a serious disease. Treatment is a real medical emergency. A child with meningitis has fever, severe headache, vomiting, and a stiff neck or stiff back. There will be no doubt that the child is very sick. With this combination of symptoms, get help

385

promptly. If you can't reach your doctor, go to the nearest hospital. Time is important!

Meningitis means inflammation, or infection, of the covering membranes of the brain. There are several different varieties caused by various kinds of infection; all are serious.

The commonly known and greatly feared "spinal meningitis" is caused by a bacterium called meningococcus. Until quite recently it was almost uniformly fatal, but with intensive hospital treatment most patients now survive and return to normal health.

POLIOMYELITIS

Incubation:	5 to 7 days, occasionally much more
Symptoms:	Fever, stiff neck, stiff back, headache, weakness
Cause:	Polio viruses
Treatment:	Nothing specific
Prevention:	Polio vaccine

This terrible disease "infantile paralysis" is now completely preventable. Everywhere in the world that the vaccine is in use the disease is controlled. The vaccine is given by mouth. No child should go without it.

Before the vaccine was developed, polio crippled and killed many thousands of children and young adults every year. There was a day when every severe headache with fever and every stiff neck quite rightly froze a parent's heart with fear. This you no longer have to face. Get the vaccine for your children and yourself.

INFECTIOUS MONONUCLEOSIS
(*Mono*)

Incubation:	Very variable
Symptoms:	Variable but usually sore throat, lack of pep, fatigue, low fever
Cause:	A virus
Treatment:	Nothing specific; rest
Prevention:	None

"Mono," the abbreviated name for this disease, is far commoner than we used to think. Many, many cases undoubtedly are undiagnosed because the symptoms are often so mild and vague. Kids don't wear labels saying, "I have mono."

The symptoms of sore throat, slightly swollen lymph glands, and a feeling of being tired all the time are common to other illnesses, but in this case they may be long-drawn-out. The fever, which is usually moderate, tends to come and go. Often there are afternoon or evening peaks and a return to normal overnight. The doctor himself is often misled by the mildness of the physical abnormalities that he can detect. The sore throat sometimes does not look very sore; the swollen glands are no more than may be seen with some colds; the occasional skin rash on the body lasts but a short time. Sometimes a doctor can feel the spleen, an abdominal organ that enlarges with this infection. If he can, it's a help in diagnosis.

Despite the general vagueness of the whole illness, the child will persist in saying he feels "lousy" or "lazy all the time" or just "blah." These are the descriptive terms that children are apt to use, for they cannot be more specific about it. The very vagueness of their symptoms should make us think of mono.

The doctor can have a blood count taken and may find one type of cells (*mono*nuclears) increased in number. There are other blood tests that become positive a little later. The results of such tests will usually clinch the diagnosis.

There is no specific medicine for this virus disease, but fortunately the children all recover. It sometimes takes several weeks, during which time the patient continues to feel below par, to have at least a little fever, and to be somewhat lacking in interest in his usual activities.

Experience shows that prolonged bedrest makes no difference. The more severe cases may need a week or two at home but can usually get back to school thereafter. Older children tend to have mono in more severe form, and an adolescent is occasionally very sick indeed. But the rule holds—they all recover.

TUBERCULOSIS

Incubation:	Weeks to many months
Symptoms:	Fever and fatigue; cough not prominent in children
Cause:	Tubercle bacillus, a very special kind of bacteria
Treatment:	Special drugs taken for a year or more
Prevention:	Removal from contacts; avoidance of serious infection depends on finding cases early by tuberculin testing

Tuberculosis in childhood can be successfully treated if it is discovered in its early stages. The definite symptoms that are usually associated with adult TB—cough, bloody sputum, fatigue, fever, loss of weight—are not often present in children. In grown-ups the disease attacks the structure of the lung, while in children it is more likely to be present in the lymph glands at the root of the lung. There it may smolder for a long time. It often heals completely without leaving anything more than a small scar visible on X ray to prove that it was there.

Occasionally, instead of healing, the infection spreads slowly to additional lymph glands and later to other structures: lungs, bones, joints, or, rarely, the membranes around the brain. During this time of slow spreading it may produce only vague symptoms such as low fever, fatigue, paleness, and failure to gain weight.

Fortunately there is a highly accurate skin test which can

reveal the presence of the disease before there are any symptoms. The skin test becomes positive about 6 to 8 weeks after TB germs enter the body. If, by means of this skin test, infection is discovered in its early stages, cure is virtually certain.

A positive skin test does not always mean that active infection is present. More often than not a healthy child will, by his own resistance, overcome the initial infection. After such healing the skin test will remain positive for a long time. Chest X rays are needed to find out whether the child with a positive skin test has an active infection or only a tiny healed scar. The skin test should come first. X rays are needed *only* when the skin test is positive. Using this sequence avoids a great many unnecessary X-ray examinations.

Whenever a child has a positive skin test it is important that all the adults in his environment be checked. The source of infection for the child is most often an unrecognized infection in an adult.

The tuberculin testing of children has led to the early discovery of many adult cases. Their treatment in turn leads to the protection of more and more children. Modern drugs make the treatment of tuberculosis so successful that even rather advanced cases are being cured. Early detection through the routine testing of children is contributing to the ultimate defeat of this disease. *A tuberculin skin test should be part of every annual health checkup throughout childhood.*

WORMS

Pinworms

The *pinworm* or *threadworm* is nearly universal among children. Despite this, the discovery of their presence seems to shock many mothers. Extensive studies have revealed that in any given classroom at any particular time, from 15 to 30 percent of the children are infested. In some areas where children are crowded together, it approaches 100 percent.

This tiny creature, usually less than ¼ inch in length and not much thicker than a piece of heavy thread, lives in the lower intestinal tract. It is generally thought of as a parasite, but it takes little or nothing from its host.

The only symptom is itching around the rectal opening and, as a result, restlessness. In girls there may also be intense itching around the vaginal area.

Unlike many parasites, the pinworm has no intermediate host. Its life cycle is simple. Female worms find their way out of the rectal opening at night and deposit myriads of tiny eggs on the surrounding skin. It is this migration from the rectum that produces the itching. The child scratches; the eggs stick to the fingers and are transferred, sooner or later, to the mouth. Once swallowed, the eggs start a new generation of worms. Because the hand-washing hygiene of children is hit-or-miss to say the least, both after toilet and at mealtime, it is not hard to see how these minute eggs find their way to infect others.

Pinworms, like all other parasites, can be acquired only from another individual, directly or indirectly. They do not come from eating dirt or too many sweets.

Treatment is simple. Your doctor may suggest that all members of the family take the necessary medication, because close contacts are usually infected. Recurrences are common while there are young children in a home.

Other parasites

Apart from the nearly universal pinworm, there are many other parasites, but their prevalence varies greatly in different parts of the world. Local medical knowledge is important for their control, as they vary in different geographic areas and different population groups. Where community hygiene is at a high level and meat and fish products are processed properly, the number of intestinal parasites of most kinds declines quite rapidly.

There is good treatment available for almost all the human parasites, as well as rapidly expanding knowledge about them. You should not try to treat children with parasitic diseases without medical help, for many of the older drugstore remedies, which were uncertain at best, have been replaced with highly potent drugs that require careful dosage and good supervision.

14
Skin Problems

RASHES

Any doctor who works with babies and children gets lots of calls about rashes. Some are very common and are limited to certain age groups, and so the doctor may even be able to tell you over the phone what it is and what to do. Easy as that sounds, successful treatment of some of the many variations is occasionally more difficult than you expect. If treatment is prescribed by phone and you do not see improvement after a couple of days, let the doctor know.

Older children present more kinds of rashes than babies, and distinguishing between them is often more difficult. The doctor may ask to see a particular rash before telling you what to do. In such cases mothers sometimes seem annoyed. "But doctor, it's just a rash. Can't you order something from the drugstore or tell me what to get?" Ten seconds of *seeing* the condition may make it easy to order the right thing. It cannot always be done without actually looking. There is more than one kind of eczema, more than one kind of diaper rash, more than one type of impetigo. Not every itchy rash on the feet is "athlete's foot."

Several of the contagious diseases of childhood have associated rashes—measles, German measles, echo virus infections, roseola, scarlet fever, some kinds of meningitis, to mention a few. It takes experience to sort them out.

On the other hand, the doctor can often tell what a rash is *not* very quickly and definitely over the phone. The following conversation is an example.

> "This is Mrs. Brown. I think Karen has measles. She has a friend at school who had them a while ago."
> "What are you using for the cough?"
> "She hasn't got a cough. She just has a rash,"
> "Then she doesn't have measles."
> "How do you know, doctor? She has a measles rash."

The doctor was sure. No cough, no measles! Definite. The rash had to be something else.

In this book there are sections about cradle cap, eczema, diaper rash, prickly heat, impetigo, measles, German measles, chicken pox, scarlet fever, hives, ringworm, poison ivy, and chemical contact rashes. These are the commoner rashes of childhood. Most are temporary and none are ordinarily serious. Some need no treatment at all and some, like eczema, may try your patience, for it can be prolonged and difficult under the best of care.

PRICKLY HEAT

This common rash usually appears shortly after the beginning of spells of hot weather. Tiny red spots appear on the forehead, behind the ears, on the neck, and sometimes down over the shoulders and stomach. When severe, almost the entire body may be covered. In some cases there are minute blisters at the center of each reddened area.

Prickly heat is usually noticed a few hours *after* a baby has been overheated. Humidity and heat combine to produce overactivity of the sweat glands. Sometimes it happens even in cold weather when babies are overdressed or covered with too many blankets in a warm house. The worst offenders in causing prickly heat in cool weather are sleeping garments that completely enclose the baby, including feet, legs, and arms. Remember, a baby cannot unzip such clothing or turn back blankets when too warm.

When it is caused by hot, humid weather, the child should be allowed to be bare or with the least possible clothes. Witch hazel lotion or cornstarch powder may be used on the skin. An old remedy is to pat on a solution of a teaspoon of baking soda (sodium bicarbonate) in a cup of water. Any of these treatments may be soothing.

Prickly heat does not seem to bother young babies very much, but older infants may be fretful and may do some scratching.

IMPETIGO

This very common skin infection begins as a little pimple or blister that later becomes scaly or crusty. Often it starts on the face, under the opening of the nose or on the chin, but it can appear anywhere on the body. It is commonest in the summer when the weather is hot and humid, but it may be seen at any season of the year. Impetigo is highly contagious for other children but less so for adults.

A crusted scabby rash on a child is likely to be impetigo. It is caused by particular kinds of staphylococcus and streptococcus which can be treated very effectively.

Unless you have experience you can easily confuse impetigo with ringworm, allergic rashes, poison ivy, and other less common skin troubles. You should let the doctor make the diagnosis and order the necessary medicine. Cure will be quite prompt. A few days at the most and the impetigo will be gone. If it has been neglected for a long time and the crusts are thick and hard, the response to treatment will be slower.

School regulations usually require that a child be kept home until impetigo is healed.

BOILS

What a nuisance boils are! These oversize pimples are caused by a germ called *staphylococcus*. Usually boils start in a hair follicle or in a tiny puncture wound. While not ordinarily dangerous, they cause much discomfort. It seems as though they select areas where they can cause maximum distress—under an arm, on the back of the neck, between the buttocks, or perhaps right where the child sits or kneels.

Rare is the child who does not have a boil or two at some time. They may occur in a whole series, a "run of boils," and still not mean that there is anything seriously wrong with the child. Some children are slow to build up resistance to the infecting staphylococcus.

Individual boils are best treated by hot wet compresses. Wring out a small towel in hot water. Fold it several layers thick and lay it over the boil. Add several layers of dry towel to hold the heat. Finally, if possible, add a partly filled hot water bottle or a heating pad to maintain warmth. Renew the compresses three or four times an hour and repeat the whole process three or more times a day. Such treatment helps bring the boil to a head. It will then discharge some pus and rapidly heal. Discard or sterilize by boiling any materials contaminated with the pus.

Overall bathing a couple of times a day with soap and running water as in a shower may reduce the chance of new infections. Surgical incision (lancing) is almost never necessary.

ACNE (ADOLESCENT PIMPLES)

Acne probably causes more worry among teen-agers than any other health problem. Their appearance is of great importance to them, and acne *is* unsightly. A face dotted with pimples does little to bolster self-esteem. Yet three quarters of all adolescents have at least a minor problem with acne.

Acne is the result of the plugging of the ducts of the sebaceous glands in the skin. This obstruction of the ducts is followed by inflammation and the formation of small abscesses or pimples.

The material that plugs the ducts of these tiny glands in the skin turns dark brown or almost black on exposure to air. The blackheads that result are *not* due to dirt. Overly vigorous efforts to remove them damages the skin and tends to aggravate the condition.

No one really knows the underlying cause of acne. There is a hereditary factor. If a child's parents had little or no acne, his chance of skipping it himself is much improved. There is clear evidence that the hormone changes occurring in the adolescent are related to it, but they are essential to normal development and can't be done away with.

Diet does not *cause* acne, but certain foods do seem to aggravate some cases. Skin specialists vary in their opinion about the role played by foods. Acne patients should probably stay away from any food that seems to aggravate their own particular case.

Tension and anxiety play a part. Periods of stress in family, school, or social activities often set off a renewed outbreak. Many a girl has known the disappointment of a crop of pimples just before the senior prom. Boys may be made worse by heavy sweating, especially if football or wrestling are involved. (Normal amounts of rest and outdoor activities seem to be helpful.)

Cosmetics, especially the cover-up or pancake type, sometimes make things worse. There are special cosmetics whose manufacturers claim that they avoid this difficulty.

Self-administered overtreatment often turns out to be harmful; picking and squeezing must be avoided. Many youngsters go through a stage of scrubbing to the point of actual damage to their skin. Thorough washing twice a day with one of the special soaps available in drugstores may be tried, but directions should be followed carefully and the soap not used more frequently than recommended.

Beyond these simple things, professional help is needed. We feel very strongly that the treatment of severe acne is not likely to be satisfactory except under close supervision. The help of a skin specialist is worthwhile in managing this trying condition. Proper early treatment will minimize the problem and reduce later scarring.

WARTS

It must be a rare child indeed—boy or girl—who grows up without having a few warts. Many of the stories about how to get rid of them border on the ridiculous and yet, as with much folklore, contain a grain of wisdom.

Warts are small, harmless, sometimes unsightly skin infections that often look like little tumors. They are all caused by a single virus to which individuals develop a variable degree of immunity over a period of time. When the body has reached a certain level of resistance, the warts disappear. That's why certain very odd treatments seem sometimes to succeed.

The appearance of warts depends upon what part of the skin is invaded. On the face they are usually flat little papules of pinhead size. Kids often call them "flat pimples." On arms, legs, and hands they are often more knobby, raised lumps from ⅛ to ¼ inch in size. On the soles of the feet, where they are called *plantar warts*, they appear much like a callus.

If you have enough patience, virtually all warts disappear without any treatment. If you happen to be using the juice of seaweed by moonlight when yours disappear, you will become a juice-of-seaweed advocate. Beyond any doubt, strong suggestion plays a part in the rapid disappearance of some patients' warts. That they can be "hexed" away is a bit of folklore that is also sometimes a fact. Witch doctors, charlatans, magicians, and hypnotists can all, at times, succeed—though how psychosomatic suggestion influences the body's resistance to the wart virus is not known.

Warts on the soles of the feet—the plantar warts—are more difficult to deal with. Perhaps this is because of the constant pressure of walking or the unusual thickness of the skin on the feet. At any rate, they seldom go away without real treatment. Neglected, they can become quite painful. There are several ways of treating plantar warts. Opinion varies sharply as to what is best. Leave it to your doctor. He'll use the means that gives the best results in his experience. If your child has a great many such warts, your doctor may wish to call on the help of a skin specialist.

RINGWORM

Ringworm is a misleading name; it has nothing to do with worms. It is an infection caused by any of several different kinds of fungus. Usually it appears as a round to oval area of redness of the skin ranging from the size of a dime to that of a half dollar. The outer edge is rough and lumpy or scaly. The center, as time goes on, becomes smooth and appears healed. When it involves the scalp, the hairs may be broken off close to the surface, leaving only a stubbly area. Fortunately there is little or no discomfort for the patient. Ringworm is not painful, seldom itches, and, except for appearances, causes almost no symptoms.

If you suspect ringworm, get your doctor to make the diagnosis and prescribe the treatment. Recovery is certain but sometimes, especially for scalp ringworm, treatment must be continued for months.

Regulations vary from place to place, but schools may exclude your child until you supply evidence that ringworm is under treatment. Although they are slow-moving, school epidemics do occur. Once adequate treatment is started, the contagiousness drops to zero.

ATHLETE'S FOOT

Athlete's foot is caused by a fungus infection of the skin, a fungus that loves heat and moisture and cannot thrive on dry surfaces. Usually it is picked up in showers, locker rooms, swimming pool areas, or other places where surfaces remain moist most of the time. The sweaty warm environment that we provide for our feet by wearing poorly ventilated shoes offers a happy hunting ground. The skin, especially between the toes, becomes soggy, cracked, itchy, and sometimes quite sore.

Remedies are available in any drugstore. They work quite well if used consistently. Socks should be changed twice a day and leather shoes dried thoroughly between wearings. Rubber footwear should be avoided because it favors sweating and hinders evaporation. If these simple measures do not produce a cure, the doctor can help. There are more potent medications available on prescription.

One very important point: If you apply medication and the condition seems to get worse instead of better, *stop the medication promptly and consult the doctor.* Several more troublesome but less common conditions may be confused with athlete's foot. Improper medication may make them much worse, so do not persist in treatment that is not promptly helpful.

POISON IVY

Poison ivy is the uninvited guest at many an idyllic picnic. The nice-looking, shiny, three-leaved plant contains an irritant poison. Not everyone is sensitive to poison ivy, but nearly everyone can become so by repeated contact. It is surely worthwhile to teach children to recognize the plant and to avoid touching it.

The rash the plant produces will appear a day or two after contact. By the time it is noticeable, nothing you put on the skin can neutralize or remove the poison. The rash is much like a second-degree burn and can create real misery. Blisters may keep developing for several days and the itching and burning persist.

There are various medications to apply to the rash, but they all provide only partial relief. Avoid greasy applications of any sort. Starch baths are cooling and helpful, especially in hot weather; use a cupful of white starch to a quarter tub of barely warm water.

If the child is very miserable and not able to sleep, or if the rash seems to involve the eyes, call the doctor. There are potent medicines that can be taken internally, but they should be used only under a doctor's supervision.

There are extracts of poison ivy available which, when taken by mouth over a period of time, are supposed to reduce skin sensitivity to the poison. Unfortunately, they do not work equally well for all patients. There are protective creams that can be applied to the skin before expected contact and then washed off. They are helpful for trained outdoor workers but not practical for children.

If you suspect that your youngster has been in contact with poison ivy, wash him promptly with lots of soap and *running* water. This helps only if done almost immediately.

When there's any chance that you are going to be in places where there may be poison ivy, be sure you know how to recognize it. Then avoid it as you would a flame and try, at least try, to teach the kids to do the same.

Poison oak and poison sumac produce very similar reactions in the skin but are usually not so severe. Neither plant is as widely distributed as poison ivy.

398

There is an allergic factor in the response to these poisonous plants. With each succeeding exposure, the reactivity may become more intense, because the skin develops an allergic response to the toxic materials in addition to its response to their purely irritating properties.

CHEMICAL CONTACT RASHES

Now and then a child's skin will react to some chemical substance with which there is some sort of contact. The rash that follows may vary from mere redness to severe blistering. Doctors call such rashes *contact dermatitis* or *dermatitis venenata*. The latter has a sort of ominous sound about it, but it is just a big descriptive word applied to a rather common condition.

These skin eruptions or rashes can be very puzzling indeed because different individuals react to a particular substance in different ways. Some represent merely a reaction to chemical irritation, while others are the result of the skin becoming gradually more and more allergic to a particular substance. (See Chapter 12.) Poison ivy belongs in the latter group.

You are not likely to recognize such rashes for what they are unless you have seen many. Of course if a child spills lye or turpentine on himself and a rash follows, the cause-and-effect relationship is quite obvious. Less obvious are those caused by contact with everyday household materials. Laundry detergents are particularly troublesome. Traces of detergent cling tenaciously to clothing even after careful rinsing. Detergent rashes are most apt to appear first where clothes rub against the skin or where there is enough perspiration to dissolve the traces of the chemical and thus bring about close contact.

Hand soaps are usually innocent, except that some contain added perfumes, dyes, antiseptics, and other chemicals to which some children react. Sometimes at fault are chemicals used in floor waxes, leather tanning, fur processing, cosmetics, insecticide sprays, paints, toothpastes, and other manufactured materials.

The essential thing in treatment is to identify what is causing the rash and eliminate it. Unfortunately, mothers rarely recognize these particular rashes for what they are, and doctors, too, are often slow in making the right diagnosis. Partly that is because such rashes may closely mimic many other skin conditions.

Be suspicious of any rash that follows a change of soap, laundry detergent, a new garment, finger paints, cosmetics (on mother's face or nails against the baby), or any other material that closely contacts the skin. Ask your doctor about it. His experience may help you find the offending material. Sometimes he knows what's going on in a community. Door-to-door sampling of a new material followed by the appearance of skin rashes may be apparent to him and may help him to spot your child's problem immediately.

There are medications that are very effective in controlling the more severe rashes while the search for the cause is made. All these medicines require a doctor's prescription.

HEAD LICE

Children do occasionally become the camping and feeding ground of these little pests. The tiny eggs of the insect are glued tightly to the individual hairs on the child's head. These eggs, called *nits*, are easier to see than the lice. They look like a smooth grain of sand stuck to the hair. Usually there is no more than one nit on a single hair. Look for them especially on hairs above the child's ears.

These pests do little damage, but they do create an itch and may keep a child awake at night. Any rash that comes is caused by the scratching and not by the lice. They really look a lot worse than they are.

A single treatment with the chemical benzene hexachloride is usually all that is needed. Apply it at night and wash it out thoroughly in the morning. You will need a doctor's prescription to get it and should follow closely any special directions he may give you.

MOLES

Almost everyone has a mole or two. Some of us have dozens. They range in color from lightest tan-pink to almost black and in shape from perfectly flat to the thickness of a miniature raspberry. Most moles are completely harmless, but sometimes a blue-black one may have the potential to become malignant. Ask the doctor about any exceptionally dark mole.

Most moles grow very slowly and in proportion to the rest of the child's growth. Any mole that begins to grow rapidly should be brought to the doctor's attention.

Moles can be removed for cosmetic reasons or if they are in a place where they are frequently irritated or injured. In childhood it is a very rare thing to have a mole make any trouble.

CANKER SORES

These little ulcers or sores in the mouth are a great bother to some children, for they can be moderately painful. Usually they are on the gums or the lining of the cheeks below tooth level. They come and go, but some children have a good many. There's no sure preventive, but it is helpful to have the child brush his teeth and rinse out his mouth at bedtime. The ulcers are apt to form where particles of food spend the night in the mouth.

Canker sores heal in a few days, whether they are treated or not. If there are many such sores at any one time or if there is a tendency for them to bleed, consult the doctor.

15
Urinary System Problems

INFECTIONS

If your child has an infection of the urinary system it may well be a mystery to you, because there may be no symptoms you can recognize as being related to this part of the body. Indeed, symptoms of urinary infections vary so greatly that it is often difficult for the doctor to make a prompt and definite diagnosis.

Infection may be signaled by rather dramatic symptoms or may be so sneaky that there are no real symptoms at all. There may be chills, high fever, restlessness, vomiting, painful urination, and abdominal pain or there may be nothing more than loss of appetite, lack of pep, or failure to gain weight over a period of time. But one thing is sure: No child is at his best while such an infection is present, whether or not it is causing any definite symptoms.

Doctors have learned to become suspicious in the case of any child whose symptoms are not otherwise explained. That suspicion, plus microscopic examination of a urine specimen, leads to recognition.

When an infection is discovered, it is very important that treatment be carried out thoroughly and for long enough to clear it up completely. A variety of medications are used. The

402

doctor will have to choose the one best suited to the particular infection. It may be necessary to give it for many weeks.

If a child has recurrences, a complete study of the whole urinary system is needed. Part of the study should be a urogram —X rays that reveal the shape and structure of the total urinary tract from upper kidney areas to outlet. Occasionally a urogram reveals some obstruction or anatomical defect that favors infection and requires correction. Such studies are important because long-standing infection may cause permanent damage to the kidneys.

We would like to emphasize one thing: If your child has a urinary infection, be sure to carry out the doctor's orders in full and for as long as necessary *even if the youngster seems to have no symptoms after treatment is started.* Over and over we have seen treatments fail and infections recur because medication was stopped too soon. Only laboratory tests of the urine can determine when the condition is finally cured.

Cystitis or pyelitis. When there is pain and urgency about voiding it is because infection is causing irritation of the bladder, a condition often called *cystitis.* When fever is present you may hear the term *pyelitis* or *pyelonephritis.* Since infection of one part of the urinary system usually means the whole system is involved, the name is of little importance. That's why most doctors simply use the term "urinary tract infection."

NEPHRITIS

Nephritis, an inflammation of the kidneys, usually begins with the passing of blood in the urine. The child may feel vaguely unwell, but at the beginning his symptoms are often minimal: a little fever, headache, loss of appetite, and constant tiredness. Usually, there will have been a streptococcal sore throat or some other strep infection about two weeks before the nephritis began, although that earlier infection may have been quite mild. Certain types of strep are apparently capable of producing substances which somehow cause this later damage in the kidneys.

Most children make a complete recovery from nephritis, but they should be under close medical supervision. There are no specific drugs for this condition, and the doctor will have to decide when healing of the kidney has progressed far enough to permit return to school.

NEPHROSIS

This uncommon kidney disease causes severe imbalance in certain body chemicals and water distribution. The most noticeable thing is great puffiness, or edema, of various parts of the body. The swelling is usually noticed first in the eyelids but it progresses rapidly and soon, with rapid weight gain, involves the whole body.

Nephrosis requires close and skillful medical supervision, often for two years or more. Treatment depends chiefly on the use of synthetic hormonelike drugs. While this disease used to be frequently fatal, the discovery of the new drugs has made the outlook for recovery quite good.

16

Less Common Troubles

APPENDICITIS

"Stomachache," that common complaint of childhood, is only occasionally due to appendicitis. It is hard for parents to decide when to call the doctor about abdominal pain, yet they are right to be concerned about acute appendicitis.

The appendix is a little structure attached to the intestine in the right lower part of the abdomen. When it becomes infected and inflamed, the child has appendicitis.

In children over 4 years of age, appendicitis behaves just as it does in adults. Usually there is pain in the abdomen which is quite constant; it does not come and go. It begins, as a rule, in the middle of the abdomen in the area around the navel.

There is loss of appetite, a little fever, and sooner or later the child throws up. Then the pain, which is not always severe, seems to move down and to the right side.

That's the usual story, but the younger the child the more variable the symptoms may be. In the child under 4 most of the typical symptoms may be missing, although complete absence of vomiting makes appendicitis very unlikely at any age. Even the most experienced physician may have a difficult time being sure of the diagnosis in the very young and may need to see the child more than once.

Surgery is the only treatment for appendicitis, once the diagnosis is reasonably certain. Otherwise, the appendix may burst and allow infected material to leak into the general abdominal space. This complication, known as *peritonitis*, used to be fatal. It can be cured today with the help of surgery and antibiotics, but convalescence is still apt to be stormy and prolonged.

It is true that a child sometimes undergoes an operation for acute appendicitis, and the appendix is found to be normal. He may have no more than some inflamed and swollen lymph glands, a condition called *mesenteric adenitis* which mimics appendicitis and does not need surgery. Nevertheless, even if the child loses a normal appendix, all it means is he will never have appendicitis in the future. Even a healthy appendix serves no important function in the body. It is not safe to delay surgery in the face of findings indicating appendicitis.

If your child has a stomachache, do *not* give a laxative. If you think his problem is caused by constipation, give him a small soapy-water enema—not more than one half to one pint of water—or use a child-size prepared enema (available in drugstores, under a variety of trade names, in disposable tubes with rectal tips). If the symptoms are relieved, well and good. If not, you will not have done any harm. If the pain continues, or if there is fever or vomiting, go no further without consulting your doctor.

CYSTIC FIBROSIS

Cystic fibrosis is an inherited defect of the function of mucus-secreting glands in various parts of the body. The genetic abnormality involved in the inheritance of this disease is a recessive trait. Both parents must carry the abnormal gene if the disease is to appear in their child. Given parents who carry the trait, we can theoretically expect 1 in 4 of their children to be affected. In the United States, about 1 child in 1,000 is involved. It is very rare among blacks and orientals.

As with so many other diseases, some children are much more severely affected than others. Sometimes the symptoms are so vague, and so like those of simpler and commoner troubles, that it is difficult to reach a diagnosis without rather complex testing.

There are two principal types of symptoms, and either or both may be present in a particular child. At the beginning there is often a moderate but stubborn diarrhea which is apt to get worse after solid foods are added to a baby's diet. The movements are exceptionally unpleasant. Most such babies are very fussy and fail to gain weight at the normal rate. Their indigestion and diarrhea result from failure of the pancreas to secrete adequate amounts of normal digestive juices.

Other cases begin with a severe and persistent cough which is worse during colds but never clears up entirely. It is caused by the production of abnormally thick and tenacious mucus by the glands in the lining of the bronchial tubes leading to the lungs. Infection gets a foothold and is very stubborn. Recurrent pneumonia is common. Most patients sooner or later have both the intestinal and the respiratory symptoms.

To make a diagnosis requires X rays of the lungs, tests that measure the amount of salt in the sweat (abnormally high), and perhaps an analysis of intestinal juices. These can be done in many hospital laboratories and in all medical centers.

It is not possible to cure cystic fibrosis at present, but with expert treatment the child can be kept comfortable and his life extended over many years. Treatment is complex, and parents of children with this condition will need to be guided in detail by the doctor in charge. Many medical centers have special services for these patients.

Parents will want to learn all they can about the subject in order to be of the greatest help possible to their child and to better face the difficult decisions about future family planning. Helpful information is available from the Cystic Fibrosis Research Foundation, 521 Fifth Avenue, New York, N.Y. 10017.

CELIAC DISEASE

Very persistent, foul-smelling, loose bowel movements and progressive weight loss are usual with celiac disease. There is often a bloated abdomen despite general thinness. Excessive irritability and a bad disposition make celiac children a real trial even to the most relaxed and devoted of parents. Fortunately, the disease is far less common than it used to be; in fact, it is quite rare wherever nutritional standards are reasonably high.

The cause lies in an inborn error of function of one or more enzymes in the intestinal lining or its secretions. Whether this is brought about by allergy or by an inherited genetic defect is not clear. Whatever the basic defect, it results in a decreased ability to digest and absorb fatty substances in the diet.

Many cases are triggered by a protein, gluten, that is present in wheat and rye. The normal child handles gluten like any other food protein, but the child with celiac disease is unable to do so. The inability to absorb fats is apparently secondary to this intolerance for gluten. In such cases the strict removal of wheat and rye from the diet may be all that is required to bring about slow but steady improvement.

Other cases do not seem to be related to gluten. These are more complex, and a period of detailed study and hospital care may become necessary. But with proper management, the outlook for these children is very good.

RHEUMATIC FEVER

Rheumatic fever is a potentially dangerous disease that follows streptococcal sore throats—usually 2 or 3 weeks after the throat discomfort is gone and all but forgotten. Though variable in onset, it usually arrives in the form of inflamed, painful joints and fever. The pain and swelling move from one joint to another: elbows, knees, ankles, wrists, and sometimes the smaller joints. While this is going on, there may be involvement of the heart. Permanent damage varies from none at all to very serious.

Naturally, if a child has fever and painful joints you will call the doctor. But rheumatic fever is sometimes sneaky, producing only excessive tiredness, low fever, vague twinges *in the joints*, and a pale sickly appearance. If your child has such symptoms and they persist, let the doctor decide what the cause may be. While we no longer accept the old idea of "growing pains," it is true that some very active children have aches in the muscles. These pains, occurring in the muscles *between* the joints, have no particular significance unless accompanied by fever.

Occasionally the nervous system is involved. When this is the case, the child develops a curious uncontrolled twitching called St. Vitus' dance, or *chorea*. This strange condition sometimes appears before any of the other symptoms of rheumatic fever. You can distinguish it from the much commoner habit spasms (such as repeated blinking or shoulder shrugging) by the fact that the motions of St. Vitus' dance are not repetitive but vary from one moment to the next. Good handwriting becomes impossible and self-feeding is difficult. These children become emotionally unstable too. Tears and laughter may alternate with little apparent cause. Caring for a child with St. Vitus' dance takes a lot of patience, but they all get well.

The important thing is not the St. Vitus' dance itself but the fact that it is a part of rheumatic fever. The patient must be carefully followed by the doctor to detect other and more threatening aspects of the underlying disease.

You may have heard that children become chronic heart invalids as a result of rheumatic fever. This can happen, but it seldom does.

Rheumatic fever is a preventable disease. It cannot be over-emphasized that rheumatic fever can be prevented by the proper diagnosis and treatment of streptococcal sore throats (see Chapter 11). Many a mother has said, "I don't want to bother you every time my kids have a sore throat." It is true that a little sore throat that comes and goes in a day or two is usually not much of a threat. But any sore throat that is severe, that is accompanied by fever, or that makes a child seem generally sick deserves medical attention.

There are many kinds of sore throats. Sometimes the doctor can distinguish the different types by their appearance, but more often he cannot. Throat cultures, easily taken in the doctor's office, are needed to separate those sore throats that represent danger from those that do not. It is infection with the hemolytic streptococcus germ that sometimes precedes the onset of rheumatic fever.

If the throat culture shows that the dangerous type of streptococcus is present, the child should be treated with penicillin for a full 10 days. To treat for a shorter time is to invite incomplete recovery. *The prevention of rheumatic fever lies in the adequate penicillin treatment of streptococcic throats.*

Even with the most severe sore throats, penicillin works well when given by mouth. It need not be injected except when vomiting is such a problem that the patient cannot retain it.

If your child has already had an episode of rheumatic fever, penicillin used in another way can protect him from further attacks: the single *preventive* dose given once a day for many years. It may be taken by mouth, provided that it is taken faithfully and without missing days. Some doctors, recognizing that even with the best of intentions people may be forgetful, prefer to give an injection of a special long-acting penicillin every two weeks. By either method, countless hearts are protected from the ravages of recurrent bouts of rheumatic fever.

Sometimes it is hard to face the expense of a visit to the doctor, plus the cost of penicillin, for what seems so simple a thing as a sore throat. It is cheaper by far than an attack of rheumatic fever with its months of treatment and the possibility of permanent heart damage.

There is better treatment for the already developed attack of the disease than was available only a few years ago. Potent drugs minimize the inflammation in the heart, and if rheumatic fever is recognized promptly and treated properly most children can be returned to full and active life. Nevertheless, despite these encouraging words, we must emphasize prevention. Here, truly, the old saying comes into its own; the ounce of prevention *is* worth a full pound of cure. Everywhere in the world that strep throats are correctly diagnosed and treated, rheumatic fever is in full retreat.

DIABETES

If you were told that your child had diabetes, you would probably feel that an absolute catastrophe had overtaken you. Endless questions would well up in your mind: "Does this mean he will have to take shots all his life? Will he grow up like the others? Can he have children? What should we do?" These deep concerns are understandable, but they are based partly on lack of knowledge. Because diabetes is so complex, parents usually understand much less about it than they do about many other illnesses.

Diabetes is an inherited disorder of the body's ability to control and use its basic fuel, glucose. Any machine that uses fuel as its source of energy must have (1) a source of fuel, (2) a means of storing fuel if intake is intermittent, and (3) a means of releasing fuel from storage in controlled amounts.

The sources of our fuel, our glucose, are the various kinds of sugars and starches in our diet. All these sugars and starches are collectively called *carbohydrate*. When you see that word, remember that it refers to those foodstuffs which are converted to glucose during the process of digestion. It is this glucose, absorbed as the carbohydrates in our food are digested, that fuels us day and night, resting or working, thinking or sleeping.

The control of glucose in the body

When we eat more sugar or starch than we need at a given moment, the excess glucose that results is absorbed into the blood and then stored in the liver and muscles in a form that can be released as needed. A delicate balance is maintained between absorption from the digestive tract and storage, so that the amount of glucose in the blood is normally kept within a constant range. When there is either too much or too little, when the blood level is too high or too low, we have trouble.

A number of different mechanisms play a part in maintaining the blood-glucose level, but the hormone called *insulin* is the one most directly in charge. When there is too little insulin, our blood-glucose level rises above tolerable limits; like a gasoline engine with a flooded carburetor, our engine begins to falter. When there is too much insulin and the blood-glucose level falls too low, our body tissues run out of usable fuel, like a gasoline engine with the throttle pedal pushed down but no fuel getting through.

Insulin is manufactured in the body by highly specialized cells in the pancreas, an abdominal organ that lies behind the stomach. The severity of diabetes depends upon the degree of inability of the pancreas to produce insulin.

It is well known that mild diabetes *in adults* can often be treated and controlled by means of medicines taken by mouth. Unfortunately, in childhood diabetes, these oral medications are almost never able to replace insulin which, because it is rapidly destroyed in the stomach, must be given by injection.

Since the discovery of insulin, the treatment of diabetic children has been very satisfactory. With the help of insulin, these children learn to take their handicap in stride and grow up into happy, productive adults.

Ideally, diabetes should be recognized before definite symptoms begin. Such discovery can result from a routine health checkup which includes a urine examination. When the blood-glucose level is higher than it should be, glucose appears in the urine, and a simple test detects its presence.

The symptoms of diabetes

The symptoms are often quite vague at the beginning. Sometimes a simple infection, such as a sore throat, accelerates the appearance of symptoms to the point where parents notice that something unusual is going on. Here are some things you might recognize:

> Weight loss despite excellent appetite
> Excessive thirst and drinking
> Excessively frequent urination
> Unusual and persistent tiredness despite normal rest
> Drowsiness and a sweet fruity odor on the breath

If your previously healthy child develops some or all of these symptoms, consult your doctor promptly. If it turns out that the child does have diabetes, the doctor will probably think it wise to hospitalize the youngster for the initial period needed to adjust the insulin dosage, diet, and activity, since this is best accomplished under closely controlled conditions.

During this hospitalization you and your child will learn a great deal about diabetes. You will be taught how to give insulin injections once or twice a day—and will discover that it is not nearly as difficult as it sounds. Most older children learn to do it for themselves. It is almost incredible how rapidly children accept and adjust to the whole program. You will also learn how to match the need for insulin against the child's daily intake of glucose-producing foods. A diabetic child usually does have some dietary restrictions, but the restrictions are simpler than they used to be. It is no longer thought necessary to keep growing, active children on very rigid diets.

Most doctors who work with diabetic children believe that it pays to keep blood-glucose levels as normal as possible. This minimizes the chances that the child will develop difficulties or complications in later years. Good modern management of diabetes leads to relatively normal life patterns and normal life expectancy.

Under some circumstances your child's doctor may wish to consult with a specialist who works almost entirely with diabetics. If he suggests this, follow his advice. There are many variables, and you will want to have the best supervision possible.

As your child grows and develops, it is of the utmost importance that, though you provide medical guidance and supervision, your child be made increasingly responsible for managing his diabetes himself. Most children can accomplish this by the age of 13 or 14 years.

Both of you must become knowledgeable about diabetes. By so doing you will avoid the feelings of confusion and fear that come from uncertainty. There are publications that can be of tremendous help to you.*

Teen-agers should have a one-to-one relationship with the supervising doctor. At this stage, the parents should remain in the background during checkup visits. Then the youngster will be brought to realize that he alone is responsible for his diabetic management. The importance of this cannot be overemphasized. It leads to far better control than continuing close parental supervision.

Many states have summer camps for diabetic children. Here,

* See, for example, *Forecast, A Magazine for Diabetics,* and other publications of the American Diabetes Association, Inc., 18 East 48th Street, New York, N.Y. 10017.

working in groups under skillful supervision, they learn very rapidly how to take care of their condition. Various special funds in most areas help with the cost if necessary.

Diabetes is a challenge, but most children can rise to meet it and gain great self-confidence while doing so.

The hereditary aspects of diabetes

The hereditary aspects of diabetes are very complex and not entirely predictable. A child who has one parent with diabetes, or even an uncle or an aunt, has a greater likelihood of developing the disease than a child with no such family history, but this development is by no means certain. However, if *two* diabetics have a child, the odds are very high that the child will have severe diabetes. Therefore, two diabetics should not have children.

EPILEPSY

Most people think of an epileptic seizure, or fit, as a sudden loss of consciousness with accompanying violent contractions of muscles, or convulsions. But not all seizures are by any means so dramatic or violent. There are many kinds, and they vary all the way from mere lapses in attention of only a second to the more violent types. These seizures usually begin after the age of 3. They are not the same thing as the fever convulsions of younger children (see Chapter 10).

What causes a seizure? Essentially it is the disruption of the normally rhythmic electrical activity patterns in the brain. In a seizure patient there are bursts of uncoordinated electrical impulses. The type of seizure depends on the exact type of electrical disturbance. Minor seizures with momentary loss of consciousness are called *petit mal*. The kind of seizure with more or less violent convulsions accompanied by unconsciousness is called *grand mal*. There are other, less common types, and some patients have more than one kind.

An instrument called an electroencephalograph, or E.E.G. for short, is used to pick up and record the electrical activity of the brain. This recording, printed out on special graph paper, is called a "brain wave tracing." Distortions of the regular rhythmic patterns are easily recognized by those trained to read these tracings.

Even when a child with epilepsy is not actually having a seizure, the tracings usually show changes that are correlated with his particular problem. Thus the E.E.G. helps the doctor to make an accurate diagnosis and to choose the medication most likely to help.

The large majority of seizures can be controlled by one or a combination of special medicines. It sometimes takes patience and persistence to find out what is exactly the best drug for the individual child, but the results are well worth the effort.

Individual epileptic seizures are self-limited. No matter how frightened you are, remember that your child's seizure will stop and he will recover. If he seems to be choking, roll him over onto his stomach and turn his head to one side.

If you have a child with seizures you will have many questions. Jot them down as they come to you and talk them over with your doctor. You will learn that three out of five epileptics can have their seizures totally controlled—but *only* if they take the necessary drugs faithfully. Most patients must keep taking their medicine for many years.

There is often, but by no means always, a family tendency to epilepsy. But epilepsy is not a family disgrace to be hidden in shame; it is a problem to be faced squarely and openly like any other health matter. That's the only road to its proper management and control. The condition should not be hidden from your child's friends or school. If a seizure occurs, it should be accepted as matter of factly as possible. It is very important not to pamper and overprotect these children. As the child grows old enough to ask, his questions should be answered honestly and in as much detail as he is capable of understanding.

Sooner or later the question of restrictions is certain to come up. It is not possible to give a rule because no two cases are alike. A child with major seizures should never swim or be around the water alone. Nor should he ride a bike in traffic or, when he grows older, drive a car, unless it is absolutely certain that the seizures are under complete control.*

LEUKEMIA

In simplest terms, leukemia is cancer of blood cells. In childhood it usually affects the white blood cells we call *lymphocytes.* Lymphocytes move with the blood throughout the body and thereby spread the disease everywhere. Without treatment, leukemia usually runs its course to its fatal outcome in just a few months. But while cure is not yet possible, great progress has been made in treatment, and life has been prolonged for years.

The disease begins, usually, when the child is between the ages of 2 and 8. Paleness and poor appetite are usually noticeable first. There may be low fever which comes and goes with no apparent reason. The youngster begins to bruise easily after the slightest injury or with no injury at all. Bleeding from the gums may follow brushing of the teeth. The child becomes irritable and may complain of pain in joints, arms, or legs. Taken by themselves, most of these symptoms have no serious significance. Pallor, poor appetite, joint pains, and fever are much more likely to be related individually to far less serious problems. Even if your child has *all* of these symptoms, don't jump to conclusions. Fortunately, most often tests prove that a child with these symptoms does not have leukemia.

But what of the unfortunate child for whom the tests are positive? What does today's treatment have to offer? Is treatment really worthwhile when a real cure is still not possible?

Drugs for the suppression of leukemia have been improved rapidly. As a result of modern drug treatment, the disease is often kept in an inactive state for 3 to 5 years or more. There are a number of cases on record in which prolonged remissions have been attained—even some apparent cures. During these remissions the child feels entirely well and lives a normal life.

Since progress has been so rapid, who is to know that a true cure is not right around the corner? Every child with leukemia deserves full treatment with modern drugs and whatever blood

* Helpful information is available from the Epilepsy United Association, Inc.; 111 West 57th Street, New York, N.Y. 10019.

transfusions are necessary. There does finally come a time when remissions end, but even then treatment can keep a child comfortable and free from suffering and pain.

Today, in every medical center, there are specialists in blood diseases who have immense resources for treatment of this disease. There are advantages in having a child with leukemia under the supervision of such a specialist if it is geographically possible. But the child should be at home during most of his illness.

Let's look at this problem through the experience of a minister whose 6-year-old boy, Robin, developed leukemia By the time the diagnosis was made, he had nearly all the symptoms. Over the years, Robin's father had seen other cases in his parish and had visited them in the hospital. He had seen the struggle to keep children alive after they had reached the point of no return. As an exceptionally well-informed man, he approached his own son's illness with great compassion for both the child and his wife.

After several conferences with their doctor, both parents determined to see that their child would enjoy the rest of his life as much as possible. And so, except for brief periods in the hospital, he was cared for at home.

The drugs brought a series of prompt and seemingly total remissions. Robin's life continued as before except for frequent blood counts to control the dosage of his medicines. The remissions lasted a full 2 years. (Today they would have lasted much longer.) His parents managed to avoid the solicitude and excessive pampering which can undermine a child's real happiness. They took little trips, had vacations on schedule, and lived their usual daily life.

The time came when Robin weakened and stayed in bed. When he asked, one day, if he would die, his mother wisely said, "Some day you will. Everyone does. But we don't have to worry about that now." Evasion, yes. Obvious deceit, no.

One day Robin had a painful hemorrhage in his knee joint. The pain was easily controlled with medication. That night in his sleep a fatal hemorrhage occurred in his brain. His parents' reaction was to be thankful that he had been granted such an easy way to go. His last years had been happy ones. Both his mother and his father had expressed their love in the finest way possible, by gently supporting him.

LOCKJAW (TETANUS)

Lockjaw, or tetanus, is a terrible but completely preventable disease. The germ that causes it is so widespread that everyone is exposed to it, but it makes no trouble unless it somehow gets into our body through a cut, burn, or other injury. Puncture wounds caused by objects that have been lying in the ground are particularly likely to be infected.

Tetanus germs grow best away from exposure to air. They multiply rapidly in the depths of a wound and produce one of the most deadly poisons known: tetanus toxin. This poison affects the nervous system. The jaw cannot be opened because of severe muscle spasm. Violent convulsions are followed by paralysis of breathing.

Modern medical facilities make cure possible, but the treatment is prolonged and difficult, and the result is by no means certain. *Prevention is the answer.* Nobody, child or adult, gets lockjaw who has ever had three doses of the preventive material plus a booster dose as needed at long intervals. (See also Immunizations in Chapter 9.)

It is too late for this kind of prevention after a wound occurs. Then it is necessary to use a serum antitoxin which is sometimes followed by unpleasant allergic reactions. Be certain that your child receives tetanus prevention. Thereafter you'll have no worries about lockjaw.

VAGINAL INFECTIONS

Little girls may have a slight vaginal discharge from time to time, most often after a bad cold, sore throat, or one of the infectious diseases like measles or chicken pox. Such discharges clear up after a few days.

Sometimes a bit of paper or a small object gets stuck in the vagina, where it causes local irritation. If this happens to your child, don't accuse her of doing something bad and don't punish her. Self-exploration by small girls is not abnormal. Besides, the discovery and removal of the foreign material that has been causing trouble will carry its own lesson.

Faulty hygiene and insufficient cleansing are occasionally responsible for irritation and discharge. Simple bathing will fix that.

For a few months before the first menstrual period most girls have a more or less constant slight discharge of mucus. It is nonirritating, causes no symptoms, and needs no treatment.

A persistent or more profuse discharge or one that is irritating or accompanied by blood should be checked by the doctor. A discharge that is thick and yellow will usually require treatment, and medical help should be sought.

INGROWN TOENAIL

This uncomfortable, troublesome, and persistent condition never need occur. It is caused by the child's wearing shoes that are too short or too narrow across the toe or, more frequently, by cutting or picking the big toenail too short at the sides. Toenails should be cut straight across. When they are not, the soft tissues at the sides may push up beneath and ahead of the nail. Then, as the nail grows forward, it tends to cut into the skin and infection starts. The toe becomes very sore and painful. After a few weeks the infection becomes difficult to cure. Very often it is necessary to have part of the nail removed. This requires at least a local anesthetic, not a pleasant experience for the child.

One treatment that often works if it is started just as soon as soreness begins is to cut out the toe of an old shoe (so there is no pressure on the child's toe), apply a generous dab of ointment containing neomycin and bacitracin, and cover it with a Band-Aid. Twice a day take the Band-Aid off and soak the foot in hot water for twenty minutes. Dry the toe gently and apply fresh ointment and Band-Aid. Continue until all soreness is gone. If the toe has not improved after 3 or 4 days of such treatment, you will need the doctor's help.

CRIB DEATHS

The usual story is of a seemingly healthy baby who went to nap, or for his night's sleep, only to be discovered dead when his mother returned. She feels guilt, but it is no fault of hers. She wonders why it happened to her child, but there is no satisfactory answer. The father may ask why the doctor could not have known and prevented it—but he could not. A crib death is a rare thing, but that is small comfort to the parents.

When autopsies are performed—and they should be done whenever possible, for they often reveal how blameless everyone was—the actual cause of death is discovered in about half the cases. Sometimes it is found that there was a defective blood vessel in a critical area and a blowout occurred; the vessel ruptured through a thin spot in its wall and a massive hemorrhage in the brain or other vital organ abruptly terminated life. In other infants there is evidence of sudden overwhelming infection by one or another type of virus against which the infant's immature defense system was powerless. Occasionally, though it is hard to prove, something disrupts the precise electrical control of the heartbeat and thereby ends life abruptly. There are other causes, but the possibilities become more and more remote as the list lengthens.

Almost never is there evidence of suffocation. Remember that: almost never. It is important to know this because most mothers seem to feel that suffocation is the most likely thing and that they could somehow have prevented it.

Be cheered by this: Crib deaths are uncommon. You hear of them only because they attract publicity. Your automobile is a far more present danger.

17
Accidents

Accidents are the number one killer throughout the early years of life.* More babies and children die as a result of accidents than from the five most common fatal diseases of childhood put together. Over sixteen thousand children, half of them pre-schoolers, die from accidents each year in the United States. About sixteen million are treated for nonfatal accidents. So though we've warned you about safety considerations already, we think they are worth repeating.

Every child will have *some* accidents. Having *little* accidents is an essential part of learning. Little accidents help to prevent big accidents. The pinched finger, the small burn, the little cut, the acid taste of something that should not have been tasted at all, the bent fender—each of these teaches, as no book can, how a similar but bigger accident could happen.

You must walk the narrow line of letting your child learn by little hurts yet protecting him from serious injury. You must not be overly protective and you must not be overly careless. You must avoid the big dangers without constantly harassing a child about the little ones from which he learns so much.

* For first aid treatment of accidents, poisonings, and emergencies, see the section printed on yellow paper at the end of the book.

You don't need to be told not to let a 2-year-old climb a high ladder or ride his cart into a busy street. But there are not-so-obvious possibilities that take many lives. We want to help you recognize and avoid those too.

We urge you to read the last chapter of this book before any accident occurs. Pay special attention to the sections on Artificial Respiration, Bleeding, and Shock. Perhaps you will never need this information, but it is best to be prepared in your mind.

AUTOMOBILE ACCIDENTS

The automobile is a prime cause of fatal and serious accidents. About fifty thousand people are killed and hundreds of thousands injured in auto accidents in the United States every year, and children are well represented as passengers in this total. It is certain that some of the six thousand children who die each year in automobile accidents could be saved by proper protection in the car.

No single type of restraint can protect children of all ages, and there are, unfortunately, many restraints on the market which have not proved to be safe and effective when properly tested. The following list suggests devices that offer good protection; there are others that may be suitable.

1. For babies up to 20 pounds:
   Infant Carrier by General Motors
2. From 12 to 25 pounds:
   Infant Harness by Rose Mfg. Co.
   Toddler Seat by General Motors
3. From 25 to 50 pounds (but under 55 inches):
   Child Seat, Shield Type, by Ford Motor Co.
4. From 55 inches up:
   Adult seat belts with shoulder harness

Automobile-pedestrian accidents. The proportion of children injured in this type accident is distressingly high. The peak age is around 3 years. Nearly half of these accidents occur between

422

3 and 6 P.M. There are nearly four times as many boy as girl victims.

It is usually the child himself who, by his unexpected and unwary presence, causes these street accidents. Every child needs careful and repeated warning about this danger. Running out between parked cars is the greatest single hazard.

After the age of 6, the location changes and there are more accidents at crosswalks and intersections. The older child knows the right place to cross but may start without looking or against a traffic light. Children repeatedly see adults crossing against lights. Can we expect them to do differently?

POISONING

In the United States nearly three thousand children under 5 years of age die of accidental poisoning each year. Nearly a million children are involved in nonfatal poisonings. It is easy to believe that carelessness on the part of parents is responsible. Certainly it is sometimes a factor, as when a toxic material is kept in a soft-drink bottle.

But slowly it has become clear that there is another very important element at work. This element is inherent in the individual child. Every doctor who works with children soon learns that *a child who is involved in one poisoning episode is very likely to be a repeater* at a later date. So often is this true that we take special pains to forewarn parents. The child who has just had his stomach pumped after eating his grandfather's heart pills is likely to try something similar again, despite the fact that stomach-pumping is an unpleasant experience. It has not been possible to identify this "type" of child before the first occurrence. But once it has happened, that child is a good candidate for a repetition. Parents are likely to think otherwise and to believe that their child has learned his lesson. They are wrong. We cannot overemphasize this point.

Many household materials are dangerous for children. The National Clearing House For Poison Control Centers has made a large amount of useful information available to hospitals

423

and doctors. Here are the twelve substances most frequently involved in home poisonings in order of frequency.*

1. Aspirin
2. Sedatives
3. Tranquilizers and stimulants
4. Mixed type medications
5. Soaps, detergents, cleaners (in large doses)
6. All "other" medications
7. Toxic plants (mushrooms, hollyberries, etc.)
8. Vitamins (in large doses)
9. Pain-killers
10. Insecticides
11. Household bleaches (in large doses)
12. Disinfectants, deodorizers

You will see at once that family medicines top the list of these accidents. There are many other household products that are highly dangerous and account for serious poisonings but in smaller numbers. These include caustic drain and oven cleaners, kerosene, gasoline, solvents, some glues and cements, moth repellants, lighter fluids, and furniture polishes.

Now you know where the dangers lie. Doing something about it is up to you. Remember, locks are cheap.

BURNS

Most burns happen in or around the home. The commonest cause is the tipping of containers of hot liquids. Fortunately, such burns, while painful and often requiring hospitalization, seldom cover enough of the body to be fatal.

As we have noted, flammable clothing often results in very serious burns or deaths. Forty to 60 percent of the serious burns in childhood are caused by clothing that has caught fire.

Gasoline burns are quite common among older boys. Gasoline does not follow the usual rules of fire. A spark or flame need only be brought *near* gasoline for sudden ignition, a great

* It should be noted that paints, plaster, and other materials containing lead are not listed because the poisoning they produce is slow and chronic and is almost never reported as an accident. (See Chronic Lead Poisoning in Chapter 4.)

forceful *whoomphf* of flame, a flash of intense heat of almost explosive suddenness. Whenever gasoline is exposed, an invisible vapor exists in the air around it. It is this vapor that ignites so easily. If one tries to touch a match to something wet with gasoline the vapor ignites before the match ever comes in contact. No boy instinctively understands this. He must be taught— or learn by bitter experience.

SUFFOCATION

Nearly two thousand children suffocate every year in home accidents. The majority choke on small objects such as peanuts, chunks of raw carrot or celery, nuts, popcorn, hard candies, beads, and buttons. Because most such accidents occur in children under 4, it is best to keep these things away until after that age. Telling children not to run and play with small things in their mouths is useless.

Mothers worry about infants suffocating in bed as a result of entanglement in pillows or blankets. The fact is that these are rarely, if ever, a cause of suffocation. On the other hand, plastic bags that are large enough to cover a child's head are extremely dangerous and should never be kept where children can get them.

DROWNING

Nearly one seventh of all accidental deaths in children are the result of drowning. Most often the victims are in the 3- to 5-year age group. Home swimming pools are particularly dangerous.

Learn how to give artificial respiration to your child (see last chapter). Your knowledge now can save his life later.

FALLS

Falls are the commonest cause of nonfatal accidents. While minor bumps and bruises are a necessary part of learning, you must beware of children's falls from high places such as windows. With young babies you must be constantly careful about falls from tables, high chairs, and bathinettes. If you have to

425

leave a young infant, put him on the floor. He can't fall there.

Babies seem to roll over for the first time at the most unexpected moments. Falls from bed or table are likely to happen while your back is turned ever so briefly. Fortunately serious damage from such falls is uncommon. The old saying, "Old folks break, babies bounce," has some truth in it, but don't count on it.

Stairway falls, which are common and look so awful, do not often produce serious injury. There just isn't enough acceleration from step to step and bump to bump to do much harm. But it's a good idea to teach toddlers to turn around and *back* down stairs until they are completely steady on their feet.

WHAT CAN YOU DO?

By this point, you know the causes of most serious children's accidents. You can adapt your daily routines and teaching to prevent most of them. It is foolish to worry, as some mothers do, about all the rare things that might happen. True, a meteor might crash through the ceiling of your baby's bedroom, but it is much more productive to be concerned and do something about the common everyday things that are likely to happen. If you carry out the following list of suggestions you will definitely prevent many of the commonest and most threatening accidents. Take it by age groups and save yourself both worry and trouble.

THE YOUNG INFANT

Never leave a baby unattended on something from which he can fall.

Keep safety pins and other sharp things out of reach.

Avoid beads or other toys with pieces small enough to cause choking.

Be sure bath water is not too hot.

Beware of your automobile; use restraints.

426

THE MIDDLE OF THE FIRST YEAR

Never leave a baby alone in his bath even for a moment.
Don't leave him even briefly except in crib or playpen.
Beware of your automobile; use restraints.

LAST HALF OF THE FIRST YEAR

Keep all hot things, tablecloth edges, and electric cords out
of reach.
Get household poisons up out of floor-level cabinets and lock
them up.
Buy safety plugs for electric outlets.
Beware of all small or sharp objects that may be lying around.
Beware of your automobile; use restraints.

THE SECOND AND THIRD YEARS

Make sure screens in windows are firm and fastened.
Keep matches out of reach.
Never leave your young child alone near water in pools, ponds,
or tubs—not even for a moment.
Lock the medicine cabinet and leave nothing out.
Lock cabinets containing insecticides, cleaners, polishes, sol-
vents, and other household poisons.
Never leave him alone outdoors unless he is fenced in.
Beware of automobiles, your own and others.

THIRD YEAR TO FIVE YEARS

Start firm teaching about road and traffic hazards.
Teach about burns and cuts.
Teach the dangers of matches and flames.
Start swimming instruction, if possible.
Watch out for knives, razors, dangerous tools, machines.
Be very careful of garage, cellar, kitchen, and medicine closet
areas.
Allow no large plastic bags to lie around.
Beware of automobiles, your own and others.

References for Further Reading

Note: Titles with asterisk (*)
are available in paperback.

Pregnancy and Childbirth

The following books may be obtained from the International Child-birth Education Association Supplies Center, 208 Ditty Building, Bellevue, Wash. 98004. They will also send a booklist on request.

Bing, Elisabeth D. *The Adventure of Birth: Experiences in the Lamaze Method of Prepared Childbirth.* New York: Simon & Schuster, 1970.

* ———. *Six Practical Lessons for an Easier Childbirth.* New York: Grosset & Dunlap, 1969.

* Chabon, Irwin. *Awake and Aware: Participating in Childbirth Through Psychoprophylaxis.* New York: Delacorte Press, 1971.

* Dick-Read, Grantly. *Childbirth Without Fear: The Principles and Practice of Natural Childbirth.* 2nd rev. ed. New York: Harper & Brothers, 1959.

———. *The Natural Childbirth Primer.* New York: Harper & Brothers, 1955.

Gelb, Barbara. *The ABC of Natural Childbirth.* New York: W. W. Norton & Co., 1954.

* Guttmacher, Alan F. *Pregnancy and Birth.* New York: Signet Books, 1962.

* Karmel, Marjorie. *Thank You, Dr. Lamaze: A Mother's Experience in Painless Childbirth.* Philadelphia: J. B. Lippincott Company, 1959.

Liley, H. M. I., and Beth Day. *Modern Motherhood.* New York: Random House, 1969.

* Wright, Erna. *The New Childbirth.* London: Tandem, 1965.

Pregnancy in Anatomical Illustrations. Los Angeles: Carnation Co.,

1968 (obtainable through your local Red Cross).

U.S. Government (Children's Bureau pamphlets):
Eat Well for You and Your Baby Who Is On the Way (1969)
Prenatal Care (rev. 1962)
When Your Baby Is On the Way (1961)

Superintendent of Documents, U.S. Government Printing Office, Washington, D.C., 20402.

Growth and Development and Child Care

* Bettelheim, Bruno. *The Children of the Dream.* New York: The Macmillan Company, 1969.

Bowen, Mary. "A Teacher's Guide to Good Discipline," *Parents' Magazine,* June, 1970, p. 50.

Carson, Ruth. *Your New Baby.* A Public Affairs pamphlet.

* Chess, Stella, Alexander Thomas, and Herbert G. Birch, *Your Child Is a Person.* New York: Simon & Schuster, 1965.

de Schweinitz, Karl. *Growing Up.* 4th ed. New York: The Macmillan Company, 1968.

* Dodson, Fitzhugh. *How to Parent.* Los Angeles: Nash Publishing Co., 1970.

* Fraiberg, Selma. *The Magic Years.* New York: Charles Scribner's Sons, 1968.

* Ginott, Haim. *Between Parent and Child.* New York: The Macmillan Company, 1965.

* ———. *Between Parent and Teenager.* New York: The Macmillan Company, 1969.

Homan, William E. *Child Sense: A Pediatrician's Guide for Today's Families.* New York: Basic Books, Inc., 1969.

* LeShan, Eda J. *Natural Parenthood.* New York: Signet Books, 1970.

Liley, H. M. I., and Beth Day. *Modern Motherhood.* New York: Random House, 1969.

Neisser, Edith G., and Fay Bauling. "The Crucial Preschool Years," *Parents' Magazine,* February, 1970, p. 49.

Riker, Audry P. *Breastfeeding.* A Public Affairs pamphlet, 1964.

* Spock, Benjamin. *Baby and Child Care.* Rev. ed. New York: Pocket Books, 1968.

Stewart, Bernice C. *Best-Fed Babies: A Guide for Nursing Mothers.* Bellevue, Wash.: International Childbirth Education Association, 1965.

Streshinsky, Shirley G.: "A Happy Mother's Guide to Successful Nursing." *Parents' Magazine,* February, 1970, p. 52.

U.S. Government (Children's Bureau pamphlets):

Infant Care (1963)
Breast Feeding your Baby (rev. 1970)
Your Baby's First Year (1963)
Your Child from One to Six (rev. 1962)
Your Child from Six to Twelve (1966)
The Adolescent in Your Family (rev. 1955)
Moving into Adolescence (1966)

Superintendent of Documents, U.S. Government Printing Office, Washington, D.C., 20402.

Nutrition and Health

Your Child's Teeth. American Dental Association, 211 East Chicago Avenue, Chicago, Ill. 60611.

Better Homes and Gardens Editors.

Casserole Cook Book (rev. ed., 1968)
Make-Ahead Cook Book (1971)
Meals in Minutes (1963)

Des Moines, Iowa: Meredith Press.

Foods for Baby and Mealtime Psychology. Gerber Products Company, Fremont, Mich. 49412.

Miller, Marjorie. *Introduction to Health Foods.* Los Angeles: Nash Publishing Co., 1971.

* Spock, Benjamin, and Miriam E. Lowenberg: *Feeding Your Baby and Child.* 2nd ed. New York, Hawthorn Books, 1967.

Sunset Editors. *Quick and Easy Dinners—Make Ahead.* Menlo Park, Cal.: Lane Books, 1971.

U.S. Government (pamphlets):

Family Food Budgeting
Food for the Family with Young Children (rev. 1970)
Foods Your Children Need (rev. 1958)
Money-Saving Main Dishes
Nutritive Value of Foods

Superintendent of Documents, U.S. Printing Office, Washington, D.C., 20402.

Accidents and Accidental Poisoning

Freese, Arthur S. *Protecting Your Family from Accidental Poisoning.* A Public Affairs pamphlet.

430

Lin-Fu, Jane S. "Childhood Lead Poisoning—An Eradicable Disease." *Children*, January-February, 1970.
Newman, Virginia H. *Teaching an Infant to Swim*. New York: Harcourt Brace Jovanovich, 1969.

U.S. Government (pamphlets):
Accidents and Children (rev. 1963)
Teach Children Fire Will Burn (1969)
Lead Poisoning in Children (1970)
Poison Prevention Packaging Act of 1970

Superintendent of Documents, U.S. Printing Office, Washington. D.C., 20402.

Sex Education

Andry, Andrew C., and Steven Schepp. *How Babies Are Made*. New York: Time-Life Books, 1968.
* Arnstein, Helene S. *Your Growing Child and Sex*. New York: Bobbs-Merrill Company, 1967.
* Barnes, Kenneth C. *He and She*. Baltimore: Penguin Books, 1970.
Gruenberg, Sidonie M. *The Wonderful Story of How You Were Born*. Rev. ed. Garden City, N.Y.: Doubleday & Company, 1970.
* Johnson, Eric W. *Love and Sex in Plain Language*. Philadelphia: J. B. Lippincott Company, 1967.
Lerrigo, Marion D., and Helen Southard. *Finding Yourself*. Sex Education Series, 1968. Distributed by the American Medical Association and the National Education Association.
Levine, Milton I., and Jean H. Seligman. *A Baby Is Born*. Rev. ed. New York: Golden Press, 1962.
Masturbation. Sex Information and Education Council of the United States. Study Guide No. 3, 1970.

Activities and Recreation

Dodds, Maryelle. *Have Fun . . . Get Well*. Ed. II. New York: American Heart Association, 1967.
Frank, Josette. *Your Child's Reading Today*. Rev. ed. Garden City, N.Y.: Doubleday & Company, 1969.
Frantzen, June. *Toys: The Tools of Children*. National Easter Seal Society for Crippled Children and Adults, 2023 West Ogden Avenue, Chicago, Ill., 1957.
Gregg, Elizabeth M., and Boston Children's Medical Center Staff. *What to Do When There's Nothing to Do*. New York: Delacorte Press, 1968.

Johnson, June. *Eight Hundred Thirty-eight Ways to Amuse Your Child.* New York: The Macmillan Company, 1970.

* Larrick, Nancy. *A Parent's Guide to Children's Reading.* Rev. ed. Garden City, N.Y.: Doubleday & Company, 1969.

Lewis, Richard. *Journeys—Prose by Children of the English-Speaking World.* New York: Simon & Schuster, 1969.

* Matterson, E. M. *Play and Playthings for the Preschool Child.* Baltimore: Penguin Books, 1967.

Nobel, Eva. *Play and the Sick Child.* Levittown, N.Y.: Transatlantic Press, 1967.

U.S. Government (pamphlets):

Handbook for Recreation (1959)
A Creative Life for Your Children (1962)

Superintendent of Documents, U.S. Printing Office, Washington, D.C., 20402.

Special Circumstances

* Benjamin, Lois. *So You Want to Be a Working Mother.* New York: Funk & Wagnalls, 1968.

Carson, Ruth. *So You Want to Adopt a Child.* A Public Affairs pamphlet.

de Hartog, Jan. *The Children: A Personal Record for the Use of Adoptive Parents.* New York: Atheneum Publishers, 1969.

Grollman, Earl, ed. *Explaining Divorce to Children.* Boston: Beacon Press, 1969.

Information on Adoption of Children of Specific Race, Color, Creed. Adoption Resource Exchange (ARENA), 44 East 23rd Street, New York, N.Y. 10010.

Questions and Answers About Nursery Schools (pamphlet)
National Association for the Education of Young Children, 104 East 25th Street, New York, N.Y. 10010.

Rowland, Florence. *Let's Go to a Hospital.* New York: G. P. Putnam's Sons, 1968.

Shay, Arthur. *What Happens When You Go to the Hospital.* Chicago: Reilly & Lee, 1969.

U.S. Government (pamphlets):

Children in Day Care with Focus on Health (1967)
Children of Working Mothers (1960)
Homemaker Service, How It Helps Children (1967)

Who Will Take Care of Your Child When You Are in Training or On the Job? (1969)

Superintendent of Documents, U.S. Printing Office, Washington, D.C., 20402.

WAIF: When You Adopt a Child from Abroad (pamphlet)

WAIF Adoption Division, International Social Service, American Branch, New York, N.Y.

The Special Child

Bettelheim, Bruno. *Love Is Not Enough: The Treatment of Emotionally Disturbed Children.* New York: The Macmillan Company, 1965.

Buck, Pearl S. *The Child Who Never Grew.* New York: John Day Company, 1950.

Faber, Nancy W. *The Retarded Child.* New York: Crown Publishers, 1968.

Finnie, Nancie R. *Handling the Young Cerebral Palsied Child at Home.* New York: E. P. Dutton & Co., 1970.

French, Edward L. and Clifford J. Scott. *How You Can Help Your Retarded Child.* Rev. ed. Philadelphia: J. B. Lippincott Company, 1967.

Greenfeld, Josh. *A Child Called Noah.* New York: Holt, Rinehart & Winston, 1972.

Hamilton, Marguerite. *Red Shoes for Nancy.* Philadelphia: J. B. Lippincott Company, 1955

Kvaraceus, William C., and E. Nelson Hayes, eds. *If Your Child Is Handicapped.* Boston: Porter Sargent, 1969.

Murray, Dorothy Garst. *This Is Stevie's Story.* Rev. ed. Nashville, Tenn.: Abingdon Press, 1967.

National Easter Seal Society for Crippled Children and Adults:

Cerebral Palsied Children Learn to Help Themselves (1962)
Self-Help Clothing for Handicapped Children (1962)

2023 W. Ogden Avenue, Chicago, Ill.

Robinson, Veronica. *David in Silence.* Philadelphia: J. B. Lippincott Company, 1965.

Ross, Alan O. *The Exceptional Child in the Family: Helping Parents of Exceptional Children.* New York: Grune & Stratton, 1964.

Spock, Benjamin M., and Marion O. Lerrigo. *Caring for Your Disabled Child*. New York: The Macmillan Company, 1965.

U.S. Government (pamphlet):

Feeding the Child with a Handicap (1970)

Superintendent of Documents, U.S. Printing Office, Washington, D.C., 20402.

Index

Canker sores, 401
Car bed, 50
Carbohydrates, 208, 411
Car travel seat, 50–51, 422
Celiac disease, 407–408
Cereals: for babies, 126; in child's diet, 210
Cerebral palsy, 262–263
Cesarian section, 68
Chairs: high, 47–48, 139; low, 48, 139
Chemical burns, 451
Chemical contact rashes, 399–400
Chicken pox, 379–380
Childbirth, 22–23, 54–69; conditions after, 68–69; contractions in, 56, 63–65; forceps in, 67; hospital, articles brought to, 58–60; hospital after birth, 69–71; labor, 64–68; natural, 55–57; psychoprophylactic, 56–57; rooming-in, 58
Child guidance clinics, 234–235
Child health stations, 121
Children: 1 to 2 years (toddlers), 149–187; preschool, 188–205; problems of childhood, 228–234; school-age, 206–235
Children, family relationships: new baby, 60–62, 72–73, 200–202; retarded child, 270, 278; toddler and baby, 151, 200–202
Children's Aid Society, 199
Children's Bureau, 184
Child Welfare League of America, 196, 250
Choking (suffocation), 425; first aid, 452
Chorea (St. Vitus' dance), 409
Chromosomes, 274
Chronic illness, 263–266
Circumcision, 82, 98
Cleaning agents, poisonous, 181–182, 456
Cleft lip, 90
Clothes: fire-resistant, 187; maternity, 32–33
Clothes for babies: dressing, 102–105; layette, basic, 51–53; washing, 105–106
Clubfoot, 90, 306
Clubs, children's, 225

Cold, common, 337–341, 371; bronchitis and, 353, 354; earache and, 348, 349; pneumonia and, 355; swollen glands and, 352
Colic, 137, 329–330
Collarbone, fracture, 455
Colostrum, 79
Congenital heart disease, 334–336
Conjunctivitis (pink-eye), 300–301
Constipation, 310–312
Convulsions: fever, 330–331, 379, 452; first aid, 452–453
County health nurses, 26
Cradle cap, 326
Cradle gym, 130
Creativity of children, 218–220
Crib, 45–46; safety in, 45–46, 120; toys strung on, 130
Crib deaths, 420
Crossed eyes, 300; of newborn babies, 78, 85
Croup, 342–344; with fever, 343–344; spasmodic, 343
Cup, drinking from, 141
Curiosity: of babies, 128, 144; about genitals, 167–168; about sex, 168–169; of toddlers, 149–150
Cuts, first aid, 453
Cystic fibrosis, 406–407
Cystic Fibrosis Research Foundation, 407
Cystitis, 403

Day care, 153–155, 193–200; cooperative nurseries, 195; group care, 133; homemaker service, 199–200; in private home, 153–155, 198–199; in your home, 197–198
Day care centers, 153, 155, 195–197
Deaf child, 260–261, 301–302
Death: in crib, 420; fear of, 172; incurable illness and, 266–268, 417–418
Dehydration, 374, 375
Delivery date, estimated, 25
Demand feeding, 71, 116
Dental care: in early childhood, 180; of school-age children, 211
Dermatitis: atopic (eczema), 369; contact (dermatitis venenata), 399–400

Housework (*continued*) 193; with newborn baby, 61, 94–95; help with while in hospital, 60–61; in pregnancy, 29–30
Husband: baby care by, 62, 71; at childbirth, 56–58, 69; housework by, 29, 30, 61, 94; with newborn baby, 94, 95
Hydrocele, 331

Illness: chronic, 263–266; incurable, 266–268, 417–418
Imaginary playmates, 192
Imagination, creative, 218–220
Imaginative play, 191–192
Immunity, allergy and, 370
Immunizations, 294–295, 377, 378, 382–386; of babies, 122; basic schedule, 295
Impetigo, 393
Incubator, 87–88
Infant seat, 49
Infectious mononucleosis, 387–388
Influenza, 372–373; vaccine, 373
Ingrown toenail, 419
Inguinal hernia, 332–333
Insect bites and stings, 450
Insulin, 411–413
Iodine in diet, 208
Iron in diet, 208
Isolette, 88
Israeli kibbutz, babies in, 133

Jealousy of new baby, 60–62, 72–73, 200–202
John Tracy Clinic, 260
Jump seat, 51

Karo corn syrup, 116–117
Knock-knees, 303–304

Labor, 22–23, 56, 64–68; false, 64; forceps in, 67; stages of, 66–67
Lamaze, Dr. Fernand, 56–57
Laryngitis (croup), 342–344
Laxatives, avoiding, 406
Layette, basic needs, list, 53–54
Lead Industry Association, 184
Lead poisoning from paint, 184–185
Learning, psychology of, 215–216

Legs, 303–306; bowlegs, 302; deformed, 261; fractures, 455; knock-knees, 303–304
Leukemia, 416–418
Lice, head, 400
Lightening in pregnancy, 63
Liley, Dr. Margaret, 135
Limbs, deformed or missing, 261
Lip, cleft, 90
Lochia, 69
Lockjaw (tetanus), 418
Low chair, 48, 139
Lowenberg, Dr. Miriam E., 175
Lower respiratory infection, 337, 353–357
Lumps, 306–308; in eyelids, 306–307; lymph glands, enlarged, 307, 352–353, 382; under nipples, 307; under scalp, 307
Lying, 228–232
Lymphatic system, 323
Lymph glands, enlarged or swollen, 307, 352–353, 382; mesenteric adenitis, 406; tuberculosis in, 388
Lymphocytes, 323, 416

Mastoid infection, 348
Masturbation, 168, 237–238
Maternity clothes, 32–33
Maternity girdles, 33
Measles, 376–377; German, *see* German measles
Meats: for babies, 126; in child's diet, 209
Meconium, 81
Medicine: breast milk affected by, 109; as poison, 182–183, 424; in pregnancy, 20, 31; safety precautions with, 182–183
Meningitis, 321, 385–386
Menstruation, 227, 236
Mental retardation, 268–282; causes, miscellaneous, 277; classes for retarded children, 281–282; Down's Syndrome (mongolism), 269, 273–275, 281; home care versus institutions, 277–281; mild, moderate, and severe, 271–272; phenylketonuria, 275–276; terms used for, 271
Mesenteric adenitis, 406

444

First Aid Treatment

First Aid Treatment

GENERAL INFORMATION

Have the following posted on or beside your phone and write them in here.

Doctor's office number _____ .

Doctor's home number _____ .

Local hospital number _____ .

Nearest Poison Information Center
  (if not listed, ask Operator) _____ .

Fire department _____ .

Police department _____ .

IN A REAL EMERGENCY, LOCAL POLICE CAN USUALLY SUPPLY
TRANSPORTATION TO NEAREST HOSPITAL

Keep a few simple first aid supplies on hand:

  Band-Aids
  Sterile gauze squares
  Adhesive tape
  Antiseptic ointment
  Local anesthetic ointment for minor burns
  2 ounces of ipecac syrup

447

Your doctor may suggest other stand-by medicines.

Certain first aid measures possible with adults are virtually impossible with small children. It is unlikely, for instance, that a small child will swallow a large dose of some bad-tasting antidote for poisoning. Advice given here has been kept to what can actually be done.

When an accident happens, try not to panic. A few moments to collect your thoughts may make your action much more effective. If you do need help, call your doctor or have someone do it for you. If you cannot get him, and you feel that time is critical, start for the nearest hospital and go directly to the emergency entrance.

Poisoning by household materials or overdoses of medicines is *very* common, but few substances cause rapid death—and those are not likely to be around your home. Therefore, take time to figure out *how much* of *what* has been swallowed before you call the doctor or go to the hospital. You will also save time if you take the time to give the child ipecac to cause vomiting whenever it's indicated. See Poisoning, p. 423.

ABDOMINAL INJURIES

When a child is hit hard anywhere on the abdomen, as by a ball bat, hard ball, handlebars, or a kick, there is some danger of damage inside. If, after such a blow, he continues to complain of pain, turns pale, sweats unusually, breathes abnormally, or is unusually thirsty you should call the doctor promptly. Internal bleeding is a possibility—and a medical emergency. In the meantime, keep the child quiet and treat for shock if necessary. See p. 458.

ARTIFICIAL RESPIRATION

Start immediately for any person not breathing. Send someone for help if possible but *start working*. Drowning, electrical shock, carbon monoxide poisoning, household gas poisoning, and attempted suicide by sedatives are the commoner causes of arrested respiration that may be reversible. Drowning is the commonest in childhood.

For drowning only:

First, place upper half of child's body in upside-down position and lay him across your lap, head near ground, for 5 to 10 seconds to drain water out of lungs. Then proceed to steps listed under "For emergencies other than drowning."

For emergencies other than drowning:

Place child flat on back. Quickly wipe out anything in mouth. A rag or just your finger will do.

Pull head back and tip chin up.

Pull lower jaw forward.

Place your mouth over child's mouth.

Pinch his nose shut—or with tiny child cover both nose and mouth with your mouth.

Blow your air into him; for a child half your size use about half your breath.

Remove your mouth and listen for air coming out.

If no air comes out, check on chin-up position.

If still no air returns, roll him over, and thump his back hard between shoulder blades to dislodge anything stuck in windpipe. Roll onto back and start again.

Repeat breath cycle 15 to 20 times per minute. For tiny tot breathe faster and with less volume.

Keep it up for at least 30 minutes or until expert help arrives.

If stomach distends with air, press on it firmly; the air will be forced out.

BITES

Animal bites. Wash briskly with soap and water. If wound is large, flush with water only. Cover with loose bandage. If wound is small, leave exposed. Gather available information on animal: If wild, capture if possible but keep alive; if a pet, find out if it has had rabies vaccine. Report to doctor. Your child may need a tetanus booster.

Human bites. Treat as for an animal bite; an antibiotic may be needed because infections frequently develop.

Snakebites. If snake was poisonous, or if you are not sure, apply moderately tight tourniquet between body and bite—tight enough to produce reddish but not blue color in the extremity. (If blue, loosen a bit.) Suck wound vigorously by mouth or by suction cups supplied with snakebite kit. Get medical help or start at once for nearest hospital if vehicle is available. Avoid exercise for patient.

Insect bites and stings. Cold compresses may help pain and swelling. Reaction to stings in local area are not dangerous, no matter how much swelling. If there is difficult breathing, stomach pain, itching, or hives in areas *other* than location of sting, get medical help or start for nearest hospital immediately.

Tick bites. Do not try to pull a tick off if the head is embedded. Apply petroleum jelly, butter, cooking oil, lighter fluid, kerosene, or turpentine and tick will drop off, including buried head. If wound later seems infected, check with doctor.

BLEEDING

BLEEDING FROM SMALL CUTS AND SCRATCHES. Bleeding from slight injuries can be stopped by simple pressure. Apply a sterile gauze pad or several layers of clean folded cloth and press firmly. Keep the pressure on for at least 3 minutes. Scalp cuts, even when small, sometimes bleed briskly, but firm pressure will stop them. *Exception:* If you think the skull under a scalp cut may be fractured, do *not* apply forceful pressure.

PROFUSE BLEEDING FROM CUTS. If a deep cut produces spurting blood, use very firm pressure over several layers of folded cloth for at least 10 minutes. If you still can't control it, get medical help promptly. Watch for signs of shock. See p. 458.

BLEEDING FROM THE EAR. Bleeding from the ear always requires examination. It is very important if it follows a head injury.

*Bleeding from the nose.** Nosebleeds in children can almost

* See Nosebleed, p. 319.

always be controlled by external pressure. Have the child sit up. Compress the nose just below the bony part. Put your thumb on one side and your index finger on the other and squeeze them together firmly. Hold for 3 minutes and then relax the pressure gradually. If bleeding starts again, repeat. If you fail to stop a nosebleed after three trials, check with the doctor.

BURNS *

Small burns. A burned area the size of the palm of your hand or smaller, unless very deep, will heal without help. Holding the area under very cold water or applying cracked ice wrapped in a clean cloth will relieve pain. So will burn ointment or sprays containing a local anesthetic, but do not apply them to large burns that are going to require medical attention. A heavy coating of Petroleum jelly will help to keep a sterile gauze bandage from sticking. Or use Telfa squares from the drugstore; they stick hardly at all. Keep burn lightly covered until healed.

Larger burns. Cover or wrap child in a clean sheet, then blankets. Call the doctor. If you do not connect promptly, start for the nearest hospital. Do not waste time. Shock starts quickly in severe and extensive burns. Do *not* apply anything to the surface. It is a waste of time and will complicate treatment at the hospital. Tetanus prevention is necessary in burns. See Shock, p. 458.

Chemical burns. Corrosive substances—acids and strong alkalis—can burn skin badly. Flush at once with large quantities of water. Then, if area is large, check with the doctor.

For chemicals in the eye, *first* have child lie down. Slowly pour a whole pitcher of water over the eye while you hold the lids apart with your fingers. Milk can be used in place of water, but be prompt. *Then* take the child to doctor or hospital.

Sunburn. Commercial sunburn creams are helpful, but if your child has a really extensive sunburn and has chills or seems sick it is best to call the doctor.

* See pp. 295 and 418 for information on tetanus prevention.

CHOKING

Turn child over your lap with his head and face down. Thump his back with the heel of your hand between his shoulder blades. If he can breathe, the thumping will not be necessary but the position will help him cough out whatever is stuck. If the child is small enough, hold him upside down by the ankles.

If something like a peanut or a bead was the cause and you *know* it's out, that's the end of it. However, if the choking was severe and nothing comes out and the child continues to cough or wheeze or to have difficulty breathing, get him to a doctor or the nearest hospital.

Foreign objects in the esophagus (swallowing tube) occasionally stick at a level below the throat. Instead of coughing and having difficulty breathing the child gags and has trouble swallowing. If you think your child has swallowed something that's stuck on the way down, get the doctor.

Most anything that gets down as far as the stomach will go on through. The narrowest part of the whole tract is about halfway from mouth to stomach.

CONVULSIONS

Convulsions are frightening but seldom dangerous. *Do not panic; the child is not dying.*

Most convulsions in children are due to sudden rise in fever and need to be treated with emergency cooling. If child is a known epileptic, see p. 414.

Uncover child. Get the clothes off. Turn on side to prevent choking. Do not worry about his catching cold. Moisten skin all over with cool water. If weather is hot, fan also. Keep applying the water. Evaporation cools, lowers temperature. Have someone call the doctor, but by the time he reaches you, seizure will probably be over. You will wonder whether doctor can believe how awful it looked to you!

Convulsions following a definite head injury or poisoning

are quite another matter. Put child on side or abdomen to prevent choking and get medical help.

You will also want to read Fever Convulsions, p. 330.

CUTS *

Small cuts or deep scratches. Little cuts do not need the doctor and will stop bleeding in a few moments. Wash thoroughly with soap and water. Flush off soap. Apply a Band-Aid or other small clean dressing. Don't use antiseptics, creams, or ointments unless you've previously checked the material with your doctor. If a small cut continues to bleed, cover with several layers of folded clean cloth and apply firm pressure for 5 to 10 minutes.

Big cuts. Larger cuts may need stitching to close them; check with the doctor. Even heavy bleeding can be stopped by very firm pressure directly over the cut with a pad of clean cloth. Press hard and keep the pressure on for 5 to 10 minutes; you won't do any damage this way. If bleeding recurs, repeat. If you still can't stop it—and that won't be often—take the child to the nearest doctor or hospital.

Scrapes or brush burns. A skinned knee or any other scraped area needs a good washing with soap and water. If dirt particles are deeply embedded, check with the doctor.

DROWNING

If child is breathing and coughing, all will be well. Place upper half of child's body in upside-down position and lay him across your lap, head near ground. He will get rid of the water and be all right.

If there is no sign of motion or breathing, DO NOT LEAVE CHILD TO GET HELP. Moments count. You are his only chance. Hold him upside down for 5 to 10 seconds to drain out the water. Then lay him flat on his back on the ground

* See pp. 295 and 418 for information on tetanus prevention.

and *start artificial respiration immediately.* Send* someone for help if possible but *start working*.

FOREIGN OBJECTS

In the windpipe or throat. See under Choking in this chapter.

In the eye. The best way to remove a particle from a child's eye is by flushing it with water. Have him lie down. Separate lids with your thumb and finger. Pour half a pint or more of water across the eye. Try to flush under lids. If you can see a particle stuck to lid or eyeball, try gentle removal with cotton or the corner of a clean handkerchief. Often this is easier said than done; if you are not successful quickly, let a doctor do it. Whenever you have doubts about an eye injury, get medical help promptly.

In the ear or nose. Kids often poke things into their ears or nose—beans, buttons, marbles, and what not. They can be difficult to remove. Let the doctor do it; you may only push it in farther and make removal still more difficult.

In the skin. Remove little splinters or other particles with a tweezer, but if you find it difficult let the doctor do it. There are definite techniques and tools. Don't keep probing, especially for a piece of glass. You may make matters much more difficult.

Sand and grit that are ground into the skin require vigorous scrubbing. If you are timid about it you'll probably need help.

FRACTURES

Without training and experience, you cannot be certain whether a bone is broken or not unless it has poked through the skin (compound fracture) or has caused obvious deformity. Every suspected break should be examined by a doctor.

If there is a skin wound over a suspected break in a bone, cover it with sterile gauze. If no sterile dressing is available, leave the wound exposed and do not let anything come in con-

---

* See Artificial Respiration, p. 448.

tact with it. *Exception:* if wound is bleeding badly, the bleeding takes precedence over other treatment. Fold a clean cloth, lay over wound, and apply firm pressure.

Before moving a child with an obviously broken bone, try to splint the area. The object is to prevent movement at the broken ends so far as possible.

Skull. Fracture of the skull of and by itself is not dangerous. See discussion that follows under Head Injuries.

Neck and back. If you suspect severe neck or back injury, do not move the child if you can get medical help. Cover him warmly while waiting. If you *must* move or transport him, roll him onto a blanket or other supporting carrier. Move slowly and carefully to avoid jarring and try to bend body as little as possible.

Arm or wrist. If no obvious deformity is present, use a simple sling for arm. Fold any large piece of cloth into a triangle and tie or pin at back of neck.

If there *is* deformity use splint *and* sling. Splints can be made of rolled magazine, newspaper, sticks. Tie to arm above and below break.

Leg and ankle. Keep the child down; no weight should be put on a broken leg. Splint by tying to other leg at several levels or splint with board, tightly rolled blanket, or broomstick. When well splinted, carry child to medical help. If there is swelling and pain at ankle and no deformity, no splint is required and child may be able to hop with help. It is difficult to tell severe sprain from break at ankle. Let the doctor decide.

Finger. Splint finger to adjacent finger with tape or use pencil or small stick.

Collarbone. Fractures here are very common in young children. Pain is in shoulder and upper arm. The child will not use arm on injured side. Use sling to support weight of arm.

HEAD INJURIES

All children have many hard bumps on the head. It is surprising how few lead to any real trouble. Most head injuries, if they do not produce at least brief unconsciousness, are not serious.

But call the doctor after any head injury that does cause even brief unconsciousness or if the child is confused, can't see right, vomits repeatedly, *or* seems unusually pale for more than a few minutes. Persistent dizziness or unusual drowsiness are other reasons for calling. The doctor may want to have the child watched in the hospital for a day or two. A severe concussion is occasionally followed by complications that are best detected by frequent checks on pulse, respiration, and blood pressure.

You may let a child rest and nap for a while, but wake him after the first hour of sleep to check on his state of consciousness.

Small scalp cuts tend to bleed very freely. Put a folded clean cloth over the cut and apply *firm* pressure for 5 minutes; repeat if necessary.

POISONING

If your child has swallowed something you know is poisonous or has taken an overdose of medicine, MAKE HIM VOMIT.

> EXCEPTIONS
> Do *not* induce vomiting for:
> Petroleum products—Kerosene—Gasoline—Solvents
> Caustics—Lye—Drain cleaners—Oven cleaners
> (because inhaling into lung or passing
> through throat a second time may
> do more harm than good)

To make child vomit, give 1 tablespoon of ipecac syrup. Follow with glass of milk or water. (One tablespoon mustard, or 1 tablespoon salt, in a glass of water can be used if ipecac is not available.) *Then* call your doctor. If you don't reach the doctor and if child does not vomit within 15 minutes, give a second tablespoon of IPECAC SYRUP (or mustard or salt solution) and another glass of milk or water. If still no vomiting after another 10 minutes, lay child face down on your lap. Insert blunt object such as spoon handle far back into mouth to cause gagging. Persist until he vomits. If this fails, start for hospital.

If your child swallows something he shouldn't but you are in doubt about whether it is poisonous see the following list of household things that are *not* dangerous in *usual* amounts. If you are then still in doubt, take the container to the phone. Call your doctor, local hospital, or nearest Poison Control Center. They will know.

If you do go to the hospital or the doctor, *take the container along*. The label often gives valuable information.

When the emergency is all over and you do have time, read the general material on poisoning in Chapter 17. *Pay close attention to what it says about repeaters.*

COMMON HOUSEHOLD ITEMS THAT ARE *NOT* VERY POISONOUS

The following materials are *not* really dangerous in the amount a child is likely to swallow.

Aftershave lotions
Airplane and other hobby glues
Ballpoint pen inks
Bath oils, afterbath lotions
Bath toys
Bleach powders
Bubble bath
Candles or paraffin (solid)
Caps for toy pistols
Colognes
Crayons (*children's*)
Dehumidifying packets
Deodorizer cakes
Glue of household types
Ink
Marking devices (felt-tip pens, etc.)
Matches
Play-doh
Polaroid picture chemicals

Putty
Sachets
Shaving creams
Silly putty
Smoke pellets for toy train
Thermometers
(This amount of mercury is not harmful)
Toothpastes
Vitamins (except *very* large doses)

SHOCK

Severe injuries are often followed by *shock,* a condition in which the body has difficulty maintaining proper blood pressure and blood circulation. Sometimes the state of shock is more dangerous than the injury that caused it; prompt medical attention is necessary.

Large burns, broken large bones, crushing injuries, and severe bleeding are very likely to be followed by shock.

Symptoms of shock are:

Cold, pale, moist skin
Generalized weakness
Thirst
Nausea and sometimes vomiting
A dull vacant look in the eyes
Irregular shallow breathing
Weak and very rapid pulse

These same symptoms often appear in children who are nauseated and about to vomit from any cause—car sickness, stomach upsets, the onset of various common illnesses. But if a child has been hurt and *then* these symptoms come on:

Have the child lie down with head a little lower than feet.
Keep him warm with blankets over *and* under him. Get medical help as soon as you possibly can.
If help must be long delayed and provided the child is not vomiting, get him to drink about ½ cupful of a solution of 1 teaspoon of salt in a pint of water about every 20 minutes.